Management of the
Unstable Shoulder

Arthroscopic and Open Repair

Management of the
Unstable Shoulder
Arthroscopic and Open Repair

Edited by:

Jeffrey S. Abrams, MD

Attending Surgeon
University Medical Center at Princeton
Department of Surgery, Section of Orthopaedics
Princeton, New Jersey

Clinical Professor
Seton Hall University
School of Health and Medical Sciences
Department of Orthopedic Surgery
Orange, New Jersey

Medical Director
Princeton Orthopaedic and Rehabilitation Associates
Sports Medicine Princeton
Princeton, New Jersey

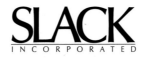

SLACK
INCORPORATED

www.slackbooks.com

ISBN: 978-1-55642-925-5

The procedures and practices described in this book should be implemented in a manner consistent with the professional standards set for the circumstances that apply in each specific situation. Every effort has been made to confirm the accuracy of the information presented and to correctly relate generally accepted practices. The authors, editor, and publisher cannot accept responsibility for errors or exclusions or for the outcome of the material presented herein. There is no expressed or implied warranty of this book or information imparted by it. Care has been taken to ensure that drug selection and dosages are in accordance with currently accepted/recommended practice. Due to continuing research, changes in government policy and regulations, and various effects of drug reactions and interactions, it is recommended that the reader carefully review all materials and literature provided for each drug, especially those that are new or not frequently used. Any review or mention of specific companies or products is not intended as an endorsement by the author or publisher.

SLACK Incorporated uses a review process to evaluate submitted material. Prior to publication, educators or clinicians provide important feedback on the content that we publish. We welcome feedback on this work.

Published by: SLACK Incorporated
                   6900 Grove Road
                   Thorofare, NJ 08086 USA
                   Telephone: 856-848-1000
                   Fax: 856-848-6091
                   www.slackbooks.com

Contact SLACK Incorporated for more information about other books in this field or about the availability of our books from distributors outside the United States.

Library of Congress Cataloging-in-Publication Data

Management of the unstable shoulder : arthroscopic and open repair / [edited by] Jeffrey S. Abrams.
     p. ; cm.
  Includes bibliographical references and index.
  ISBN 978-1-55642-925-5 (alk. paper)
 1. Shoulder joint--Endoscopic surgery. 2. Shoulder joint--Surgery. 3. Arthroscopy. I. Abrams, Jeffrey S.
  [DNLM: 1. Shoulder Dislocation--surgery. 2. Arthroscopy--methods. 3. Joint Instability--surgery. 4. Shoulder--surgery. 5. Shoulder Joint--surgery. WE 810]
  RD557.5.M36 2011
  617.5'720597--dc22
                                          2010049052

Printed in the United States of America.

Last digit is print number: 10 9 8 7 6 5 4 3 2 1

DEDICATION

To my first lady, Kathleen, for your guidance and encouragement. To Matthew for your dedication to playing sports at the highest level. To Kimberly for your warm smile, sense of humor, and devotion to hard work. I am proud to share life with you.

CONTENTS

Dedication .... *v*

Acknowledgments .... *ix*

About the Editor .... *xi*

Contributing Authors .... *xiii*

Foreword by James R. Andrews, MD .... *xvii*

Foreword by Richard J. Hawkins, MD.. *xix*

Introduction .... *xxi*

SECTION I   **ARTHROSCOPIC TECHNIQUES TO TREAT THE UNSTABLE SHOULDER** 1

Chapter 1   Patient Selection: Nonoperative, Arthroscopic, and Open Options 3
Matthew Bollier, MD and Robert A. Arciero, MD

Chapter 2   Patient's Preparation, Positioning, and Portals for Arthroscopic
Stabilization.. 23
Part I: Advantages of the Lateral Decubitus Position 23
Jason Sullivan, MD and Guido Marra, MD
Part II: Advantages of the Beach Chair Position.................................. 34
CDR Matthew T. Provencher, MD, MC, USN; ENS Sean McIntire, MC, USN;
Tistia Gaston, PA-C; and Daniel J. Solomon, MD

Chapter 3   Arthroscopic Bankart Repair: A Reproducible Technique.................. 45
Richard Ryu, MD and Jeffrey S. Abrams, MD

Chapter 4   Knotless Suture Anchor Techniques to Repair
the Unstable Shoulder 59
Raymond Thal, MD

Chapter 5   When We Should Consider Posterior Plication Sutures
and Interval Plication.. 77
Mark T. Wichman, MD

Chapter 6   Techniques to Repair the Multidirectionally Unstable Shoulder 89
Marcus S. Briones, MD; Michael J. Pagnani, MD;
William J. Mallon, MD; and John H. Flint, MD

Chapter 7   Posterior Shoulder Instability: Recognition and
Arthroscopic Treatment 101
Richard L. Angelo, MD

SECTION II   **SPECIAL SITUATIONS IN SHOULDER INSTABILITY** 111

Chapter 8   The Best Treatment for the First-Time Dislocator 113
Drew Fehsenfeld, MD, PhD and Robert A. Arciero, MD

Chapter 9   Treatment Decisions in the Elite Athlete 127
Todd C. Moen, MD and Gordon W. Nuber, MD

Chapter 10   Assessment of Bone Loss in the Chronic, Recurrent,
Unstable Shoulder 135
Anshu Singh, MD; Travis G. O'Brien, BA; Jianhua Wang, MD;
and Jon J. P. Warner, MD

Contents

Chapter 11   Applying a Soft Tissue Repair in a Chronic Unstable Shoulder
With Bone Loss 149
Robert T. Burks, MD

Chapter 12   Arthroscopic Latarjet Graft Technique 155
Laurent Lafosse, MD and Simon Boyle, MSc, FRCS (Tr and Orth)

Chapter 13   Treatment of Superior Labral Tears in the Unstable Shoulder 171
Joseph P. DeAngelis, MD and John E. Kuhn, MD

Chapter 14   Arthroscopic Revision Surgery and Treatment of
Complications in Shoulder Stabilization 181
Jeffrey S. Abrams, MD

Section III   Arthrotomy and Repair of the Unstable Shoulder 197

Chapter 15   Bankart Repair and Capsule Shift 199
J. Douglas Haltom, MD and Gary W. Misamore, MD

Chapter 16   Subscapularis Tears and Capsular Deficiency
in Shoulder Instability 209
Bojan Zoric, MD and Peter J. Millett, MD, MSc

Chapter 17   Techniques to Bone Graft the Deficient Anterior Glenoid Rim 223
*Michael J. DeFranco, MD; Monica Morman, MD; Travis G. O'Brien, BA;
Laurence D. Higgins, MD; and Jon J. P. Warner, MD*

Chapter 18   Hill-Sachs Injuries of the Shoulder: When Are These Important
and How Should I Manage Them? 235
*CDR Matthew T. Provencher, MD, MC, USN; LT Matthew Rose, MD,
MC, USN; and William Peace, MD*

Chapter 19   Mini-Open and Arthroscopic Repair of the Humeral
Anterior Capsular Avulsion 253
*Drew Fehsenfeld, MD, PhD; Augustus D. Mazzocca, MS, MD;
and Robert A. Arciero, MD*

Chapter 20   Open Surgical Approach for Posterior Stabilization 263
Luke S. Oh, MD and Scott P. Steinmann, MD

Section IV   Rehabilitation of the Athlete 275

Chapter 21   Dislocation During the Athletic Season: Treatment Options 277
Daniel D. Buss, MD and Aimee S. Klapach, MD

Chapter 22   A Dynamic Approach to a Postoperative Rehabilitative
Program for the Surgically Stabilized Shoulder 285
John M. Tokish, MD and Erick J. Kozlowski, ATC

Financial Disclosures 299
Index 303

ACKNOWLEDGMENTS

I have been taught by many educators, and the challenge of teaching young individuals is a formidable task. Dr. James R. Andrews and Dr. Richard J. Hawkins are two world-renowned surgeons who have devoted their lives to the treatment of individuals wishing to pursue an active lifestyle. These two individuals had been my fellowship instructors and they taught me the importance of listening to our patients and providing a logical approach to their shoulder problems. It is their inspiration and enthusiasm that motivate me to approach every day as a new opportunity to learn and to provide personalized attention to patients. For this I thank them.

I also want to extend a special thanks to acquisitions editor, Carrie Kotlar, and project editor, Debra Toulson, for their devoted assistance in maintaining a schedule and assembling this textbook. Thank you to Linda Dreyer for her secretarial assistance transcribing and assembling individual chapters in this text.

About the Editor

Jeffrey S. Abrams, MD graduated with honors from the Rensselaer Polytechnic Institute and received his MD degree from SUNY, Upstate Medical Center in Syracuse, New York. He served his surgical internship at Santa Barbara Cottage Hospital, and his orthopaedic residency at Thomas Jefferson University Hospital in Philadelphia, Pennsylvania.

Dr. Abrams has served on the staff of Alfred I. DuPont Institute in Wilmington, Delaware, doing research on childhood cervical, hip, and knee disorders. He has completed a Shoulder Fellowship at the University of Western Ontario under the direction of Richard J. Hawkins, MD a Sports Medicine Fellowship in Aspen, Colorado, and the Hughston Sports Medicine Hospital in Columbus, Georgia under Dr. James R. Andrews.

Since moving to Princeton, New Jersey, Dr. Abrams continues to be involved in education on shoulder injuries and sports medicine. He lectures internationally and has been invited to lecture and perform surgery in Canada, South America, Asia, and Europe. He has served on the Continued Medical Education Committee for American Academy of Orthopaedic Surgeons, is on the Board of Directors for the Arthroscopy Association of North America, and is President-elect of the American Shoulder and Elbow Surgeons.

Dr. Abrams is among the first surgeons to perform rotator cuff repairs and stabilization surgery using arthroscopy. As an inventor, he has assisted multiple surgical companies on equipment designs to perform minimally-invasive surgery. He has served on the Board of Directors for arthroscopy education at the Orthopaedic Learning Center in Chicago. He is currently on the editorial staff of four orthopaedic periodicals, section editor for *Orthopaedic Knowledge Update*, has written over 50 chapters in orthopedic textbooks, and is editor of *Arthroscopic Rotator Cuff Surgery: A Practical Approach to Management*.

Dr. Abrams has served as a program chairman for the American Shoulder and Elbow Surgeons Summer Institute, Biennial Meeting, Comprehensive Meetings; Arthroscopy Association of North America Annual Meeting, and the Orthopaedic Learning Center. As a co-chairman with Dr. Robert Arciero, the Management of the Unstable Shoulder: Arthroscopic and Open Repairs occurred in October 2008 at the Orthopaedic Learning Center.

Dr. Abrams is currently an attending surgeon in the Department of Surgery at the University Medical Center at Princeton in Princeton, New Jersey. He is a Clinical Professor at Seton Hall University School of Graduate Medicine, Department of Orthopaedic Surgery in Orange, New Jersey. He joined Princeton Orthopaedic and Rehabilitative Associates in 1986, and headed up shoulder surgery at Sports Medicine Princeton. He continues to serve as an orthopaedic consultant to Princeton University, College of New Jersey, Mercer Community College, as well as local public and private schools. In addition, he is a consultant to the National Hockey League, National Football League, Major League Baseball, International Skating Federation, and the United States Tennis Association.

Contributing Authors

Richard L. Angelo, MD (Chapter 7)
Clinical Professor, Orthopedics
University of Washington
Seattle, Washington
Evergreen Orthopedic Clinic
Kirkland, Washington

Robert A. Arciero, MD (Chapters 1, 8, 19)
Professor, Department of Orthopaedic
  Surgery
Director, Orthopaedic Sports Medicine
  Fellowship
Orthopaedic Team Physician
University of Connecticut
Farmington, Connecticut

Matthew Bollier, MD (Chapter 1)
Assistant Clinical Professor
Department of Orthopaedic Surgery
University of Iowa
Iowa City, Iowa

Simon Boyle, MSc, FRCS (Tr and Orth)
  (Chapter 12)
Consultant Upper Limb Surgeon
York Teaching Hospital
York, England

Marcus S. Briones, MD (Chapter 6)
OrthoCarolina
Monroe, North Carolina

Robert T. Burks, MD (Chapter 11)
Professor, Orthopedic Surgery
University of Utah
Salt Lake City, Utah

Daniel D. Buss, MD (Chapter 21)
Sports and Orthopaedic Specialists, PA
Edina, Minnesota

Joseph P. DeAngelis, MD (Chapter 13)
Instructor, Department of Orthopaedic
  Surgery
Harvard Medical School
Beth Israel Deaconess Medical Center
Boston, Massachusetts

Michael J. DeFranco, MD (Chapter 17)
Orthopedic Surgeon
Lenox Hill Hospital
New York, New York

Drew Fehsenfeld, MD, PhD (Chapters 8, 19)
Advanced Orthopaedics and Sports
  Medicine
Houston, Texas

John H. Flint, MD (Chapter 6)
Flagstaff Bone and Joint
Flagstaff, Arizona

Tistia Gaston, PA-C (Chapter 2, Part II)
Department of Orthopaedic Surgery
Naval Medical Center San Diego
Division of Shoulder, Knee, and Sports
  Surgery
San Diego, California

J. Douglas Haltom, MD (Chapter 15)
West Tennessee Bone & Joint Clinic
Jackson, Tennessee

Laurence D. Higgins, MD (Chapter 17)
Chief, Sports Medicine and Shoulder
  Service
Co-Chief, Harvard Shoulder Service
Brigham and Women's Hospital
Boston, Massachusetts

Aimee S. Klapach, MD (Chapter 21)
Sports and Orthopaedic Specialists, PA
Women's Orthopaedic Center
Edina, Minnesota

Erick J. Kozlowski, ATC (Chapter 22)
The United States Air Force Academy
Colorado Springs, Colorado

John E. Kuhn, MD (Chapter 13)
Associate Professor
Chief, Shoulder Surgery
Vanderbilt University Medical School
Nashville, Tennessee

Laurent Lafosse, MD (Chapter 12)
Alps Surgery Institute
Clinique Générale d'Annecy
Annecy, France

William J. Mallon, MD (Chapter 6)
Medical Director
Triangle Orthopaedic Associates
Durham, North Carolina

Guido Marra, MD (Chapter 2, Part I)
Associate Professor
Department of Orthopaedic Surgery
Loyola University Medical Center
Maywood, Illinois

Augustus D. Mazzocca, MS, MD (Chapter 19)
Associate Professor, Orthopedic Surgery
Shoulder and Elbow Surgery
Director, The Human Soft Tissue
    Research Laboratory
Assistant Director, Orthopaedic
    Residency Program
Orthopedic Team Physician, University of
    Connecticut Athletic Department
University of Connecticut
Farmington, Connecticut

ENS Sean McIntire, MC, USN (Chapter 2, Part II)
Department of Orthopaedic Surgery
Naval Medical Center San Diego
Division of Shoulder, Knee, and Sports
    Surgery
San Diego, California

Peter J. Millett, MD, MSc (Chapter 16)
Director, Shoulder Surgery
Shoulder, Knee, Sports Medicine
The Steadman Clinic
Vail, Colorado

Gary W. Misamore, MD (Chapter 15)
Methodist Sports Medicine Center
Indianapolis, Indiana

Todd C. Moen, MD (Chapter 9)
Fellow, Shoulder and Elbow Surgery
Columbia University Medical Center
New York, New York

Monica Morman, MD (Chapter 17)
Orthopedic Specialist of Wyoming
Campbell County Memorial Hospital
Gillette, Wyoming

Gordon W. Nuber, MD (Chapter 9)
Professor, Clinical Orthopedic Surgery
Northwestern University Medical School
Chicago, Illinois

Travis G. O'Brien, BA (Chapters 10, 17)
Research Assistant
The Harvard Shoulder Service
Boston, Massachusetts

Luke S. Oh, MD (Chapter 20)
Massachusetts General Hospital
Boston, Massachusetts

Michael J. Pagnani, MD (Chapter 6)
Director, Nashville Knee & Shoulder
    Center
Nashville, Tennessee

William Peace, MD (Chapter 18)
Department of Orthopaedic Surgery
Naval Medical Center San Diego
Division of Shoulder, Knee, and Sports
    Surgery
San Diego, California

CDR Matthew T. Provencher, MD, MC, USN *(Chapters 2, Part II; 18)*
Associate Professor, Surgery, Orthopedics, USUHS
Director, Orthopedic Shoulder, Knee, and Sports Surgery
Naval Medical Center San Diego
San Diego, California

LT Matthew Rose, MD, MC, USN *(Chapter 18)*
Department of Orthopaedic Surgery
Naval Medical Center San Diego
Division of Shoulder, Knee, and Sports Surgery
San Diego, California

Richard Ryu, MD *(Chapter 3)*
Santa Barbara, California

Anshu Singh, MD *(Chapter 10)*
Shoulder and Elbow Surgeon
Kaiser Permanente
San Diego, California

Daniel J. Solomon, MD *(Chapter 2, Part II)*
Department of Orthopaedic Surgery
Naval Medical Center San Diego
Division of Shoulder, Knee, and Sports Surgery
San Diego, California

Scott P. Steinmann, MD *(Chapter 20)*
Professor, Orthopedic Surgery
Mayo Clinic
Rochester, Minnesota

Jason Sullivan, MD *(Chapter 2, Part I)*
Loyola University
Maywood, Illinois

Raymond Thal, MD *(Chapter 4)*
Town Center Orthopaedic Associates
Reston, Virginia

John M. Tokish, MD *(Chapter 22)*
Orthopedic Surgery
Sports Medicine
Tripler Army Medical Center
Honolulu, Hawaii

Jianhua Wang, MD *(Chapter 10)*
Orthopedic Surgeon
Sixth Peoples Hospital
Shanghai, China

Jon J. P. Warner, MD *(Chapters 10, 17)*
Chief, Harvard Shoulder Service
Massachusetts General Hospital
Boston, Massachusetts

Mark T. Wichman, MD *(Chapter 5)*
Director, Sports Medicine
Aurora Advanced Healthcare
Milwaukee, Wisconsin

Bojan Zoric, MD *(Chapter 16)*
Team Physician
US Women's National Soccer Team
Stetson Powell Orthopedics and Sports Medicine
Burbank, California

FOREWORD

When I began my career as an orthopedic sports medicine physician in 1973, successful surgical treatment of the athlete's shoulder was uncommon. However, arthroscopic surgery was in its infancy and about to change orthopedic surgery forever. The debate raged in orthopedics as to whether the arthroscope could be an acceptable tool for treatment of shoulder lesions. Thirty-seven years later that question has long since been answered in the positive.

Around the world, the media are filled daily with the exploits of patients who have been returned to their jobs or sport at the same or improved skill level they enjoyed prior to their injury by the skilled hands of orthopedic surgeons.

In this country, this happy state of affairs was made possible by the introduction of the arthroscope by early pioneers such as Bob Jackson, Robert Metcalf, and Lanny Johnson, among others. These clinicians recognized the special need for instruments and techniques for shoulder care. The arthroscope has been the number one advancement in shoulder surgery in the last 40 years. Its use was pioneered by such greats as Howard Sweeney, Dick Caspari, and others. Their efforts to define shoulder treatment issues and provide understanding led to the application of arthroscopic surgical technology in a wide range of acute and chronic problems. A variety of previously career-ending pathologies are now routinely resolved with minimal intervention.

Orthopedic management of unstable shoulders continues to march along. Keeping up with recent developments is a task unto itself. Previous authors have produced an abundance of excellent texts addressing anatomic regions, arthroscopy, open procedures, and frequently both. My former fellow, Jeff Abrams, and his contributors have produced an outstanding body of updated knowledge with this current work, *Management of the Unstable Shoulder: Arthroscopic and Open Repair.*

This comprehensive work will serve as a great shoulder treatment adjunct or a reference guide. It is structured in 4 sections and 22 chapters, supplemented by 14 videos that demonstrate proven successful surgical techniques. It is a clear and concise text, generously illustrated with excellent color photos describing both arthroscopic and open techniques, indications and contraindications, technical alternatives, and pitfalls. In addition, it provides guidelines for postoperative rehabilitation.

Management of the Unstable Shoulder: Arthroscopic and Open Repair is an exceptional and unrivaled contribution to the continuing evolution of unstable shoulder management and treatment. I believe it will be an indispensable and informative addition to orthopedic libraries everywhere.

James R. Andrews, MD
Medical Director, The American Sports Medicine Institute
Birmingham, Alabama
The Andrews Institute
Gulf Breeze, Florida
Andrews Sports Medicine and Orthopaedic Center
Birmingham, Alabama
Clinical Professor, University of Virginia School of Medicine
Charlottesville, Virginia
Clinical Professor, University of South Carolina
Columbia, South Carolina
Clinical Professor, University of Alabama at Birmingham
Birmingham, Alabama
Clinical Assistant Professor, Florida State University
Tallahassee, Florida

FOREWORD

It is indeed a pleasure and an honor to write a Foreword for this text for my very good friend, Jeffrey Abrams. I have known Jeffrey for 25 years and we together have been through the smiles and trials as we learn and teach about the shoulder.

This excellent textbook is organized and focused on a single subject, which it covers in a comprehensive manner, that being arthroscopic and open surgery for shoulder instability. Years ago when Jeffrey was a fellow and we did a shoulder instability procedure, it would almost always be through an open incision. As the years have gone by, we have now developed arthroscopic procedures that can treat most of our patients with shoulder instability. Dr. Abrams and others who have contributed to this book have been pioneers in developing these arthroscopic techniques. There still, however, remains a roll to do open surgery in the unstable shoulder, particularly in the face of glenoid and humeral head bone deficiency. This excellent text describes these various techniques with effective illustrations and state of the art video demonstrations. The book is easy to read with a consistent format throughout.

As a reference text, it would be perfect to consult the description of a procedure you are performing the following day and see the technique in video format to take you step by step through the procedure. It is also an excellent resource text dealing with the philosophy of shoulder instability. It is divided into arthroscopic techniques, open techniques, and a section on specialized problems in shoulder instability. A chapter on rehabilitation at the end of the book is included to complete the picture of shoulder instability. If you want to see world renown surgeons instruct arthroscopic posterior shoulder plication, a reproducible Bankart repair, or an arthroscopic Latarjet, they are easily accessible in this new textbook.

All the authors should be congratulated for their effective and comprehensive contributions and Jeffrey Abrams congratulated for putting together such a text. As surgeons, we are all students of the shoulder and we appreciate the teaching that all these authors, who are also students of the shoulder, share with us. As a shoulder surgeon, when it comes to dealing with shoulder instability, we need to be familiar with multiple pathologies, complex situations, and these state of the art techniques. This book is a must to keep in your office or library.

Richard J. Hawkins, MD
Clinical Professor of Orthopedic Surgery, University of South Carolina
Columbia, South Carolina
Director, Steadman Hawkins Clinic of the Carolinas
Greenville, South Carolina and Spartanburg, South Carolina
Attending Surgeon, Greenville Hospital System University Medical Center
Greenville, South Carolina
Team Physician, Denver Broncos
Denver, Colorado
Team Physician, Colorado Rockies
Denver, Colorado

INTRODUCTION

Treatment for the unstable glenohumeral joint continues to be a challenge for physicians, therapists, and athletic trainers. This is a common injury for young athletic individuals, and outcomes can have far reaching consequences. Successful treatment no longer is considered successful if the athlete is unable to return to physical activities due to overconstraint. A successful return to sports places the individual at risk for instability recurrence.

On October 3-4, 2008, a group of renowned educators came together in Rosemont, Illinois to instruct a program on the unstable shoulder. Here, experts from American Shoulder and Elbow Surgeons, Arthroscopy Association of North America, and American Academy of Orthopedic Surgeons combined surgical skills and laboratory instruction with a didactic lecture program under the leadership of Drs. Robert Arciero and myself. Recognized experts presented state-of-the art techniques, debated pros and cons of open and arthroscopic management, and reviewed short- and long-term results, making this a unique educational experience.

Long-term outcome studies have identified this population to be at risk for developing degenerative arthritis. This dilemma has been demonstrated in nonoperative and operated patients. Radiographic changes have been seen in patients following a single instability event within a decade or two. Unfortunately, these patients are still young and middle-aged at the onset of these degenerative changes. The goals of early surgical treatment include creating an anatomical repair that stabilizes the shoulder, allows return to athletics and physical activities, and minimizes the risk of arthritis. Treating physicians must be familiar with multiple surgical approaches to correct the unstable shoulder. Patient selection, surgical techniques, and postoperative management are the goals for each chapter.

The textbook is designed to cover important aspects for managing the unstable glenhumeral joint. Technique chapters include a narrated video that can be replayed on your personal computer using the proper access codes supplied within the front cover. Understanding the subtleties of surgical decisions may define success and failure in our active patients. This project is designed for trating surgeons, team physicians, therapists, athletic trainers, and orthopedic surgeons who work with athletes.

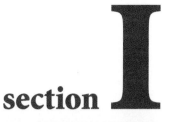

Arthroscopic Techniques to Treat the Unstable Shoulder

1

Patient Selection
Nonoperative, Arthroscopic, and Open Options

Matthew Bollier, MD and Robert A. Arciero, MD

For the shoulder joint to function properly, the humeral head must remain centered on the glenoid throughout a full range of motion by the coordinated interaction of static, dynamic, and bony structures.[1,2] When the humeral head is not maintained in its reduced position, it becomes unstable. Shoulder instability is one of the most common conditions affecting the shoulder and may result from disruption or deficiency of the labrum, capsule, glenohumeral ligaments, rotator cuff musculature, or the normal articular-bony anatomy. The incidence of shoulder instability in a high-demand population is 2.9% with more than 80% of shoulder dislocations being anterior.[3] Instability often becomes recurrent and compromises athletic participation and performance. In patients younger than 20 years, recurrence rates have been reported between 64% and 90%.[4-7] Several factors have been found to affect recurrence rates, including age of the patient, participation in contact sports, hyperlaxity, and significant bone loss.[8,9]

Evaluation and management of shoulder instability has evolved significantly over the years with advances in diagnostic imaging, arthroscopy, and surgical techniques. With a multitude of varying approaches and algorithms available, it is difficult to know how best to evaluate and treat patients with shoulder instability. This chapter will focus on the pathoanatomy of shoulder instability, present 3 common clinical scenarios, and highlight decision-making strategies in the evaluation and management of shoulder instability.

PATHOANATOMY

The humeral head is maintained in a centered position by active and passive forces (muscles, ligaments, concavity-compression, negative intra-articular pressure) compressing it against the concave glenoid. Deficiencies in any of these structures lead to an unstable shoulder. Static stabilizers include the glenoid, labrum, glenohumeral ligaments, capsule, and rotator interval. The glenoid provides a platform for humeral

Abrams JS. *Management of the Unstable Shoulder: Arthroscopic and Open Repair* (pp. 3-22).
© 2011 SLACK Incorporated

head translation and rotation. Adequate bony cross-sectional area and diameter are essential in maintaining a centered humeral head.

The concavity of the glenoid is an essential component of shoulder stability and relies on thicker peripheral cartilage and an intact labrum to deepen the socket.[10] The labrum provides sites of attachment for the glenohumeral ligaments, functions as a bumper to limit translation, and increases the depth of glenoid concavity. A deeper glenoid and labral concavity will have more resistance to humeral head translation. In addition, the tight fit between the concave socket and convex humeral head works as a suction cup through the negative intra-articular pressure in the glenohumeral joint, providing additional stability.[11]

Glenohumeral joint motion involves a delicate balance between mobility and stability. The analogy of a golf ball on a tee provides a useful visual reference of the humeral head on the glenoid. Without adequate bony glenoid support and static and dynamic constraints compressing the humeral head into the glenoid concavity, instability results. The joint capsule and glenohumeral ligaments function as checkreins at the extremes of shoulder motion when they develop increasing tension.[10] Increased tension provides a compressive force and limits excessive humeral head rotation. The inferior glenohumeral ligament complex is the primary static restraint in 90 degrees of abduction. The anterior band is the essential anterior stabilizer in the abducted, externally rotated position. The superior and middle glenohumeral ligaments resist inferior and anteroposterior (AP) translation with the arm at the side and during early abduction. The rotator interval tissues prevent inferior humeral head translation when the arm is at the side, and the inferior capsule and ligaments provide stability against inferior dislocation when the arm is abducted to 90 degrees.

During the mid-range of shoulder motion, the ligaments are lax, but the humeral head remains centered because of the dynamic muscular forces working in a coordinated fashion to compress the humeral head into the glenoid concavity. The subscapularis functions as an anterior compressor, the supraspinatus as a superior compressor, and the infraspinatus as a posterior compressor. These muscles have decreased force production at the extremes of shoulder motion when the length-tension relationship is suboptimal, and shoulder stability is increasingly dependent on the capsuloligamentous structures. Working in a reciprocal way, normal capsular and ligamentous tension and function prevent the rotator cuff musculature from being overstretched and injured. These structures also become more important in areas without muscle (rotator interval, inferior capsule).

The normal concavity-compression mechanism can be disrupted in several ways, leading to shoulder instability. Loss of dynamic compression from the rotator cuff muscles can occur with tendon rupture, denervation, or muscle imbalance. Instability typically occurs in the direction of the insufficient tendon. Capsuloligamentous injury (Bankart lesion, humeral avulsion of the glenohumeral ligaments) decreases glenohumeral stability in several ways. Loss of inferior glenohumeral ligament tension allows the humeral head to obtain positions of extreme rotation without adequate checkreins. At the limits of shoulder motion, the rotator cuff is not able to maintain sufficient compression to provide adequate stability. In addition to loss of ligament tension, capsulolabral detachment (Bankart lesion) results in loss of the labral bumper, and labral resection has been found to decrease the resistance to translation by 20%.[12,13] Similarly, patulous redundant capsule from hyperlaxity or repetitive microtrauma does not provide adequate static compression to maintain stability.

When glenoid or humeral head bone deficiency is present in association with labral detachment, the normal glenoid articular arc is decreased, and shoulder stability is

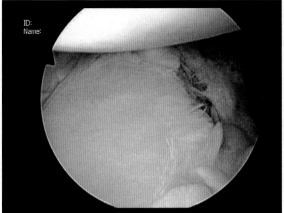

Figure 1-1. Arthroscopic view of anteroinferior glenoid bone loss when viewing through an anterosuperior arthroscopy portal.

greatly decreased. With a "significant" amount of bone deficiency, the humeral head is able to dislocate anteriorly with only minimal amounts of translation. There has been much debate on how much bone loss is needed for a "significant" defect. Burkhart and De Beer found a 4% recurrence rate after arthroscopic Bankart repair without the presence of significant bone defects (more than 25% loss of inferior glenoid diameter or engaging Hill-Sachs lesion) and a 67% recurrent instability rate in athletes with significant bone defects (more than 25% loss of inferior glenoid diameter or engaging Hill-Sachs lesion; Figure 1-1).[14] Gerber and Nyffeler reported a greater than 30% loss of resistance to anterior shoulder dislocation when the length of the anteroinferior rim defect was more than half of the maximal AP inferior glenoid diameter.[15] Itoi and colleagues performed sequential osteotomies in cadaver shoulders of the anteroinferior glenoid and found that stability to anterior translation was significantly less with a bony defect greater than 21% of the diameter of the glenoid.[16] It is clear that increasing glenoid bone defect size correlates with decreased stability of the glenohumeral joint.[15-17] An "inverted-pear" has been used to describe the glenoid appearance with anteroinferior bone loss and an abnormally narrowed inferior half of the glenoid (see Figure 1-1).[14] Although there is no agreement on the exact amount of bone loss needed for a significant lesion, most experts suggest between 20% and 30%.

Hill-Sachs lesions involve an impression defect in the posterolateral humeral head when the soft humeral head contacts the hard glenoid rim during an anterior shoulder dislocation (Figure 1-2). Lesions less than 20% of the humeral head curvature typically are not significant causes of instability and do not typically cause an "engaging" Hill-Sachs lesion.[2,18] An engaging Hill-Sachs lesion occurs when the humeral head falls into the anteroinferior glenoid defect with the arm in an abducted, externally rotated position (Figure 1-3).[19,20] Hill-Sachs lesions greater than 40% are considered large and directly correlate with the presence of recurrent instability.[2,21] Hill-Sachs defects between 20% and 40% may be significant, but depend on the location, orientation, and engagement of the lesion with the anteroinferior glenoid. Isolated soft tissue stabilization in the presence of an engaging Hill-Sachs lesion has a high rate of failure.[14]

Patients complaining of shoulder instability present with a wide variation in pathoanatomy and can be viewed along a spectrum.[22] At one end of the spectrum is the patient with acute traumatic instability and a Bankart lesion who typically needs surgical stabilization.

At the other end is the patient with congenital laxity and a trivial event, without a specific traumatic event leading to the symptoms of instability. The anatomic finding in

Figure 1-2. AP radiograph of a Hill-Sachs lesion.

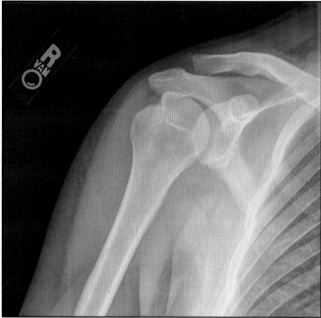

Figure 1-3. Arthroscopic view of an engaging Hill-Sachs lesion when viewing from posterior portal.

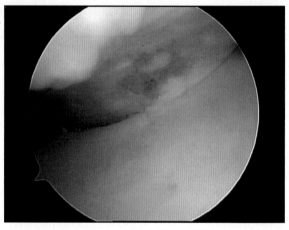

these patients is a loose patulous inferior capsule resulting in a global increase in capsular volume. These patients usually present with atraumatic instability and can often be managed nonoperatively. If they do not respond to rehabilitation, arthroscopic or open surgery can be performed to address the capsular redundancy. In the middle of the spectrum are patients with some degree of ligamentous laxity and some element of structural injury. These patients require labral reattachment and reduction in capsular volume.

HYPERLAXITY

Excessive shoulder laxity can be acquired through repetitive microtrauma, secondary to congenital hyperlaxity, or a combination of both. Patients who perform activities or play sports that constantly force the shoulder into extreme positions will consistently place the capsule and ligaments under excessive tension. Over time, the cumulative effect of repetitive trauma and stretch lead to increased laxity. Patients with congenital hyperlaxity demonstrate evidence of multidirectional shoulder laxity and increased laxity in other joints as well. A major or minor traumatic episode can trigger one shoulder to become symptomatic, but symptoms often develop with no particular injury. This may occur when the dynamic muscular restraints fatigue and are unable to keep the humeral head centered.[23]

Multiple definitions of multidirectional instability have been proposed, but it can be simplified to at least one direction of instability (anterior, posterior, or inferior) with evidence of multidirectional hyperlaxity.[23-25] It is important to distinguish hyperlaxity from instability. Shoulder laxity can be defined as physiologic passive translation of the humeral head on the glenoid, while instability involves symptomatic excessive translation leading to dislocation, decreased function, or pain. The initial evaluation of these patients can be frustrating because they often present with vague, ill-defined complaints. Symptoms can be divided into 3 main categories: pain, intermittent neurologic symptoms (numbness or tingling), or instability.[23] These vary widely between patients, occur with normal activities, and can be quite disabling. Pain, not instability, is the most common complaint in patients with hyperlaxity and varies from sharp intermittent pain to diffuse constant achiness.[26] Although some patients may describe specific shoulder dislocation events, this is rare unless a traumatic labral avulsion occurred in association with underlying laxity. Often, they report a sense of the shoulder slipping, particularly in the mid-range of shoulder motion. When dislocations do occur, they often happen atraumatically and can be reduced by the patients themselves. Determining the mechanism and arm position that causes pain or instability can provide information regarding the direction of humeral head translation.

Physical examination should initially focus on shoulder girdle muscle symmetry and scapular mechanics. A specific assessment of signs of generalized ligamentous laxity includes knee, elbow, and thumb hyperextension. Because there is wide range of normal shoulder laxity, the presence of asymmetry when compared to the contralateral side is important to determine.

The load and shift test may identify the direction of instability, especially if this maneuver provokes symptoms, and must be performed in the plane of the scapula with the scapula stabilized (Figure 1-4). A load is applied so that the humeral head is compressed into the center of the glenoid. The humeral head is then shifted in an anterior and posterior direction. Translation can be graded by assessing movement of the humeral head over the glenoid rim: 1+ to the rim, 2+ over the rim, and 3+ translation. Pain and apprehension may be present in association with increased laxity. Apprehension with the shoulder in an abducted, externally rotated position relieved by a posterior-directed force (relocation test) signifies anterior instability. A sulcus sign of greater than 2 cm indicates the presence of inferior laxity and a loose rotator interval. Apprehension with the arm in forward flexion and internal rotation is associated with posterior instability.[27,28] If the shoulder is brought from flexion to extension, a palpable clunk may be appreciated with posterior laxity (jerk test).

Imaging studies should include standard AP, scapular Y, and axillary radiographs. In hyperlax patients without a significant traumatic episode, these are often normal. Magnetic resonance imaging (MRI) may reveal a large patulous capsule but can be nonspecific. In true nontraumatic hyperlax patients with multidirectional instability, the labrum will be intact without tearing or avulsion. Diagnostic imaging can rule out other shoulder pathology, but the diagnosis of multidirectional instability is primarily a clinical one.

Figure 1-4. Load and shift test.

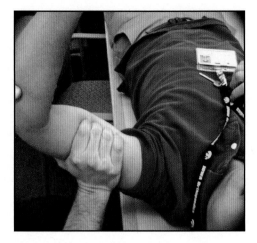

Management

Treatment of ligamentously lax patients without a significant traumatic shoulder injury primarily consists of nonoperative modalities. Rehabilitation involves physical therapy directed at strengthening the scapular and rotator cuff muscles. Improved muscle strength, coordination, and proprioception can enhance the concavity-compression mechanism and keep the humeral head centered during range of motion. One study reported 88% good to excellent results with this approach in patients with atraumatic multidirectional instability.[29] Operative intervention is reserved for those patients who fail at least 6 months of nonoperative treatment. Neer and Foster described the open capsular shift in 1980, and that was the standard treatment for many years.[25] More recently, arthroscopic capsular plication with the use of either labral tissue or anchors has been advocated to reduce capsular volume. We will perform arthroscopic capsular plication when good tissue quality is present, the patient is a throwing athlete, and in cases with associated traumatic labral lesions. Open capsular shift is considered in revision cases, contact athletes, and in patients with extreme hyperlaxity or deficient capsular tissue. In patients with primarily posterior instability associated with multidirectional instability, a concealed labral lesion (Kim lesion) may be present without frank labral detachment.[30] A superficial crack at the chondrolabral junction often indicates a deep labral avulsion that can't be seen on direct inspection. The posterior-inferior labrum becomes flat with relative retroversion of the chondro-labral glenoid. Good results can be obtained with takedown and repair of the posterior labrum in addition to a capsular shift.[30]

The rotator interval has traditionally been closed in patients with increased capsular volume to decrease inferior translation in the adducted arm.[23,25] Some authors have recommended rotator interval closure if excessive inferior translation remained after anterior and posterior capsular placation,[24,31] while others recommend closure of the rotator interval in all patients with excessive capsular laxity.[32] Several recent studies have highlighted the differences between open and arthroscopic rotator interval closure and have suggested that arthroscopic rotator interval closure does not reduce posterior or inferior humeral head translation.[33-35] We perform our standard arthroscopic anterior and posterior capsular plication and then reassess the amount of residual inferior laxity by performing an arthroscopic sulcus sign in neutral and 30 degrees of external rotation. If inferior laxity remains, we close the rotator interval arthroscopically. When we perform open capsular shift, the rotator interval is closed because these are typically revision cases or patients with severe capsular redundancy.

TRAUMATIC ANTERIOR SHOULDER DISLOCATION

First-Time Dislocation

The natural history of a first-time anterior shoulder dislocation has been clearly established with up to 80% to 90% of young, active individuals sustaining a recurrent dislocation.[4-6,36] In addition to age, other proposed prognostic factors include type of sport, activity level, associated pathology, and the presence of glenoid or humeral head bone defects. A focused history will reveal a significant traumatic episode. Important questions include the need for reduction, arm position at the time of dislocation, and disability after the instability event. Physical examination in patients with acute shoulder dislocations should include inspection of shoulder girdle symmetry and muscle atrophy, generalized ligamentous laxity exam, documentation of range of motion, rotator cuff strength testing, position, and axillary nerve function. In addition, load and shift testing is performed to examine laxity in the anterior and posterior directions. It is also important to assess for a sulcus sign in neutral and in 30 degrees of external rotation and compare findings bilaterally. Apprehension, relieved with the relocation test, when the shoulder is in an abducted, externally rotated position signifies anterior shoulder instability. It is important to separate feelings of pain from instability.

Radiographic assessment should include AP, scapular Y, and axillary views. Anteroinferior glenoid bony defects , posterolateral humeral head Hill-Sachs lesions, or glenoid rim fractures may be identified. MRI has become the gold standard in evaluating the specific site of soft tissue disruption and typically shows an anteroinferior capsulolabral injury. Other MRI indications of anterior instability include anterior capsular redundancy, humeral avulsion of the glenohumeral ligament (HAGL lesion), large Hill-Sachs, and anteroinferior glenoid bony defects. MRI evaluation with the patient's shoulder in a position of abduction and external rotation has been found to increase the ability to evaluate the anterior capsulolabral attachments (Figure 1-5).[37]

Management

Although nonoperative treatment is often implemented as first-line treatment for a primary anterior shoulder dislocation, it has been shown to have little effect on preventing recurrence in young active individuals. The duration of immobilization has not been shown to change the rate of recurrent instability, but there have been several reports of decreased recurrence with immobilization in external rotation compared to internal rotation.[38] External rotation has been proposed to increase the contact force between the detached labrum and the glenoid, theoretically resulting in better healing of the capsulolabral avulsion. However, the results have not been consistently reproduced, and patient compliance issues continue to be a concern.[39] Braces that limit the shoulder from being placed in an abducted, externally rotated position only play a small role in the treatment of anterior shoulder instability. They are primarily used so that athletes can finish their current season without recurrence but are quite restricting to overhead athletes. In a study of 30 in-season athletes with acute shoulder dislocations, 26 of the 30 were able to return to their sport at an average of 10 days and complete the season.[40] Ten of the 30 athletes had a recurrence during the season.

There have been many reports supporting arthroscopic stabilization of primary dislocations in young contact or overhead athletes.[41-43] The ideal patient for primary operative treatment of anterior shoulder instability is a young contact or overhead athlete who sustained a traumatic glenohumeral dislocation, has adequate capsulolabral tissues, and has a clearly defined direction of instability. A Bankart lesion has

Figure 1-5. Gadolinium enhanced shoulder MRI in abducted externally rotated position.

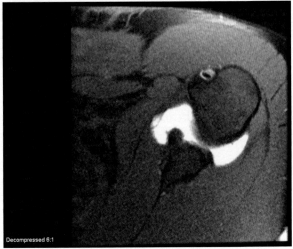

been found to be present in more than 95% of traumatic anterior shoulder dislocations. Bottoni and colleagues found that 75% of young, active patients treated nonoperatively had a recurrence, compared with only 11% of those undergoing immediate stabilization.[43] A systematic review of the literature identified 3 well-designed, prospective, randomized, Level 1 studies comparing nonoperative treatment with early surgery.[44] When the endpoint of treatment is simply recurrence, these studies demonstrate superior results with immediate stabilization. A recent randomized, double-blind trial attempted to address these issues and reported that the risk of recurrence was reduced by 82% with primary arthroscopic stabilization versus arthroscopy and lavage alone.[41] More importantly, they also found improved functional scores, lower treatment costs, and higher patient satisfaction with immediate repair. Other advantages of immediate stabilization include a technically easier repair, better capsulolabral tissues, and decreased risk of extending the labral lesion or creating bone deficiencies from recurrent subluxation or dislocation.

While it is clear that a particular subset of patients (15- to 25-year-old athletes participating in a contact or overhead sport) experiences an unacceptably high rate of recurrent dislocations, it is important to have a thorough discussion of the advantages and disadvantages of primary stabilization versus a trial of nonoperative treatment. As previously stated, the recurrence rate among young, active individuals approaches 90%. However, there are still some patients who do not experience another instability event or patients who are willing to modify their activities. There is no current way to consistently predict which patients will have a recurrence and which will not.

The risk of further intra-articular damage with recurrent instability events has also been cited as a reason for immediate stabilization. Increased bone loss of the glenoid and humeral head articular damage, rotator cuff injury, progressive capsular attenuation, and labrum and biceps damage are potential risks with nonoperative treatment. Habermeyer and colleagues have shown that progressive damage to supporting structures occurs with recurrent instability events.[45]

In addition, a higher risk of osteoarthritis is associated with recurrent dislocations.[46] Significant bony deficiencies and severe capsular attenuation are less common with immediate stabilization. However, the amount of repeated dislocations needed to compromise a delayed repair is unknown. Immediate stabilization may allow associated pathology to be addressed acutely and prevent further damage to the joint, labrum, or capsule.

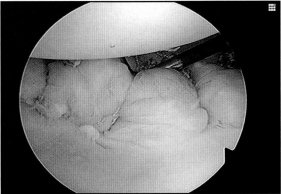

Figure 1-6. Arthroscopic Bankart repair.

When immediate stabilization is chosen in patients with a first-time shoulder dislocation, we recommend arthroscopic capsulolabral evaluation and repair (Figure 1-6). Bone deficiency and poor tissue quality are very rare in these patients, and an arthroscopic approach has several advantages. A complete diagnostic glenohumeral evaluation can be performed, and the morbidity of subscapularis takedown and repair is eliminated. We prefer to perform shoulder instability surgery in the lateral decubitus position, and the anatomy and pathology are clearly defined in acute cases. We usually perform the arthroscopic Bankart repair without capsular plication stitches or rotator interval closure.

Recurrent Instability

Almost all patients who experience recurrent anterior dislocation or subluxation events report significant disability in sports, work, and activities of daily living. Complaints include apprehension, avoidance of activities that position the arm in provocative positions, pain, and decreased athletic performance. Initial evaluation should include a complete history of the onset, chronology, and frequency of dislocations. Other important information includes the position of the arm at the time of dislocation and nonoperative or operative treatments to date. The ease and frequency of instability episodes increases the likelihood of significant bone defects. Shoulder instability that occurs with activities of daily living, sleep, or at lower arm abduction angles is associated with glenoid or humeral head lesions. In addition, bone deficiency is suspected in patients who have failed arthroscopic capsulolabral reconstruction and in patients who report many dislocation events in a short period of time. Patients with an engaging Hill-Sachs lesion may report crepitus or catching as the humeral head falls into the glenoid rim defect when the arm is abducted and externally rotated. Physical examination in patients with recurrent shoulder instability should include a complete evaluation of range of motion, strength, and direction of apprehension. When load and shift testing is performed, decreased resistance, grinding, or crepitus will be felt with a defect in the anterior glenoid rim or humeral head. Patients who present with apprehension and guarding at lower degrees of abduction are more likely to have significant bone deficiencies.[47]

Glenoid and humeral head bone deficiencies can be assessed with plain radiographs, computed tomography (CT) scans, and at the time of arthroscopy. While MRI is valuable in assessing the location and degree of soft tissue injury, it often underestimates the size of bone lesions. AP, trans-scapular lateral, and axillary radiographs

Figure 1-7. (A) West Point axillary radiograph. (B) Technique for West Point axillary radiograph. (Reprinted with permission from Itoi E, Lee SB, Amrami KK, Wenger DE, An KN. Quantitative assessment of classic anteroinferior bony Bankart lesions by radiography and computed tomography. *Am J Sports Med*. 2003;31:112-118.)

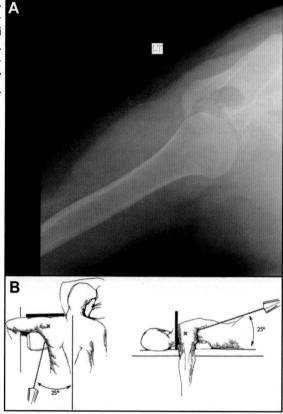

may confirm the direction of dislocation, associated bone defects, or fracture. A modified axillary radiograph, the West Point view, specifically examines glenoid bone loss (Figure 1-7A). Itoi and colleagues have reported that the West Point view demonstrates a high correlation with CT in estimating glenoid bone loss.[48] The patient is positioned prone with the head turned to the contralateral side and the x-ray beam is angled 25 degrees from the midline and is directed through the axilla (Figure 1-7B).

CT scan provides the most information in evaluating bone deficiencies. Indications for obtaining a CT include significant apprehension in lower levels of abduction, instability with minimal provocation, multiple instability events, revision surgery, and any bone loss detected on plain radiographs. Many authors now advocate the use of 3-D CT with digital subtraction of the humeral head (Figure 1-8).[1,49,50] The anteroinferior bone defect can be quantified as a percentage of the inferior glenoid surface area. A circle outlining the inferior two-thirds of the glenoid is drawn, and the amount of bone missing from the circle is calculated as a percentage of the total surface area of the circle.[1,51] In addition, the length of the anteroinferior glenoid defect can be calculated on the sagittal cuts, and if this lesion is greater than the normal AP radius of the inferior glenoid, a 30% loss of resistance to anterior dislocation can be expected with concern for soft tissue reconstruction failure.[15] Hill-Sachs lesions can be quantified on either the coronal or axial cuts by dividing the defect arc with the humeral head arc to obtain a percentage of bone loss.[24]

Significant glenohumeral bone loss can be identified at arthroscopy by looking for the "inverted-pear" glenoid (greater than 25% loss of the inferior glenoid diameter) or an engaging Hill-Sachs lesion. The glenoid bone defect can be assessed

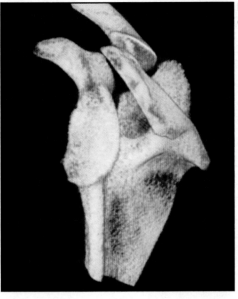

Figure 1-8. Three-dimensional CT scan of glenoid with digital subtraction of humeral head.

arthroscopically with the camera in the anterior superior portal. The distances from the posterior glenoid to the bare area and from the bare area to the anterior rim are measured. In the normal glenoid, the anterior and posterior rims are equidistant from the central bare area. Anteroinferior glenoid bone loss can be determined by dividing the distance from the bare area to the anterior rim by 2 times the distance from the bare area to the posterior rim.[1,52] During diagnostic arthroscopy, the arm can be taken out of traction and put through a range of motion. If the humeral head falls into the anteroinferior glenoid defect with the arm in an abducted, externally rotated position, an engaging Hill-Sachs lesion is present.

Management

Most would agree that recurrent anterior glenohumeral instability is difficult to manage nonoperatively and open or arthroscopic stabilization is recommended in young, active individuals. The exact procedure depends on the quality of tissue, presence of bone defects, and location of the pathology (Figure 1-9). Open repair through the deltopectoral interval has been the traditional treatment of choice, with reported recurrence rates between 3% and 5% (Figure 1-10). Arthroscopic management of anterior shoulder instability has evolved significantly in the past 20 years. Newer techniques and equipment, better skills, and increased knowledge have led to outcomes comparable to open stabilization without the morbidity of an open approach and subscapularis takedown.[31,53-57]

Arthroscopic soft tissue repair alone is appropriate in the presence of a nonengaging Hill-Sachs lesion (continuous contact of the articular surfaces as the humeral head passes across the anterior glenoid) and glenoid bone loss less than 20%. In an attempt to preoperatively predict success or failure with arthroscopic soft tissue repair, Balg and Boileau recently reported the Instability Severity Index Score.[58] It is based on a preoperative questionnaire, clinical examination, and review of radiographs. Patients are given 2 points if they are younger than 20 years, participate in a competitive sport, have a Hill-Sachs lesion visible on an AP radiograph in external rotation, or have loss of glenoid contour on an AP radiograph. They are given 1 point if they participate in a contact or overhead sport or have shoulder hyperlaxity. Patients with a score greater

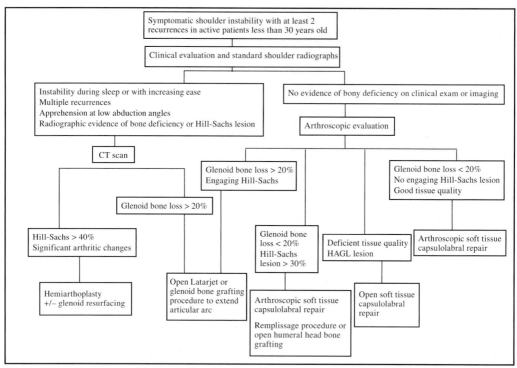

Figure 1-9. Recurrent shoulder instability algorithm.

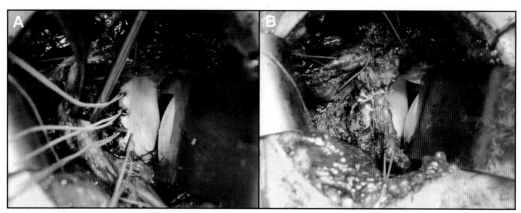

Figure 1-10. Open Bankart procedure.

than 6 points had a recurrence rate of 70% with soft tissue repair alone.[58] In patients with a score greater than 6 points, an open procedure to address the bony defect is recommended.

In the presence of significant glenoid bone deficiency, the anterior soft tissue structures may not be able to resist the displacing force. Burkhart and De Beer reported a 67% recurrence rate after soft tissue stabilization in athletes with significant bone defects.[14] They noted an 89% failure rate in contact athletes with bone defects and soft tissue repair. Other authors reported good outcomes with arthroscopic stabilization for recurrent instability in the presence of glenoid bone defects.[59,60] Mologne and colleagues reported a 14% failure rate of arthroscopic stabilization in 21 patients with more than 20% anteroinferior bone loss.[60] Each of their failures had attritional bone

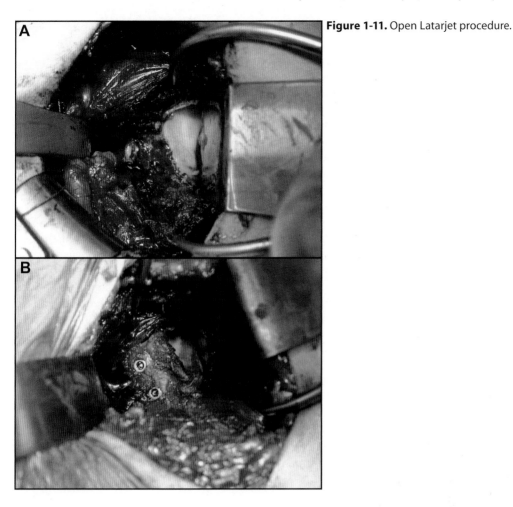

Figure 1-11. Open Latarjet procedure.

loss without a specific detached fragment. The success of arthroscopic stabilization in the presence of bone loss is higher when the bony fragment can be incorporated into the repair.[1,51] Pagnani had a 2% overall recurrence rate after open capsular repair in the presence of bony deficiency.[59] However, only 4% of patients had severe (>20%) bone defects.

Indications for an open bony procedure to extend the glenohumeral articular arc include anteroinferior bone loss greater than 20%, an engaging Hill-Sachs lesion, or Instability Severity Index Score greater than 6 with special consideration given to the collision athlete who is younger than 20 years old. Transfer of the coracoid tip and conjoined tendon (Bristow procedure) has been used historically as a bone block to resist anterior glenohumeral translation. Successful long-term results can be achieved in preventing recurrent anterior instability, but concerns exist regarding the development of arthropathy and loss of external rotation.[1,49,61-63] Current recommendations include the Latarjet procedure or iliac crest bone graft.[14,20,64] The Latarjet procedure involves osteotomizing the coracoid process at its base, rotating the graft 90 degrees, passing it through a split in the subscapularis, and securing it flush to the anterior glenoid with screws (Figure 1-11). This increases the arc of motion by extending the glenoid margin, restores bony architecture, and provides tension to the lower subscapularis. Iliac crest autograft and allograft and distal tibia allograft have also been described to address glenoid bone deficiency.[64-67] Similar to the Latarjet procedure, these techniques extend the glenoid arc to increase the amount of translation or excursion needed for dislocation. These grafts may be better for larger glenoid lesions, but lower union rates may be a concern.

Outcomes after bony stabilization procedures have been encouraging. Burkhart and colleagues reviewed outcomes on 102 patients treated with the modified Latarjet procedure for glenoid bone loss greater than 25%. Four percent of patients sustained a recurrent dislocation, 5% had instability complaints, and there was an average of 5 degrees of loss of external rotation with the arm adducted.[20] Auffarth and colleagues reported no recurrences and one traumatic graft failure with iliac crest bone graft transfer to the glenoid rim.[64] Allain and colleagues reported on 56 patients followed for an average of 14 years after the Latarjet procedure.[68] They had no recurrent dislocations, and 12% of patients complained of recurrent instability.

When an engaging Hill-Sachs lesion is discovered, there is often associated anteroinferior glenoid bone deficiency. It is important to provide bony stability so that the arc of motion between the humerus and glenoid is sufficient in the patient's desired range of motion. An open bony procedure can be performed to address the glenoid bone loss and increase the glenoid articular arc to prevent an otherwise engaging Hill-Sachs lesion from translating anteriorly. In the presence of a small Hill-Sachs lesion (<30%), the humeral head does not typically need to be addressed directly. A moderate Hill-Sachs lesion (30% to 40%) often requires either the Remplissage technique, autograft or allograft bone grafting, or focal prosthetic resurfacing.[49,69-73] The Remplissage technique involves securing the infraspinatus tendon and posterior capsule to the abraded bony surface of the Hill-Sachs lesion with suture anchors (Figure 1-12).[70] This prevents the Hill-Sachs lesion from engaging the glenoid with shoulder abduction and external rotation. Humeral head bone grafting can be performed through a deltopectoral or posterior approach.[69,73] With either approach, the humeral head defect is fully exposed and débrided. A humeral head allograft is cut and shaped to fit the Hill-Sachs lesion and is secured with counter-sunk screws (Figure 1-13). Hemiarthroplasty is recommended for large Hill-Sachs lesions (>40%).

MIDDLE-AGED ATHLETE WITH SHOULDER DISLOCATION

The incidence of shoulder instability is lower in middle-aged patients, and they often have different structural pathology and natural history than younger patients.[74,75] In the younger patient, isolated capsulolabral avulsion is the most common lesion identified in an acute shoulder dislocation. In the older patient, the rotator cuff will have prior degenerative weakening and typically ruptures. In the middle-aged athlete, a rotator cuff tear and a Bankart lesion can be present concurrently. Associated neurovascular injury is also more common in the older patient at the time of shoulder dislocation than in a younger individual.[76-79] As in the younger patient, questions regarding mechanism of injury, arm position, need for a reduction, and quantity of dislocations are important. Other important questions include associated numbness or tingling, shoulder weakness, night pain, and pain with overhead activities. A complete shoulder exam will usually reveal the direction of instability. Special focus on the neurovascular exam is crucial to document any abnormalities. The axillary nerve provides sensation to the lateral upper arm and motor to the deltoid and teres minor and is the most frequently injured nerve in an anterior shoulder dislocation. Manual muscle strength testing of the supraspinatus, subscapularis, and infraspinatus may reveal weakness or pain when an associated rotator cuff tear is present.

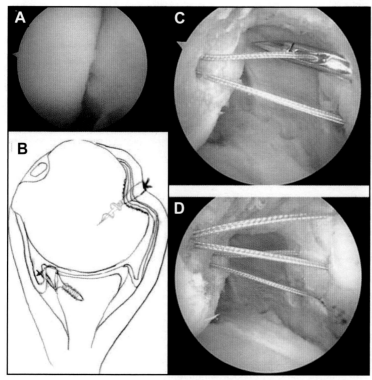

Figure 1-12. Remplissage technique. (Figure B is reprinted from *Arthroscopy*, 24(6), Purchase RJ, Wolf EM, Hobgood ER, Pollock ME, Smalley CC, Hill-Sachs "Remplissage": an arthroscopic solution for the engaging Hill-sachs lesion, pp 723-726, copyright (2008), with permission from Elsevier.)

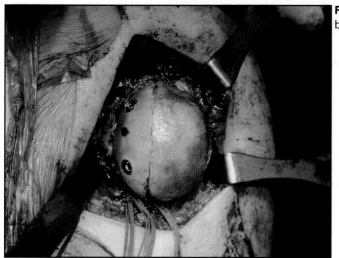

Figure 1-13. Humeral head allograft bone grafting.

Management

Less active older patients have lower recurrence rates with nonoperative treatment than younger patients who participate in contact sports or are involved in overhead occupations or activities.[80] Although many studies show unacceptably high recurrence rates among young individuals, other series report much lower rates in patients older than 30 years.[81,82] Hovelius found only a 12% recurrence rate among patients over the age of 30.[81] Treatment of the middle-aged patient with a shoulder dislocation should focus on rotator cuff pathology and neurologic injury. If a nerve injury is present, an electromyogram (EMG) should be ordered 3 weeks after the injury as a baseline exam. Typically, these injuries are neuropraxias that resolve with time, but they should be closely followed with repeat EMG and serial exams. An MRI is recommended to evaluate the rotator cuff. When no rotator cuff tear is present, even in the presence of an obvious Bankart lesion, nonoperative treatment results in low recurrence rates. A brief period of shoulder immobilization should be followed by a therapy program to regain motion and strength. If a rotator cuff tear is discovered, patients should be counseled regarding the natural history and expected outcomes of both nonoperative and operative treatment of rotator cuff pathology. When operative treatment is elected, we often find that attention is more focused on the rotator cuff pathology than the instability issue.

REFERENCES

1. Piasecki DP, Verma NN, Romeo AA, Levine WN, Bach BR Jr, Provencher MT. Glenoid bone deficiency in recurrent anterior shoulder instability: diagnosis and management. *J Am Acad Orthop Surg.* 2009;17:482-493.
2. Chen AL, Hunt SA, Hawkins RJ, Zuckerman JD. Management of bone loss associated with recurrent anterior glenohumeral instability. *Am J Sports Med.* 2005;33:912-925.
3. Owens BD, Duffey ML, Nelson BJ, DeBerardino TM, Taylor DC, Mountcastle SB. The incidence and characteristics of shoulder instability at the United States Military Academy. *Am J Sports Med.* 2007;35:1168-1173.
4. Robinson CM, Howes J, Murdoch H, Will E, Graham C. Functional outcome and risk of recurrent instability after primary traumatic anterior shoulder dislocation in young patients. *J Bone Joint Surg Am.* 2006;88:2326-2336.
5. Rowe CR. Prognosis in dislocations of the shoulder. *J Bone Joint Surg Am.* 1956;38A:957-977.
6. McLaughlin H, Cavallaro W. Primary anterior dislocation of the shoulder. *Am J Surg.* 1950;80:615-621.
7. te Slaa RL, Wiffels MP, Brand R, Marti RK. The prognosis following acute primary glenohumeral dislocation. *J Bone Joint Surg Br.* 2004;86B:58-64.
8. Urayama M, Itoi E, Sashi R, Minagawa H, Sato K. Capsular elongation in shoulders with recurrent anterior dislocation. Quantitative assessment with magnetic resonance arthrography. *Am J Sports Med.* 2003;31:64-67.
9. Wang RY, Arciero RA. Treating the athlete with anterior shoulder instability. *Clin Sports Med.* 2008;27:631-648.
10. Matsen FA 3rd, Chebli CM, Lippitt SB. Principles for the evaluation and management of shoulder instability. *Instr Course Lect.* 2007;56:23-34.
11. Gibb TD, Sidles JA, Harryman DT 2nd, McQuade KJ, Matsen FA 3rd. The effect of capsular venting on glenohumeral laxity. *Clin Orthop Relat Res.* 1991;268:120-127.
12. Hsu HC, Luo ZP, Cofield RH. Influence of rotator cuff tearing on glenohumeral instability. *J Shoulder Elbow Surg.* 1997;6:413-422.
13. Bankart AS, Cantab MC. Recurrent or habitual dislocation of the shoulder-joint. *Clin Orthop Relat Res.* 1993;291:3-6.
14. Burkhart SS, De Beer JF. Traumatic glenohumeral bone defects and their relationship to failure of arthroscopic Bankart repairs: significance of the inverted-pear glenoid and the humeral engaging Hill-Sachs lesion. *Arthroscopy.* 2000;16:677-694.
15. Gerber C, Nyffeler RW. Classification of glenohumeral joint instability. *Clin Orthop Relat Res.* 2002;400:65-76.
16. Itoi E, Lee SB, Berglund LJ, Berge LL, An KN. The effect of a glenoid defect on anteroinferior stability of the shoulder after Bankart repair: a cadaveric study. *J Bone Joint Surg Am.* 2000;82:35-46.
17. Montgomery WH Jr, Wahl M, Hettrich C, Itoi E, Lippitt SB, Matsen FA 3rd. Anteroinferior bone-grafting can restore stability in osseous glenoid defects. *J Bone Joint Surg Am.* 2005;87:1972-1977.
18. Taylor DC, Arciero RA. Pathologic changes associated with shoulder dislocations. Arthroscopic and physical examination findings in first-time, traumatic anterior dislocations. *Am J Sports Med.* 1997;25:306-311.
19. Burkhart SS, Danaceau SM. Articular arc length mismatch as a cause of failed Bankart repair. *Arthroscopy.* 2000;16:740-744.

20. Burkhart SS, De Beer JF, Barth JR, Cresswell T, Roberts C, Richards DP. Results of modified Latarjet reconstruction in patients with anteroinferior instability and significant bone loss. *Arthroscopy.* 2007;23:1033-1041.
21. Boileau P, Villalba M, Hery JY, Balg F, Ahrens P, Neyton L. Risk factors for recurrence of shoulder instability after arthroscopic Bankart repair. *J Bone Joint Surg Am.* 2006;88:1755-1763.
22. Matsen FA 3rd, Thomas S. *Glenohumeral Instability.* 2nd ed. Philadelphia, PA: W.B Saunders; 1998.
23. Schenk TJ, Brems JJ. Multidirectional instability of the shoulder: pathophysiology, diagnosis, and management. *J Am Acad Orthop Surg.* 1998;6:65-72.
24. Baker CL 3rd, Mascarenhas R, Kline AJ, Chhabra A, Pombo MW, Bradley JP. Arthroscopic treatment of multidirectional shoulder instability in athletes: a retrospective analysis of 2- to 5-year clinical outcomes. *Am J Sports Med.* 2009;37:1712-1720.
25. Neer CI, Foster C. Inferior capsular shift for involuntary inferior and multidirectional instability of the shoulder: a preliminary report. *J Bone Joint Surg Am.* 1980;62:897-908.
26. Hawkins RJ, Abrams JS, Schutte J. Multidirectional instability of the shoulder: an approach to diagnosis. *Orthop Trans.* 1987;11:246.
27. Kim SH, Park JC, Park JS, Oh I. Painful jerk test: a predictor of success in nonoperative treatment of posteroinferior instability of the shoulder. *Am J Sports Med.* 2004;32:1849-1855.
28. Kim SH, Park JS, Jeong WK, Shin SK. The Kim test: a novel test for posteroinferior labral lesion of the shoulder—a comparison to the jerk test. *Am J Sports Med.* 2005;33:1188-1192.
29. Burkhead WZ, Rockwood CA. Treatment of instability of the shoulder with an exercise program. *J Bone Joint Surg Am.* 1992;74:890-896.
30. Kim SH, Ha KI, Yoo JC, Noh KC. Kim's lesion: an incomplete and concealed avulsion of the posteroinferior labrum in posterior or multidirectional posteroinferior instability of the shoulder. *Arthroscopy.* 2004;20:712-720.
31. Gartsman GM, Roddey TS, Hammerman SM. Arthroscopic treatment of anterior-inferior glenohumeral instability. Two to five-year follow-up. *J Bone Joint Surg Am.* 2000;82-A:991-1003.
32. Treacy SH, Savoie FH, Field LD. Arthroscopic treatment of multidirectional instability. *J Shoulder Elbow Surg.* 1999;8:344-349.
33. Provencher MT, Mologne TS, Romeo AA, Bradley JP. The use of rotator interval closure in the arthroscopic treatment of posterior shoulder instability. *Arthroscopy.* 2009;25:109-110.
34. Provencher MT, Mologne TS, Hongo M, Zhao K, Tasto JP, An KN. Arthroscopic versus open rotator interval closure: biomechanical evaluation of stability and motion. *Arthroscopy.* 2007;23:583-592.
35. Mologne TS, Zhao K, Hongo M, Romeo AA, An KN, Provencher MT. The addition of rotator interval closure after arthroscopic repair of either anterior or posterior shoulder instability: effect on glenohumeral translation and range of motion. *Am J Sports Med.* 2008;36:1123-1131.
36. DeBerardino TM, Arciero RA, Taylor DC. Arthroscopic stabilization of acute initial anterior shoulder dislocation. The West Point Experience. *J South Orthop Assoc.* 1996;5(4):263-271.
37. Cvitanic O, Tirman PF, Feller JF. Using abduction and external rotation of the shoulder to increase the sensitivity of MR arthrography in revealing tears of the anterior glenoid labrum. *Am J Roentgenol.* 1997;169:837-844.
38. Itoi E. Immobilization in external rotation after shoulder dislocation reduces the risk of recurrence. *J Bone Joint Surg Am.* 2007;89:2124-2131.
39. Finestone A, Milgrom C, Radeva-Petrova DR, et al. Bracing in external rotation for traumatic anterior dislocation of the shoulder. *J Bone Joint Surg Br.* 2009;91:918-921.
40. Buss DD, Lynch GP, Meyer CP, Huber SM, Freehill MQ. Nonoperative management for in-season athletes with anterior shoulder instability. *Am J Sports Med.* 2004;32:1430-1433.
41. Robinson CM, Jenkins PJ, White TO, Ker A, Will E. Primary arthroscopic stabilization for a first-time anterior dislocation of the shoulder. A randomized, double-blind trial. *J Bone Joint Surg Am.* 2008;90:708-721.
42. DeBerardino TM, Arciero RA, Taylor DC, Uhorchak JM. Prospective evaluation of arthroscopic stabilization of acute, initial anterior shoulder dislocations in young athletes. Two- to five-year follow-up. *Am J Sports Med.* 2001;29:586-592.
43. Bottoni C, Wilckens JH, DeBerardino TM. A prospective randomized evaluation of arthroscopic stabilization versus non-operative treatment in patients with acute, first-time shoulder dislocation. *Am J Sports Med.* 2002;30:576-580.
44. Kuhn JE. Treating the initial anterior shoulder dislocation: an evidence-based medicine approach. *Sports Med Arthrosc Rev.* 2006;14:192-198.
45. Habermeyer P, Gleyze P, Rickert M. Evolution of lesions of the labrum-ligament complex in posttraumatic anterior shoulder instability: a prospective study. *J Shoulder Elbow Surg.* 1999;8:66-74.
46. Hovelius L, Saeboe M. Neer Award 2008: Arthropathy after primary anterior shoulder dislocation—223 shoulders prospectively followed up for twenty-five years. *J Shoulder Elbow Surg.* 2009;18:339-347.

47. Bushnell BD, Creighton RA, Herring MM. The bony apprehension test for instability of the shoulder: a prospective pilot analysis. *Arthroscopy*. 2008;24:974-982.

48. Itoi E, Lee SB, Amrami KK, Wenger DE, An KN. Quantitative assessment of classic anteroinferior bony Bankart lesions by radiography and computed tomography. *Am J Sports Med*. 2003;31:112-118.

49. Bushnell BD, Creighton RA, Herring MM. Bony instability of the shoulder. *Arthroscopy*. 2008;24:1061-1073.

50. Chuang TY, Adams CR, Burkhart SS. Use of preoperative three-dimensional computed tomography to quantify glenoid bone loss in shoulder instability. *Arthroscopy*. 2008;24:376-382.

51. Sugaya H, Moriishi J, Kanisawa I, Tsuchiya A. Arthroscopic osseous Bankart repair for chronic recurrent traumatic anterior glenohumeral instability. *J Bone Joint Surg Am*. 2005;87:1752-1760.

52. Lo IK, Parten PM, Burkhart SS. The inverted pear glenoid: an indicator of significant glenoid bone loss. *Arthroscopy*. 2004;20:169-174.

53. Stein DA, Jazrawi L, Bartolozzi AR. Arthroscopic stabilization of anterior shoulder instability: a review of the literature. *Arthroscopy*. 2002;18:912-924.

54. Stein DA, Jazrawi LM, Rosen JE, Loebenberg MI. Arthroscopic stabilization of anterior shoulder instability: a historical perspective. *Bull Hosp Joint Dis*. 2001;60:124-129.

55. Mazzocca AD, Brown FM Jr, Carreira DS, Hayden J, Romeo AA. Arthroscopic anterior shoulder stabilization of collision and contact athletes. *Am J Sports Med*. 2005;33:52-60.

56. Owens BD, DeBerardino TM, Nelson BJ, et al. Long-term follow-up of acute arthroscopic Bankart repair for initial anterior shoulder dislocations in young athletes. *Am J Sports Med*. 2009;37:669-673.

57. Taylor DC, Nelson BJ. Anterior shoulder stabilization in collision athletes: arthroscopic versus open Bankart repair. *Am J Sports Med*. 2007;35:148.

58. Balg F, Boileau P. The instability severity index score. A simple pre-operative score to select patients for arthroscopic or open shoulder stabilisation. *J Bone Joint Surg Br*. 2007;89:1470-1477.

59. Pagnani MJ. Open capsular repair without bone block for recurrent anterior shoulder instability in patients with and without bony defects of the glenoid and/or humeral head. *Am J Sports Med*. 2008;36:1805-1812.

60. Mologne TS, Provencher MT, Menzel KA, Vachon TA, Dewing CB. Arthroscopic stabilization in patients with an inverted pear glenoid: results in patients with bone loss of the anterior glenoid. *Am J Sports Med*. 2007;35:1276-1283.

61. Schroder DT, Provencher MT, Mologne TS, Muldoon MP, Cox JS. The modified Bristow procedure for anterior shoulder instability. *Am J Sports Med*. 2006;34:778-786.

62. Hovelius L, Sandstrom B, Sundgren K, Saebo M. One hundred eighteen Bristow-Latarjet repairs for recurrent anterior dislocation of the shoulder prospectively followed for fifteen years: study I—clinical results. *J Shoulder Elbow Surg*. 2004;13:509-516.

63. Hovelius L, Sandstrom B, Saebo M. One hundred eighteen Bristow-Latarjet repairs for recurrent anterior dislocation of the shoulder prospectively followed for fifteen years: study II—the evolution of dislocation arthropathy. *J Shoulder Elbow Surg*. 2006;15:279-289.

64. Auffarth A, Schauer J, Matis N, Kofler B, Hitzl W, Resch H. The J-bone graft for anatomical glenoid reconstruction in recurrent posttraumatic anterior shoulder dislocation. *Am J Sports Med*. 2008;36:638-647.

65. Kropf EJ, Sekiya JK. Osteoarticular allograft transplantation for large humeral head defects in glenohumeral instability. *Arthroscopy*. 2007;23:322, e1-5.

66. Provencher MT, Ghodadra N, LeClere L, Solomon DJ, Romeo AA. Anatomic osteochondral glenoid reconstruction for recurrent glenohumeral instability with glenoid deficiency using a distal tibia allograft. *Arthroscopy*. 2009;25:446-452.

67. Warner JJ, Gill TJ, O'Hollerhan JD, Pathare N, Millett PJ. Anatomical glenoid reconstruction for recurrent anterior glenohumeral instability with glenoid deficiency using an autogenous tricortical iliac crest bone graft. *Am J Sports Med*. 2006;34:205-212.

68. Allain J, Goutallier D, Glorion C. Long-term results of the Latarjet procedure for the treatment of anterior instability of the shoulder. *J Bone Joint Surg Am*. 1998;80:841-852.

69. Miniaci A, Berlet G, Hand C, Lin A. Segmental humeral head allografts for recurrent anterior instability of the shoulder with large Hill-Sachs defects: a 2 to 8 year follow up. *J Bone Joint Surg Br*. 2008;90 Supplement I:86.

70. Purchase RJ, Wolf EM, Hobgood ER, Pollock ME, Smalley CC. Hill-Sachs "Remplissage": an arthroscopic solution for the engaging Hill-sachs lesion. *Arthroscopy*. 2008;24:723-726.

71. Ochoa E Jr, Burkhart SS. Glenohumeral bone defects in the treatment of anterior shoulder instability. *Instr Course Lect*. 2009;58:323-336.

72. Toro F, Melean P, Moraga C, Ruiz F, Gonzalez F, Vaisman A. Remplissage: infraspinatus tenodesis and posterior capsulodesis for the treatment of Hill-Sachs lesions: an all intraarticular technique. *Tech Shoulder Elbow Surg*. 2008;9:188-192.

73. Bushnell BD, Creighton RA, Herring MM. Hybrid treatment of engaging Hill-Sachs lesions: arthroscopic capsulolabral repair and limited posterior approach for bone grafting. *Tech Shoulder Elbow Surg.* 2007;8:194-203.

74. Araghi A, Prasarn M, St Clair S, Zuckerman JD. Recurrent anterior glenohumeral instability with onset after forty years of age: the role of the anterior mechanism. *Bull Hosp Joint Dis.* 2005;62:99-101.

75. Porcellini G, Paladini P, Campi F, Paganelli M. Shoulder instability and related rotator cuff tears: arthroscopic findings and treatment in patients aged 40 to 60 years. *Arthroscopy.* 2006;22:270-276.

76. Hawkins RJ, Bell RH, Hawkins RH, Koppert GJ. Anterior dislocation of the shoulder in the older patient. *Clin Orthop Relat Res.* 1986:192-195.

77. Neviaser RJ, Neviaser TJ. Recurrent instability of the shoulder after age 40. *J Shoulder Elbow Surg.* 1995;4:416-418.

78. Neviaser RJ, Neviaser TJ, Neviaser JS. Concurrent rupture of the rotator cuff and anterior dislocation of the shoulder in the older patient. *J Bone Joint Surg Am.* 1988;70:1308-1311.

79. Neviaser RJ, Neviaser TJ, Neviaser JS. Anterior dislocation of the shoulder and rotator cuff rupture. *Clin Orthop Relat Res.* 1993:103-106.

80. Sachs RA, Lin D, Stone ML, Paxton E, Kuney M. Can the need for future surgery for acute traumatic anterior shoulder dislocation be predicted? *J Bone Joint Surg Am.* 2007;89:1665-1674.

81. Hovelius L. Anterior dislocation of the shoulder in teenagers and young adults. *J Bone Joint Surg Am.* 1987;69:393-399.

82. Simonet WT, Cofield RH. Prognosis in anterior shoulder dislocation. *Am J Sports Med.* 1984;12:19-24.

2

Patient's Preparation, Positioning, and Portals for Arthroscopic Stabilization

Part I: Advantages of the Lateral Decubitus Position

Jason Sullivan, MD and Guido Marra, MD

There are 2 primary positions commonly employed for arthroscopic shoulder surgery: the lateral decubitus position and the beach chair position. Other patient positioning techniques described are hybrids of these 2 positions. The purpose of this chapter is to review the lateral decubitus position for shoulder arthroscopy, with an emphasis on the advantages of lateral decubitus positioning in regard to patient safety, portal placement, and special intraoperative considerations.

PATIENT SELECTION

A careful history and physical evaluation of the patient should be performed prior to making the decision to proceed with arthroscopic shoulder surgery. Relative contra-indications to arthroscopic surgery include dermatologic skin conditions or infections

Abrams JS. *Management of the Unstable Shoulder: Arthroscopic and Open Repair* (pp. 23-44).
© 2011 SLACK Incorporated

near the surgical site, as well as medical comorbidities that supersede the need for elective shoulder surgery. Patients should also understand and be willing to consent to an open surgical procedure should it be warranted during the case. Open communication with the patient regarding how he or she will be positioned during surgery will not only help answer some of the patient's questions, but will also help promote a thorough discussion during the consenting process regarding potential complications.

Few patients are contraindicated for the lateral decubitus position; however, congestive heart failure patients represent one group that should be approached with caution. Congestive heart failure can result in venous congestion in the dependent lung due to poor cardiac function. Palermo and colleagues found that as a patient lies on his or her side, greater lung deterioration occurs in patients with enlarged hearts.[1] In addition, this effect on lung function can be exacerbated by phrenic nerve paralysis if an interscalene anesthetic is used. For this reason, opting for a different position in patients with congestive heart failure should be strongly considered.

Lateral acromion morphology has been suggested as a potential selection criterion by Baechler and Kim.[2] Arthroscopic access to the superior glenoid using lateral portals becomes more difficult with increased lateral coverage of the humeral head by the acromion. Using coronal oblique magnetic resonance imaging (MRI), they proposed that a 25-degree minimum vertical arc is necessary between the humerus and lateral acromion for arthroscopic instrumentation of the superior glenoid (Figure 2-1). The authors stated that some patients require minimal or no traction at all to achieve this desired corridor and using the beach chair position would not compromise access to the superior glenoid. However, patients who require inferior displacement of the humeral head equal to or greater than 25% of the humeral head diameter to achieve this optimal 25 degrees arc of vertical clearance may benefit from the lateral decubitus position due to the advantage of continuous traction.

PREOPERATIVE SET-UP MATERIALS

Shoulder arthroscopy can be performed under general anesthetic with or without regional nerve block. A preoperative interscalene block helps to decrease the amount of analgesic used during the case along with pain control postoperatively. After induction of anesthesia, it is important to examine the patient's shoulder in the supine position to allow comparison to the contralateral shoulder. Range of motion and shoulder stability should be documented and correlated with prior clinical assessment to confirm final operative plan.

The patient is positioned with the nonoperative shoulder in the dependent position. An axillary roll is placed from posterior to anterior slightly distal to the true axilla, padding the thorax to protect compression of the brachial plexus and improve ventilation throughout the case (Figure 2-2). The radial artery of the dependent limb should then be palpated to detect any vascular compromise due to positioning.

Improper positioning of the axillary roll can lead to severe complications. Keyurapan and colleagues reported that 3 out of 896 patients over a 10-year period developed the equivalent of stage III pressure ulcers of the thorax after arthroscopic or combined open and arthroscopic shoulder surgery.[3] Patients' average age was 35 years, case length averaged 107 minutes, and in all cases an intravenous fluid bag was used as the axillary roll. The authors felt that the ulcers were caused by inadequate security of the patient, leading to ulcer formation from skin shear.

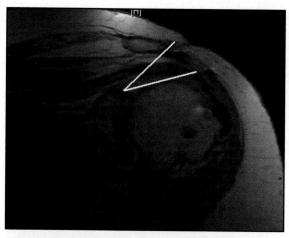

Figure 2-1. A coronal oblique MRI of the shoulder demonstrating the angle described by Baechler and Kim. In this case, the angle measures more than 25 degrees, allowing a large enough corridor of access for instrumentation in either the lateral decubitus or the beach chair position.

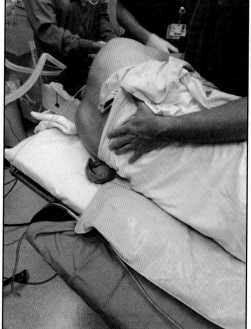

Figure 2-2. Patient positioned in the lateral decubitus position with an axillary roll in position.

Optimal patient stability can be achieved through the use of a vacuum bean bag device, which allows for secure position and minimizes contact pressure points (Figure 2-3). A peg board or other positioning devices can be used as long as the patient is resting securely. Pillows or foam padding should be placed under the dependent leg at the knee and ankle to protect the peroneal nerve and lateral malleolus, respectively (Figure 2-4). Pillows, blankets, or foam can be placed between the legs and secured to the operating table. The patient's head should be positioned in neutral alignment, taking care to avoid lateral bending of the neck. The nonoperative upper extremity should be padded appropriately and secured to an arm board. The patient's eyes must be protected and the endotracheal tube secured along the length of the table anterior to the patient and connected to the ventilator at the patient's feet. The anesthesiologist and anesthesiology equipment are at the foot of the bed to allow complete access to the surgical site by the surgeon.

Figure 2-3. Patient stabilized in the lateral decubitus position with a vacuum bean bag.

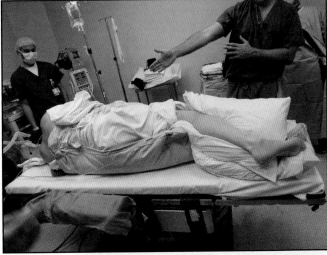

Figure 2-4. Padding of the legs with pillows during preparation prior to surgery.

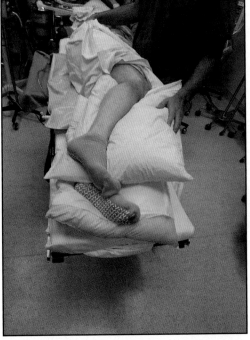

The extremity is draped in a sterile fashion while the arm is being abducted. It is important to achieve a water-tight seal around the surgical site so that irrigation used during arthroscopy does not invade the drapes and soak the patient. The hand is then placed in a sleeve that is wrapped with Coban and hooked at the end into the traction device. The surgeon and assistant will stand posteriorly to the patient.

MODIFICATIONS

In 1985, Gross and Fitzgibbons described a modification to the straight lateral decubitus positioning that included rolling the patient 20 to 30 degrees posteriorly.[4] This compensated for normal glenoid version, making it parallel with the floor. Advantages to this positioning included the need for less traction, accentuation of labral tears, and improved access to the inferior third of the glenoid labrum and capsule.

The La Jolla beach chair position is a hybrid between beach chair and lateral decubitus positioning, with the patient in a 45-degree lateral position, hips flexed, and the back of the table elevated 30 degrees. This position affords most of the same advantages as those associated with the lateral decubitus position, but with the anatomy in a more upright position, according to Hoenecke and colleagues.[5]

TRACTION

Consistent traction in the lateral decubitus position is an important advantage that should be used appropriately. Klein and colleagues performed a cadaveric assessment of strain on the brachial plexus using longitudinal traction in different combinations of flexion-abduction arm positions.[6] They further analyzed how these different arm positions affected glenohumeral joint visibility. Cadaveric specimens were placed in the lateral decubitus position with gauges placed on the 3 trunks of the brachial plexus. Minimal strain was noted at 90 degrees of flexion and 0 degrees of abduction, though with poor visibility. Positions that maximized visibility while minimizing strain were 45 degrees of forward flexion and 90 degrees of abduction along with 45 degrees of forward flexion and 0 degrees of abduction. Many surgeons prefer positioning of 45 to 70 degrees of abduction and 20 to 30 degrees of forward flexion, which provided for the best visibility of the glenohumeral joint in this study, but at the expense of increased strain. Straying from ideal positioning of the limb requires greater attention to length of operation and weight of traction applied to avoid traction neuropathies of the brachial plexus.[7] The operative extremity should be removed from traction when closing to minimize time under tension.

Jerosch and colleagues described the ideal position of the shoulder as abducted and externally rotated concerning maximizing the distance between the axillary nerve and the glenoidal/humeral capsule insertion.[8] This arm position causes the axillary nerve to be in its most native position while tightening the glenohumeral capsule, thus increasing the distance between portal entry sites and the axillary nerve. The continuous traction during lateral decubitus positioning can be used to mimic the described safer position of the shoulder.

The exact amount of traction should be no more than 10 to 15 pounds and should be tailored to the physique of the patient. Pitman and colleagues studied somatosensory evoked potentials (SEPs) of the musculocutaneous nerve, ulnar nerve, and either the radial or median nerve in 20 patients undergoing arthroscopic shoulder surgery.[9] In all patients, the musculocutaneous nerve had abnormal SEPs, and 75% of these occurred when traction was applied to the limb. Abnormal SEPs occurred 55% of the time with placement of longitudinal traction greater than 12 pounds and 30% of the time with vertical traction greater than 7 pounds. There were varying combinations of radial, median, and ulnar nerve involvement. Ten percent developed a transient neuropraxia with traction equal to or greater than 15 pounds in both cases. No changes in SEPs were seen when less than 12 pounds was used for longitudinal traction or less than 7 pounds was used for vertical traction.

Once satisfactorily positioned and prior to placement in traction, the wrist padding should be adequate. Ellman attributed inadequate wrist padding as the cause of transient dysesthesias of the radial sensory nerve to the thumb in 3 patients placed in the lateral decubitus position.[10] If the operative extremity is improperly placed in traction, the device may act like a partial or complete venous tourniquet, causing decreased oxygen tissue perfusion. Hennrikus and co-workers used pulse oximetry on the operative arms of 30 patients in 3 different positions: longitudinal traction only, the addition of vertical traction with a 2-inch sling, and the addition of a 4-inch sling.[11] Simple longitudinal traction ablated oxygen saturation in only 3% of patients. The addition of vertical traction with only a 2-inch sling caused ablation of oxygen saturation 83% of the time compared to only 23% of the time with a 4-inch sling. Their conclusion was that using a 4-inch sling was necessary if vertical traction was used during shoulder arthroscopy in the lateral decubitus position. Pulse oximetry is a helpful adjunct toward monitoring oxygen tissue perfusion pressure of the operative extremity.

PORTAL PLACEMENT

There are many described portals for shoulder arthroscopy that can be easily confused. It is advised to mark out the anatomical structures of the shoulder, including proposed portal placement, prior to starting the case. Drawing out the clavicle, acromion, and coracoid process will promote successful portal establishment, especially later in the case as fluid extravasation increases and soft tissues distend. Prior to portal establishment, joint distension can be performed with approximately 20 cc. With confirmation of backflow, approximately 30 to 60 mL of normal saline can be injected in the glenohumeral joint.[12] Distension of the glenohumeral joint may help prevent iatrogenic chondral injury upon introducing a trocar into the joint.

The posterior portal remains the primary portal for entry in the glenohumeral joint. The proposed entry site is a soft spot upon palpation that represents the interval between the infraspinatus and teres minor. Internal and external rotation of the humerus is beneficial to assess the appropriate angle to aim the blunt tip probe. The entry point is usually 2 cm inferior and 1 cm medial to the posterolateral tip of the acromion. Understanding the version of the glenoid on preoperative imaging may help with minute variations in the chosen angle of posterior portal entry. After a vertical incision, the blunt trocar is passed through skin and aimed at the coracoid process anteriorly. The posterior portal can be used to diagnose pathology, provide access to both the glenohumeral and subacromial space, and introduce new portals under direct visualization. If anticipating subacromial decompression, then the posterior portal can be made slightly superior, allowing for the scope to be parallel to the undersurface of the acromion. A cadaveric study by Meyer and colleagues showed the posterior portal to be safe from injuring the axillary nerve and suprascapular artery and nerve with distances of 49, 27, and 29 mm, respectively. Injury to the teres minor or infraspinatus occurred in 1 of 12 cadavers.[13]

Variations of the posterior portal are specifically used to gain better access to the glenoid labrum as the direct posterior portal is parallel to the glenoid surface. The low posterolateral portal is described as 2 to 4 cm lateral and 4 to 5 cm inferior to the posterolateral corner of the acromion. This portal is obtained via an "outside-in" technique and provides a more optimal angle for anchor placement and suture passage through the posterior and inferior labrum. Nord and colleagues reported no complications in 17 patients using this portal.[14] Five cadaveric specimens were used and determined that the axillary nerve and posterior humeral circumflex artery were 13.8 and 13.4 mm, respectively, from the low posterolateral portal. Similarly, the 7 o'clock posteroinferior portal was found to be safe in evaluating the inferior capsular recess of the glenohumeral joint. Davidson and Rivenburgh demonstrated a safer distance from neurovascular (axillary and suprascapular nerves) structures by approximately 5 mm, using the "inside-out" technique as opposed to the "outside-in."[15]

The axillary pouch portal is placed 2 cm inferior to the anterior lateral border of the acromion and 21.3 mm lateral to the posterior viewing portal. The spinal needle should be angled medially by 30 degrees and 5 degrees inferiorly. With the use of both 30- and 70-degree arthroscopes, the inferior glenohumeral ligament complex can be evaluated, specifically humeral avulsion of glenohumeral ligament (HAGL) lesions.

Finally, Hoenecke and Fronek[16] studied the posteromedial portal with proposed benefits of suture anchor placement posterior to the biceps insertion when addressing posterosuperior labral pathology. Traditional anterior superior portals or trans-supraspinatus portals traverse through the rotator cuff, whereas the posterior medial portal does not. The initial posterior viewing portal must be placed 1 to 2 cm lateral from its usual position, allowing a safe distance from the posteromedial portal, which is described as 3 cm directly medial of the viewing portal. An 18-gauge spinal needle can be used for accurate placement. This portal is 2 cm lateral to the spinoglenoid notch and suprascapular nerve.

Multiple anterior portals have been described in the literature. Understanding the goals of the surgery will dictate precise portal entry. Most commonly, the anterior portal is established using a needle placed halfway between the coracoid and the anterolateral corner of the acromion. By visualizing the needle placement, the established anterior portal can be achieved exactly as planned. Matthews and colleagues described the anterior portal to be located about 1:30 to 2 o'clock in relation to the glenoid between the triangle formed by the biceps tendon, glenoid rim, and humeral head.[17] Wolf further described a portal at 3 o'clock at the superior border of the subscapularis.[18]

The anterior superior portals are difficult to use when trying to address anterior inferior instability, such as a Bankart lesion. This pathology often requires interosseous fixation, which is difficult to achieve at an acute angle. In a cadaveric study, Davidson and Tibone proposed the 5 o'clock portal for direct access to anteroinferior glenoid.[19] The portal was created using an "inside-out" technique with the humerus maximally adducted. They described the portal placement in relationship to the axillary (24.4 mm) and musculocutaneous (22.9 mm) nerves along with cephalic veins. They concluded that safe placement of the portal was achieved with the arm adducted, achieving portal placement lateral to the conjoined tendon; however, it does course through the subscapularis. The cephalic vein and anterior humeral circumflex arteries were not injured with use of blunt instruments. This portal is very useful in shoulder stabilization procedures due to its easy access to the inferior glenoid neck.

The lateral portal is often used for instrumentation and visualization of the subacromial bursa. This portal passes through the deltoid 2 to 3 cm distal to the lateral border of the acromion. Superior portals piercing the trapezius have also been described. In 1987, Thomas Neviaser described the superior medial portal, which is bordered by the clavicle, acromioclavicular joint, and spine of the scapula.[20] The cannula is inserted 15 to 20 degrees from vertical and aimed laterally and anteriorly. The portal pierces the trapezius; however, Baker and Souryal showed the joint may be entered without violating the supraspinatus with the arm in 30 degrees of abduction.[21] The modified Neviaser uses essentially the same entry point, 1 cm medial to the medial border of the acromion, though it is designed to pierce the supraspinatus. Both portals are useful in repair of the supraspinatus. Last, the subclavian portal is found 1 to 2 cm medial to the acromioclavicular joint and directly inferior to the clavicle. This portal is slightly medial and superior to the coracoid and typically is best used after acromial decompression to allow smooth passage into the subacromial space.

ADVANTAGE

The lateral decubitus position facilitates glenohumeral surgery through the use of vertical and horizontal traction. Free access of the scapula is an added benefit of the lateral decubitus position that is more difficult to achieve in the beach chair position due to constraints of the operating table.

No assistant is necessary to hold the limb or distract it during the case due to the use of continuous traction. Previously, this was a significant downside of the beach chair position, which required an assistant to achieve different amounts of traction and different positions of the limb. The introduction of mechanical arm holders has made traction and adequate positions of the limb much easier to attain in the beach chair position. However, these devices do not quantify the amount of traction applied as opposed to the consistent and continuous traction of the lateral decubitus position.

In addition, lateral decubitus positioning keeps the brain collinear with the heart, leading to uniform tissue perfusion pressures throughout the case. A blood pressure cuff reading on the patient's contralateral arm or leg provides an adequate representation of the blood pressure supplying the cerebral vasculature.

In comparison, blood pressure measurements in the beach chair position differ greatly from head to toe, due to hydrostatic pressure. In the *Journal of Clinical Anesthesia*, Pohl and Cullen reported 4 catastrophic cases of ischemic brain and spinal cord injury after shoulder surgery in the beach chair position.[22] The 4 people were 47, 53, 54, and 57 years old, and none had a history of tobacco use or hypertension. The only risk factors identified for stroke were a family history of coronary artery disease in 1 patient, male gender in 2 patients, and hyperlipidemia in 1 patient. They postulated the cause of these events was related to critical positioning of the head, potentially leading to mechanical blockage of major arteries or veins of the neck, postural hypotension, and/or intraoperative monitoring of blood pressure.

The effect of position can be compounded by the use of hypotension to assist in intraoperative visualization. When in the beach chair position, it is essential to understand the relationship of blood pressure cuff measurements in relation to the cerebral blood pressure. Papadonikolakis and colleagues provided a concise review of different cuff positions during surgery related to the catastrophic complications of cerebral ischemia (Table 2-1).[23] Often, during arthroscopic shoulder surgery, the blood pressure cuff will be placed on the patient's calf due to intravenous access in the nonoperative arm. In the beach chair position, the hydrostatic pressure gradient can account for as much as a 94 mm Hg greater blood pressure reading in the calf as opposed to the arm. If this large pressure gradient is not taken into consideration when attempting to use controlled hypotension in the beach chair position, then dangerously low cerebral perfusion may result. Comparatively, the pressure difference from arm to calf in the lateral decubitus position is a more negligible difference of 5 mm Hg. To avoid complications, they suggested using the heart as the gold standard for referencing blood pressure monitoring, using the brachium for the cuff or an arterial line and aggressively treating perioperative hypotension. Thus, the lateral decubitus position alleviates the need for meticulous calculations of intraoperative blood pressure, allowing for safer and more controlled intraoperative hypotension and thus safer visualization.

Table 2-1

BLOOD PRESSURE MONITORED IN DIFFERENT POSITIONS WITH CUFF AT ARM AND CALF

	BLOOD PRESSURE (MM HG)	
POSITION	*CUFF AT BRACHIUM*	*CUFF AT CALF*
Supine	111/72	110/70
Beach chair	116/82	168/87
Standing	114/78	209/139

Note: In the beach chair position, the blood pressure at the calf is roughly 23 inches or 58 cm below the heart, or 43 mm Hg higher than the blood pressure at the brachium. The resting systolic blood pressure of a normotensive individual is shown in different positions. The systolic blood pressure in the beach chair position is 116 mm Hg at the brachium and 168 mm Hg at the ankle. If the blood pressure cuff is placed at the calf and the surgeon requests a blood pressure of 100 mm Hg, then the blood pressure at the arm will be 48 mm Hg and the blood flow to the brain will be extremely low. On the contrary, in the lateral position the blood pressure at the cuff can only be 5 mm Hg higher than the blood pressure at the brachium. Thus the danger of reducing the blood pressure to critical values is minimized.

Reprinted from *Arthroscopy*, 24(4), Papadonikolakis A, Wiesler ER, Olympio MA, Poehling GG, Avoiding catastrophic complications of stroke and death related to shoulder surgery in the sitting position, 481-482, copyright (2008), with permission from Elsevier.

DISADVANTAGES/COMPLICATIONS

Arthroscopic shoulder surgery is thought to be minimally invasive and less aggressive than open shoulder surgery. However, it is not free of complications. It is difficult to quantify complication rates due to alleged under-reporting, as noted by both Berjano and colleagues and Bigliani and co-workers.[24,25]

Multiple disadvantages of the lateral decubitus position exist, such as complications caused by improper padding during positioning, as described earlier in this chapter. The most fundamental difference between the lateral decubitus and beach chair positions is the spatial disorientation of the anatomy. Contrary to beach chair position, where the anatomy and the effects of gravity are in a normal upright position, lateral decubitus positioning rotates the orientation and changes the effects of gravity on structures such as the labrum and biceps tendon.

The use of continuous traction on the arm can result in neurologic injuries postoperatively if there is excessive weight applied or increased operative time. Cutaneous,[26] motor, and sensory nerve lesions[27] after arthroscopic shoulder surgery have been described in the literature. Though most are neuropraxias and are self-limited, neurologic injury after arthroscopic shoulder surgery is reported to be as high as 30% by McFarland and colleagues.[28] Rodeo and colleagues reviewed neurologic complications and found reports of injury to all of the following: the musculocutaneous, median, radial, ulnar, and axillary nerves.[26] There are also isolated reports of medial pectoral nerve and anterior interosseous nerve injuries. These injuries are most likely explained by local tissue distension and subsequent compression to the nerves. However, no definitive conclusion has been reached. Weber and colleagues, in a review of complications related to shoulder arthroscopy, concluded that, despite increasing complexity and prevalence of procedures performed, the complication rates have not dramatically increased.[29]

Berjano and colleagues reported one complication of respiratory distress and reintubation attributed to liquid diffusion from the subacromial space.[24] He also reported 2 cases of cubital nerve neuropraxias out of 141 arthroscopic shoulder surgeries in the lateral decubitus position. These were attributed to the wrapping around the elbow because the traction never exceeded 2 kg.

Hoenecke and Fronek made the observation that conversion from a lateral decubitus shoulder arthroscopy to an open procedure, particularly an anterior one, can be more difficult than conversion from the beach chair position.[16] In addition, set-up—though simple and routine—is user specific and potentially time consuming. Both the surgeon and anesthesiologist must coordinate in setting up due to the increased distance from the airway to the anesthesiologist. Last, the monetary value of having a traction system should not be overlooked and can cost thousands of dollars.

CONCLUSION

The lateral decubitus position is popular due to advantages of continuous traction, improved exposure to intra-articular glenohumeral pathology and decreased concerns for severe intraoperative complications such as stroke. Though set up is more time consuming, its benefits over the beach chair position need to be considered. The lateral decubitus position has proven to be an effective positioning technique for shoulder arthroscopy.

REFERENCES

1. Palermo P, Cattadori G, Bussotti M, Apostolo A, Contini M, Agostoni P. Lateral decubitus position generates discomfort and worsens lung function in chronic heart failure. *Chest.* 2005;128:1511-1516.
2. Baechler MF, Kim DH. Patient positioning for shoulder arthroscopy based on variability in lateral acromion morphology. *Arthroscopy.* 2002;18:547-549.
3. Keyurapan E, Hu SJ, Redett R, McCarthy EF, McFarland EG. Pressure ulcers of the thorax after shoulder surgery. *Knee Surg Sports Traumatol Arthrosc.* 2007;15:1489-1493.
4. Gross RM, Fitzgibbons TC. Shoulder arthroscopy: a modified approach. *Arthroscopy.* 1985;1:156.
5. Hoenecke HR, Fronek J, Hardwick M. The modified beachchair position for arthroscopic shoulder surgery: the La Jolla beachchair. *Arthroscopy.* 2004;20:113-115.
6. Klein AH, France JC, Mutschler TA, Fu FH. Measurement of brachial plexus strain in arthroscopy of the shoulder. *Arthroscopy.* 1987;3:45-52.
7. Phillips BB. Arthroscopy of upper extremity. In: Canale ST, ed. *Campbell's Operative Orthopaedics.* Vol 3. 10th ed. Philadelphia, PA: Mosby; 2003:2614-2615.
8. Jerosch J, Filler TJ, Peuker ET. Which joint position puts axillary nerve at lowest risk when performing arthroscopic capsular release in patients with adhesive capsulitis of the shoulder. *Knee Surg Sports Traumatol Arthrosc.* 2002;10:126-129.
9. Pitman MI, Nainzadeh N, Ergas E, Springer S. The use of somatosensory evoked potentials for detection of neuropraxia during shoulder arthroscopy. *Arthroscopy.* 1988;4:250-255.
10. Ellman H. Arthroscopic subacromial decompression: analysis of one- to three-year results. *Arthroscopy.* 1987;3:173-181.

11. Hennrikus WL, Mapes RC, Bratton MW, Lapoint JM. Lateral traction during shoulder arthroscopy: its effect on tissue perfusion measured by pulse oximetry. *Am J Sports Med.* 1995;23:444-447.
12. Stanish WD, Peterson DC. Shoulder arthroscopy and nerve injury: pitfalls and prevention. *Arthroscopy.* 1995;11:458-466.
13. Meyer M, Gravelearu N, Hardy P, Landreau P. Anatomic risks of shoulder arthroscopy portal: anatomic cadaveric study of 12 portals. *Arthroscopy.* 2007;5:529-536.
14. Nord KD, Brady PC, Yazdani RS, Burkhart SS. The anatomy and function of the low posterolateral portal in addressing posterior labral pathology. *Arthroscopy.* 2007;9:999-1005.
15. Davidson PA, Rivenburgh DW. The 7-o'clock posteroinferior portal for shoulder arthroscopy. *Am J Sports Med.* 2002;30(5):693-696.
16. Hoenecke HR, Fronek J. The posterior-medial portal. *Arthroscopy.* 2006;2:232e1-3.
17. Matthews LS, Zarins B, Michael RH, Helfet DL. Anterior portal selection for shoulder arthroscopy. *Arthroscopy.* 1985;1:33-39.
18. Wolf EM. Anterior portals in shoulder arthroscopy. *Arthroscopy.* 1989;5:201-208.
19. Davidson PA, Tibone JE. Anterior-inferior (5 o'clock) portal for shoulder arthroscopy. *Arthroscopy.* 1995;11:519-525.
20. Neviaser TJ. Arthroscopy of the shoulder. *Orthop Clin North Am.* 1987;18:361-372.
21. Baker CL, Souryal TO. Anatomy of the supraclavicular fossa portal in shoulder arthroscopy. *Arthroscopy.* 1990;6:297-300.
22. Pohl A, Cullen DJ. Cerebral ischemia during shoulder surgery in the upright position: a case series. *J Clin Anesth.* 2005;17:463-469.
23. Papadonikolakis A, Wiesler ER, Olympio MA, Poehling GG. Avoiding catastrophic complications of stroke and death related to shoulder surgery in the sitting position. *Arthroscopy.* 2008;24(4):481-482.
24. Berjano P, Gonzalez BG, Olmedo JF, Perez-Espana LA, Munilla MG. Complications in arthroscopic shoulder surgery. *Arthroscopy.* 1998;14:785-788.
25. Bigliani LU, Flatow EL, Deliz ED. Complications of shoulder arthroscopy. *Orthop Rev.* 1991;20(9):743-751.
26. Rodeo SA, Forster RA, Weiland AJ. Neurologic complications due to arthroscopy. *J Bone Joint Surg.* 1993;75A:917-926.
27. Segmuller HE, Alfred SP, Zilo G, Sales AD, Hayes MG. Cutaneous nerve lesions of the shoulder and arm after arthroscopic shoulder surgery. *J Shoulder Elbow Surg.* 1995;4:254-258.
28. McFarland EG, O'Neill OR, Hsu CY. Complications of shoulder arthroscopy. *J South Orthop Assoc.* 1997;6:190-196.
29. Weber SC, Abrams JS, Nottage WM. Complications associated with arthroscopic shoulder surgery. *Arthroscopy.* 2002;18:88-95.

SUGGESTED READING

Bhatia DN, De Beer JF. The axillary pouch portal: a new posterior portal for visualization and instrumentation in the inferior glenohumeral recess. *Arthroscopy.* 2007;23(11):1241.e1-5.
Gelber PE, Reina F, Caceres E, Monllau JC. A comparison of risk between the lateral decubitus and the beach-chair position when establishing an anteroinferior shoulder portal: a cadaveric study. *Arthroscopy.* 2007;23:522-528.
Ho E, Cofield RH, Balm MR, Hattrup SJ, Rowland RM. Neurologic complications of surgery for anterior shoulder instability. *J Shoulder Elbow Surg.* 1999;8:266-270.
Mohommed KD, Hayes MG, Saies AD. Unusual complications of shoulder arthroscopy. *J Shoulder Elbow Surg.* 2000;9:350-353.
Nord KD, Mauck MM. The new subclavian portal and modified Neviaser portal for arthroscopic rotator cuff repair. *Arthroscopy.* 2003;9:1030-1034.

Part II: Advantages of the Beach Chair Position

*CDR Matthew T. Provencher, MD, MC, USN; ENS Sean McIntire, MC, USN;
Tistia Gaston, PA-C; and Daniel J. Solomon, MD*

The beach chair and lateral decubitus positions are both reliable methods to accomplish effective arthroscopic shoulder procedures. Each has its own merits and drawbacks for specific cases involving the shoulder joint. Almost every type of shoulder arthroscopy case can be performed in either the beach chair or lateral decubitus position; however, surgeon training, joint positioning, and orientation may favor one position over the other. The beach chair position remains a versatile and well-accepted manner in which to accomplish both open and arthroscopic procedures involving all aspects of the shoulder joint. Not only are open shoulder cases easier in the beach chair position, but also the anatomy and ease of set-up make this a very attractive option for all aspects of shoulder surgery. This also includes cases in which an arthroscopic procedure is converted to an open case. Regardless, with either shoulder position, it is absolutely paramount that the patient is positioned carefully with proper padding, properly balanced suspension forces, and proper head set-up in order to minimize the chances of well-described and potentially devastating positioning complications.

ADVANTAGES OF THE BEACH CHAIR POSITION

The beach chair position with the arm free allows for ease of anatomic orientation and ease of access to the glenohumeral joint itself with the body position of the patient anatomically positioned. Arthroscopic visualization of the glenohumeral structures as well as the subacromial and anterior shoulder spaces is excellent. These factors create an easy and progressive learning curve for self-improvement as well as instruction of assistants in the operating room, such as residents, fellows, and other assistants. Patient placement in this position is easily accomplished because no additional equipment is required. However, specially designed bed attachments can improve access to the shoulder, and additional arm holders are available, which ease arm positioning and increase traction leading to improved visualization of certain aspects of the glenohumeral joint and subacromial space. For ease of application and monetary concerns, a standard operating room table can easily adjust to the beach chair position. The beach chair arm-free position is the best option for transition to open shoulder work, especially the deltopectoral approach, open instability approach, and for arthroplasty cases.[1] In addition, the beach chair position provides more flexibility if a conversion from an arthroscopic to open procedure is required, such as during an instability case with significant glenoid bone loss.[1-4]

In addition to the ease of open approach in the beach chair position, rotational control of the upper extremity is both precise and optimal. This is often difficult to achieve with the patient in the lateral decubitus position. Rotational control can be especially important in cases of subscapularis tears, certain areas of rotator cuff tears (very posterior—infraspinatus), and in exact positioning during rotator interval closure. It also may be imperative to obtain an exact position of external rotation or precise tensioning of the inferior glenohumeral ligament (IGHL) and capsule. A padded operative mobile table (Mayo stand) may be used to hold the arm in position, with the feet of the mobile stand placed under the table to allow ease of surgeon access. An assistant or a clamp that is attached to a padded arm holder (such as a padded arm wrap) and hooked to the drapes is also an effective manner in which to obtain sufficient arm control. In addition to its precise positioning advantages, the beach chair position can also easily accommodate awake anesthesia with the regional shoulder-blocked patient who has appropriate blood pressure control.

The beach chair with a mounted arm positioner approach allows for precise control of arm rotation and provides for additional glenohumeral and subacromial distraction during the case. This also removes the need for an assistant to manipulate the arm.[2] This position also allows for traction in multiple planes, especially inferior, such as when performing subacromial work. However, not all arthroscopic shoulder cases require the precise positioning and traction afforded by the arm-mounted devices. Traction devices also allow for precise positioning of the glenohumeral joint, such as if the shoulder is subluxated anteriorly. In this circumstance (usually associated with anterior instability), the glenohumeral joint can be easily reduced into the glenoid, providing easier access to anterior soft tissue structures for instrumentation access and repair.

One of the disadvantages of the beach chair arm-mounted position is that the set-up time can be longer. In addition, sterility can be an issue. In order to maintain sterility of the device, additional drapes and multiple attachments are required. A nitrogen supply is also necessary for the pneumatic arm holders. In general, the use of a commercial arm holder adds both time and overall cost to the case.

Another drawback of the beach chair position is that the surgeon's arms are abducted at the glenohumeral joint for the majority of the case. This potentially increases the fatigue factor, which is generally not seen in the lateral decubitus position. It is also difficult to provide good glenohumeral distraction without an assistant or arm positioner device. If the arm is left free, an assistant is also required, or well-positioned supports are needed to keep the arm in position during the entire case. It has also been suggested that the beach chair position provides less visualization and instrumentation access of the posterior and posteroinferior aspects of the glenohumeral joint, although this may be improved with adequate gentle distraction techniques.

BEACH CHAIR SET-UP

The first and foremost concern when setting up the patient using the beach chair position is to avoid injury to other structures while allowing for an ease of surgical exposure to complete the shoulder case successfully.

Tips for Successful Positioning (Arm Free)

Regional anesthesia (ie, interscalene block) may permit the patient to stay awake and sit in the beach chair position. If the patient is awake during the case, this facilitates safe and comfortable positioning with the active participation of the patient. However, blood pressure control must be optimal for safety and to facilitate visualization. In the awake monitored anesthetic care (MAC) patient, there are the obvious advantages of decreased postoperative pain medications, shorter postoperative stay, and less nausea, all of which are available in the beach chair position with the patient awake or lightly sedated.

Figure 2-5. (A) Patient is placed supine in beach chair ensuring buttocks and greater trochanter are positioned at the main break in the operating table. This will avoid sacral and decubitus pressure ulcers. (B) Foam padding is placed at the thorax positioners to avoid pressure sores.

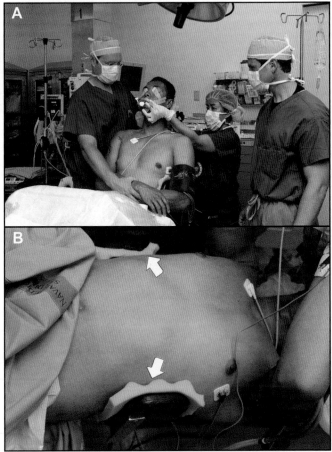

For initial beach chair positioning, the patient is placed supine with his or her buttocks and greater trochanter positioned at the main break in the operative table (Figure 2-5). A common mistake that occurs at this point is to position the patient too inferior, allowing a large space between the back of the table and the buttocks. This causes increased pressure on the back and sacrum, predisposing the patient to pressure ulcers and nerve injuries. After adequate anesthesia is administered, the operative table is lowered maximally, and the back is elevated to the desired level. For arthroscopic cases, the elevation is usually maximal at 60 to 80 degrees, and for open and arthroplasty cases, it is generally less at 20 to 50 degrees (Figure 2-6).

The patient is slid to the edge of the table on the operative side, or slightly off the table depending upon body habitus, to allow free and easy access to the posterior aspect of the shoulder (at least to the mid-scapula). A wedge-pad may be used underneath the thighs to facilitate the sitting position to avoid slouching and pressure sores during the case. A kidney rest can be useful to keep the patient from leaning toward the operative side.

Next, one or two towels are placed posterior to the medial scapular spine against the table. This is very important, as the towels not only stabilize the scapula, but they also serve to decrease the retroversion of the scapula such that direct anterior access to the glenoid is accomplished with a stable glenoid/scapular platform (Figure 2-7).

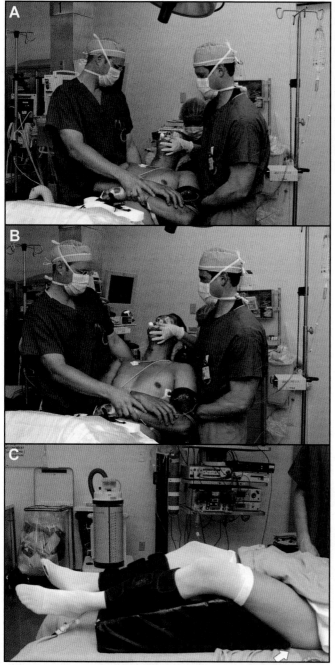

Figure 2-6. Once positioned correctly on the beach chair, elevate the back end (A) 20 to 50 degrees (for open cases) and (B) 60 to 80 degrees (for arthroscopic cases). (C) A wedge-pillow is placed under the knees to facilitate the sitting position and to avoid pressure sores. It is key to have the wedge pillow placed up to the buttock and under the thighs to facilitate correct positioning and to avoid pressure sores (white arrow).

Commercially available beach chair attachments replace part of the standard operating room table and allow ease of access to the posterior shoulder and attach to the standard operative table. There are often retractable flaps posteriorly on the operative side that retract to allow this access as well.

At this point, confirming neck and head position is paramount. Care must be taken to ensure a neutral neck position both in the coronal and sagittal planes to avoid airway obstruction,[5,6] cerebral vascular insults,[7,8] and brachial plexus traction (Figure 2-8).

Figure 2-7. (A) Commercially available beach chairs are equipped with (B) retractable flaps (white arrow) for posterior access to the shoulder (Tenet Medical Engineering, Calgary, Alberta, Canada). A blue towel is placed under the medial edge of the scapula to help stabilize the shoulder.

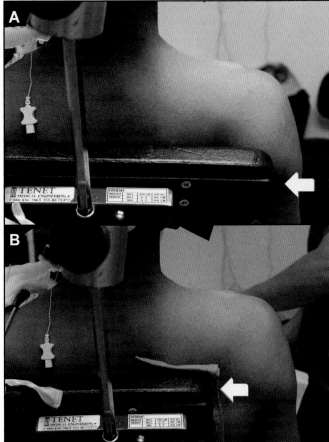

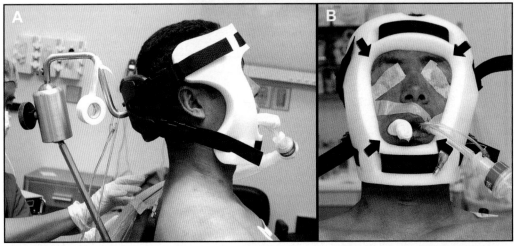

Figure 2-8. Ensure correct c-spine alignment in (A) both coronal and (B) sagittal planes to prevent nerve and vascular complications. The ear and mucosal surfaces of the lips should be free and not in contact with the foam head holder (black arrows). When securing the head, ensure that there is not contact of the straps or padding with the eyes, ears, and lips to reduce the threshold of nerve injury (black arrows).

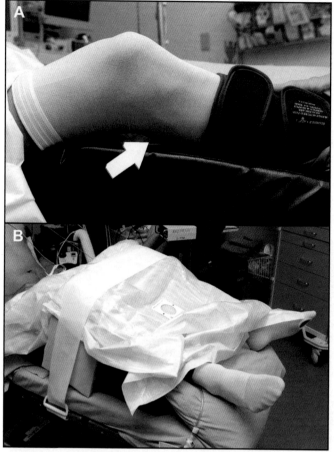

Figure 2-9. (A) Place pillows and padding near the extremity to protect the peroneal nerve (white arrow). (B) A strap is secured over the padding to hold it loosely in place.

Nerve and vascular complications have been reported, including hypoglossal dysfunction and cerebral vascular insults felt to be caused by carotid kinking and suboptimal positioning.[7-10] It is important to ensure that the head is in a neutral position, not extended, and in good coronal and sagittal alignment. Head positioners are also available, which have a variety of straps and gel-foam to hold the head in place. When securing the head, it is necessary to make sure that there is no contact of straps or padding on the ears, the eyes, and the lips. All of these mucosal and submucosal areas are very sensitive and have a low threshold for sensory nerve problems. Alternatively, towels, tape, and/or elastofoam may be used to gently secure the head in a neutral position.

The next step is to flex the table to accommodate the hips and ensure that the legs are level. It is very important to place pillows and/or padding at the knees to avoid peroneal nerve pressure injuries (Figure 2-9). The nonoperative limb is either placed on a well-arm holder or strapped to the body after being placed in a well-padded foam splint or on several pillows taped to the table (Figure 2-10).

The table may be turned 45 degrees to the room to facilitate surgeon access to the anterior, lateral, and posterior aspects of the shoulder. The arm may be wrapped in a protective sterile sock/stockinette and/or elastofoam and secured to well-positioned drapes with a hemostat (Figure 2-11).

Figure 2-10. The nonoperative arm is padded well with either gel padding or foam to protect the ulnar nerve. The nonoperative arm should be in a neutral position.

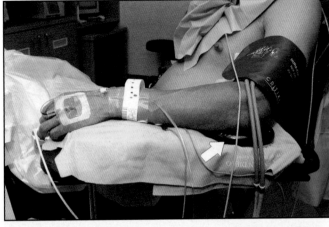

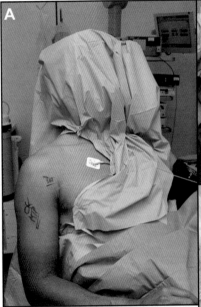

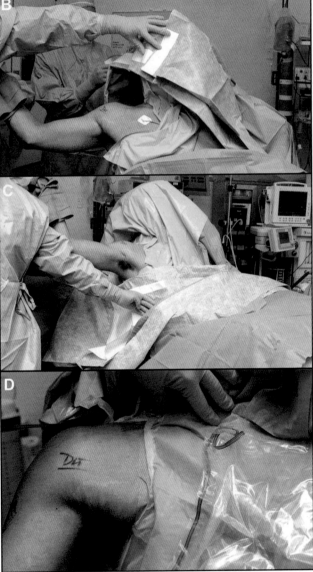

Figure 2-11. The table is rotated to allow ease of surgeon access, and then the operative limb is prepped and draped.

Tips for Successful Positioning (Arm Mounted)

In addition to the method previously described, several commercially available arm positioners may be used to secure the forearm of the operative limb. Several positioners are available, including the pneumatic-operated Spyder (Tenet Medical Engineering, Calgary, Canada) and the manually operated with manual lock McConnell (McConnell Orthopaedics, Greenville, TX). One pearl is to place the forearm in the holder prior to attachment to the fixed pole for the arm holder.

This allows for ease of arm placement in the holder and brings the arm to the holder, rather than the holder to the arm, making assembly quicker and simpler. Care is taken to ensure that the hand and arm holder are well padded, especially at the wrist and elbow, which are potential nerve compression sites. A gentle fist around the metal palm rod should be held in place with provided foam and velcro straps (Figure 2-12).

The operating room staff passes the nonsterile, arm-holding rod to the scrubbed operating room technician who attaches the sterile drapes provided with the device. The arm is held in neutral position during the start of glenohumeral arthroscopy and then adjusted as necessary. Inferior traction is applied through the device prior to starting subacromial work.

OTHER PITFALLS/COMPLICATIONS

Brachial plexus strain is the most common complication related to positioning the shoulder. Care should be taken to avoid excessive traction; subclinical neuropraxia is often higher than recognized.[2,10] Other nerve injuries include axillary nerve problems; however, abduction, external rotation, and perpendicular traction increase the zone of safety for the axillary nerve during capsulolabral repair in the inferior aspect of the shoulder joint.[11] The surgeon should avoid positions of extreme extension and abduction in the lateral decubitus position to avoid nerve stretch, especially of the musculocutaneous nerve.[4] Other potentially reported complications include hypoglossal nerve injury,[10] vasovagal episodes,[7] visual loss and ophthalmoplegia,[9] and cerebral ischemia.[8]

CONCLUSION

Beach chair positioning provides optimal access for open shoulder cases, allows for ease of conversion from an arthroscopic to an open procedure, and provides for anatomic orientation that facilitates assistant participation in the case. With careful attention to positioning and protection of the head, airway, mucosal surfaces, and common nerve compression points throughout the body, the beach chair position offers a safe and reliable access to all areas of the glenohumeral joint and subacromial space.

The views expressed in this article are those of the authors and do not reflect the official policy or position of the Department of the Navy, Department of Defense, or the US government.

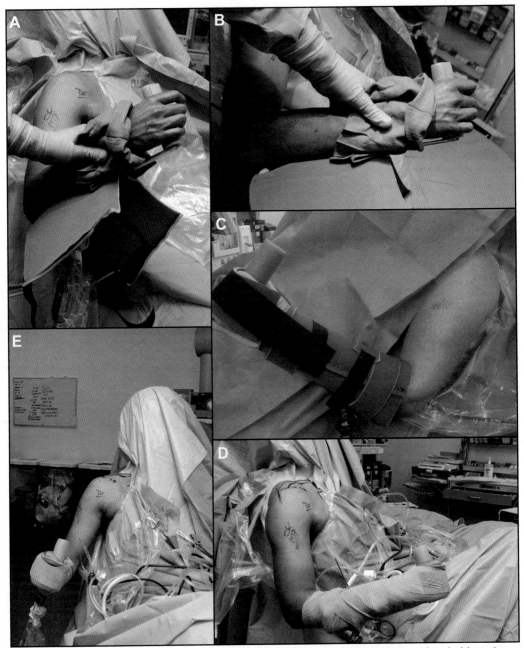

Figure 2-12. (A) Placement of the operative arm in pneumatic device, Spyder, in a Velcro holder prior to attaching to fixed pole. (B, C) Wrap fingers around metal palm rod making a fist and strap down with Velcro straps or elastic wrap. (D, E) The final operative prepping and positioning is shown for a glenohumeral and subacromial arthroscopy.

REFERENCES

1. Skyhar MJ, Altchek DW, Warren RF, Wickiewicz TL, O'Brien SJ. Shoulder arthroscopy with the patient in the beach-chair position. *Arthroscopy*. 1988;4(4):256-259.
2. Rodeo SA, Forster RA, Weiland AJ. Neurological complications due to arthroscopy. *J Bone Joint Surg Am*. 1993;75:917-926.
3. Struzik S, Glinkowski W, Gorecki A. Shoulder arthroscopy complications. *Ortop Traumatol Rehabil*. 2003;5(4):489-494.
4. Weber SC, Abrams JS, Nottage WM. Complications associated with arthroscopic shoulder surgery. *Arthroscopy*.2002;18(2 Suppl 1):88-95.
5. Dietzel DP, Ciullo JV. Spontaneous pneumothorax after shoulder arthroscopy: a report of four cases. *Arthroscopy*. 1996;12(1):99-102.
6. Hynson JM, Tung A, Guevara JE, Katz JA, Glick JM, Shapiro WA. Complete airway obstruction during arthroscopic shoulder surgery. *Anesth Analg*. 1993;76(4):875-878.
7. Kahn RL, Hargett MJ. Beta-adrenergic blockers and vasovagal episodes during shoulder surgery in the sitting position under interscalene block. *Anesth Analg*. 1999;88(2):378-381.
8. Pohl A, Cullen DJ. Cerebral ischemia during shoulder surgery in the upright position: a case series. *J Clin Anesth*. 2005;17(6):463-469.
9. Bhatti MT, Enneking FK. Visual loss and ophthalmoplegia after shoulder surgery. *Anesth Analg*. 2003;96(3):899-902.
10. Mullins RC, Drez D Jr, Cooper J. Hypoglossal nerve palsy after arthroscopy of the shoulder and open operation with the patient in the beach-chair position. A case report. *J Bone Joint Surg Am*. 1992;74(1):137-139.
11. Uno A, Bain GI, Mehta JA. Arthroscopic relationship of the axillary nerve to the shoulder joint capsule: an anatomic study. *J Shoulder Elbow Surg*. 1999;8(3):226-230.

3

Arthroscopic Bankart Repair
A Reproducible Technique

Richard Ryu, MD and Jeffrey S. Abrams, MD

INTRODUCTION

There have been significant evolutions in technique, resulting in the current technique of suture anchor arthroscopic anterior stabilization. The goal of surgical stabilization is to re-establish normal anatomy by repairing the Bankart lesion and retensioning the elongated inferior glenohumeral ligament. Today, the results of stabilization are comparable to the results of open soft tissue repairs.[1-3] The desired outcome of surgical intervention is to not only achieve a stable shoulder, but also to restore function and preserve glenohumeral range of motion.

There was early enthusiasm in using the arthroscope to visualize articular structures and determine the pathoanatomy following a shoulder dislocation.[4,5] Instrumentation and implants were developed that can reliably repair the essential lesions. Surgical approaches that would divide or detach the subscapularis can be avoided, and the injured overhead shoulder athlete is the ideal patient to consider for arthroscopic stabilization. The success has spread to repairing first-time dislocators who engage in high-risk activities at an age where recurrence is high, as well as to patients with failed prior open and arthroscopic repairs. Today, the stabilization rates are anticipated to be higher than 90%, and return to sports and employment are likely.[6-8]

PATIENT SELECTION

At the early developmental stages of arthroscopic stabilization, the indications for choosing arthroscopy were limited due to recurrence rates exceeding those of open repair. As fixation techniques improved, the recurrence rate has become comparable to the open Bankart repair. Success today not only emphasizes stability of the shoulder but also return to prior athletics. The overhead athlete has been challenging due to the demands of the combined need for stability while maximizing range of motion.

Abrams JS. *Management of the Unstable Shoulder:
Arthroscopic and Open Repair* (pp. 45-58).
© 2011 SLACK Incorporated

The arthroscope has become the procedure of choice for stabilization in the overhead athlete. Combining the preservation of the subscapularis insertion while directly repairing multiple quadrants of capsular and labral injury has contributed to the success of the arthroscopic reconstructive approach.

The indications today for arthroscopic stabilization include 1) recurrent subluxation and dislocation, 2) initial or first-time dislocation in a high-risk young athlete, 3) glenoid rim fracture following an instability event displaced medially or inferiorly, 4) shoulder dysfunction due to instability in the overhead athlete, 5) patient with limiting apprehension due to injury to the anterior capsule and labral structures, and 6) failed prior stabilization due to soft tissue injury.

The most common reason for surgical repair in an athlete or worker is recurrent dislocation or subluxation. Instability recurrence has been considered a likely outcome of nonoperative treatment in young individuals who continue to participate in contact or collision activities. Following multiple events of instability, there are permanent changes to the static restraints including capsule, labrum, and bone. There has been reported an increased failure rate following a soft tissue arthroscopic repair if there is significant glenoid bone loss and/or an engaging Hill-Sachs lesion. Early publications identified this factor as the most common reason for failure in a contact or collision athlete.[9] Multiple techniques to evaluate patients preoperatively can be used to identify and inform patients of options including open and arthroscopic techniques.[10,11]

Cases where bone deficiency is excessive need alternative treatment. There may be cases where arthroscopy is used to evaluate structures intraoperatively and formulate the best plan to help the athlete or worker. Today, additional procedures are being incorporated into an arthroscopic Bankart repair that may extend the applications of arthroscopy to the chronically unstable shoulder. These procedures include posteroinferior plication, rotator interval closure, infraspinatus insertion into the humeral head defect, and bone grafting procedures to the anterior glenoid. Results from these additional procedures are pending and may be considered in patients who prefer an arthroscopic approach.

The first-time dislocator has raised interest in immediate arthroscopic repair.[12-14] This may be considered in a young athlete who wishes to continue to participate in activities that place their shoulder at risk. Studies, both military and civilian, suggest recurrences, when treated nonoperatively, exceeding 60% in these patients.[15-18] The appeal of an early repair is the increased successful return to activities and the reduced risk of recurrence. High stabilization rates may be due to the reduction of bone loss and capsular injuries. Studies reviewing the success of surgery repairing first-time dislocators have indicated that 25% of the patients choose surgery after recurrence, 25% do not choose surgery in spite of recurrence, and 50% make lifestyle changes to avoid the chance of recurrence.[19,20] This does not take into account the potential for greater degrees of bone loss that may jeopardize future attempts at repair.

Glenoid rim fractures that are displaced can be identified with radiographs and computerized scans.[21] Suture anchor repairs can predictably reduce and fix these injuries. Malunited fractures can be addressed with either fracture mobilization or transferring the soft tissue restraints to stabilize the shoulder.

Failed shoulder stabilization can be multifactional. A well-performed arthroscopic or open stabilization can fail due to additional trauma. This may create a recurrent Bankart lesion or failure at an additional location. Arthroscopy has been successful in identifying multiple areas of failure that may have resulted from the recurrent trauma. There is also a number of stabilized shoulders that have failed following a relatively minor event. Shoulders that have had a previous extra-articular procedure (ie, a Bristow transfer) may have subluxation recurrences due to a persistent capsulolabral defect not addressed at the index surgery. In these cases, arthroscopic revision surgery has been successful in restoring stability without risking neurologic injury while mobilizing the transferred coracoid and short head of the biceps.

A similar argument can be made when considering options for an atraumatic recurrence following a well-performed arthroscopic stabilization. Repeating a similar surgery may not have the same success as considering an open approach.[22] Additional soft tissue reinforcement may be a consideration when selecting a reconstructive procedure, particularly after failed surgery.

A number of workers and athletes may injure their capsule following a traumatic dislocation. Capsular detachments from the humeral head, also known as a humeral avulsion glenohumeral ligament (HAGL) lesion, have been identified as a risk factor for recurrence. Reattachment of the capsule is an important factor in restoring stability. While midcapsular tears can be repaired arthroscopically by placing side-to-side sutures, for patients requiring humerus reattachment, the proximity of neurologic structures may make anchor placement into the anterior aspect of the humeral head challenging. Patients with a HAGL lesion may choose a miniopen approach to reduce risk of injury.

Surgical Stabilization

The goal of surgical stabilization is to re-establish normal anatomy by repairing the Bankart lesion and retensioning the elongated inferior glenohumeral ligament.[23,24] The desired outcome of this surgical intervention is to not only achieve a stable shoulder, but to also restore full function while preserving glenohumeral range of motion.

Arthroscopic Bankart Technique

1. This procedure can be performed under a general anesthetic and/or with a regional nerve block. Neurological sequelae, although uncommon with experienced anesthesiologists, should be discussed in detail with patients preoperatively. Interscalene nerve blocks can enhance intraoperative muscle relaxation, blood pressure control, and perioperative pain management.

2. The lateral decubitus position is the preferred position for anterior stabilization procedures. Unencumbered access to the anterior and posterior aspects of the shoulder facilitates the procedure and is ergonomically desirable as well. Placing the anesthesiologist and equipment at the foot of the table is easily achieved (Figure 3-1).

3. Examination under anesthesia of the involved and uninvolved shoulders should be performed as a matter of routine. Grading and documenting the degree of instability can also be helpful if further surgery is necessitated. With the shoulder in neutral rotation, load-and-shift testing is performed to determine the predominant direction and degree of instability. This examination provides confirmation of the preoperative diagnosis and if not, the role of stabilization must be reassessed. The arm is placed in a padded arm holder with 8 to 10 pounds of axial balanced suspension, counterbalanced by a second force attached to the upper sleeve of 8 to 10 pounds. This dual traction set-up promotes improved intra-articular visualization and the ability to manipulate tissue in the inferior pouch. The arm is slightly forward flexed (10 degrees) in an internally-rotated position. At this time, the table can be rotated such that the glenoid is parallel to the floor, which assists in orientation while inserting instruments and implants.

Figure 3-1. Lateral decubitus position with gentle traction and lateral distraction.

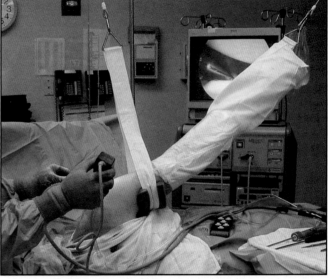

Figure 3-2. Posterior viewing portal inferior to angle of acromion and scapular spine.

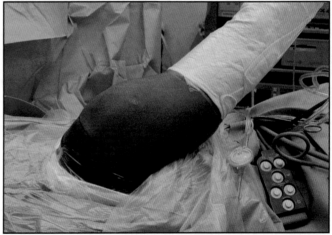

4. Arthroscopy is initiated with a standard posterior portal slightly lateral to the glenohumeral joint line. This initial viewing portal will become a working portal and must be placed such that instruments are lateral to the posterior glenoid rim and easy to manipulate (Figure 3-2; also see Chapter 3 video).

   While viewing from the posterior portal, dual anterior portals are established at the inferior and superior margins of the rotator interval (Figure 3-3) using an inside-out technique with a Wissinger rod. Maximizing the distance between the 2 anterior portals facilitates instrumentation without "crowding." The anteroinferior working portal typically requires an 8.25 mm cannula to allow for passage of suture hooks used in the repair, and should be created slightly superior and lateral to the superior border of the subscapularis. Use of a spinal needle to verify a satisfactory angle of approach to the inferior glenoid can be helpful prior to establishing the anteroinferior working portal. The anterosuperior portal becomes the viewing portal, while the posterior portal is converted to a working portal.

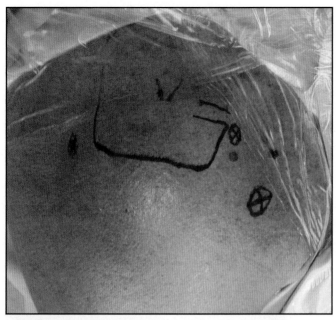

Figure 3-3. Right shoulder anterior portals: anteroinferior working portal lateral to coracoid process, superior viewing portal.

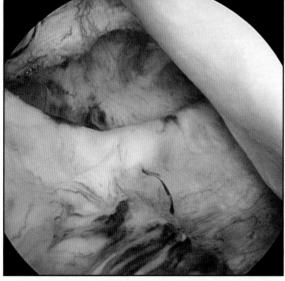

Figure 3-4. Humeral avulsion of glenohumeral ligament (HAGL lesion).

5. Utilizing a probe from the anteroinferior portal, a comprehensive diagnostic arthroscopy is performed. The inferior capsular pouch and humeral insertion of the ligaments are visualized to rule out a HAGL lesion (Figure 3-4). Associated superior labrum from anterior to posterior (SLAP) or rotator cuff pathology is documented and treated concomitantly, if indicated. If a Hill-Sachs lesion is encountered, engagement of the humeral head on the anterior glenoid rim should be assessed as the shoulder is positioned in an abducted externally-rotated position (Figure 3-5). If contact occurs, the possibility of a bony solution must be considered, since the failure rate for arthroscopic Bankart repair is considerably greater under these circumstances (see Chapter 3 video).

Figure 3-5. Large humeral head Hill-Sachs lesion when positioned in external rotation and mid abduction.

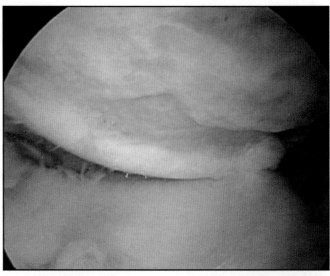

Figure 3-6. Anterior view of right shoulder allows evaluation of glenoid bone loss anterior to bare spot.

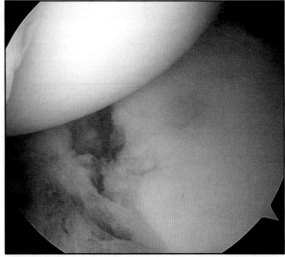

6. A bony deficiency of the glenoid can be assessed arthroscopically. Measuring from the "bare spot," which usually represents the center of the glenoid, the radius of the glenoid can be measured, and the lengths of the anterior and posterior radii compared (Figure 3-6). Bone loss measuring greater than 20% may necessitate a bony solution, especially in conjunction with an "engaging" Hill-Sachs lesion.

7. The arthroscope is then switched to the anterosuperior portal for viewing. With anterior instability cases, the humeral head can be seen to subluxate anteriorly (Figure 3-7). Assessing for an "engaging" Hill-Sachs lesion can also be evaluated from this viewing portal. Centering of the humeral head should be verified at the conclusion of the stabilization procedure. Attention is now directed toward mobilization of the Bankart lesion. An angled periosteal elevator or radiofrequency device is used to develop the plane between the glenoid and capsulolabral complex (see Chapter 3 video). In order to retension the inferior glenohumeral ligament, a thorough release must be accomplished so that the defect can be closed and the tissue sequentially shifted inferior to superior with each anchor. The capsulolabral

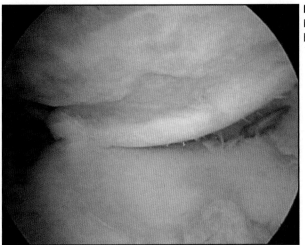

Figure 3-7. Anterior view of engaging Hill-Sachs lesion due to combined glenoid bone loss.

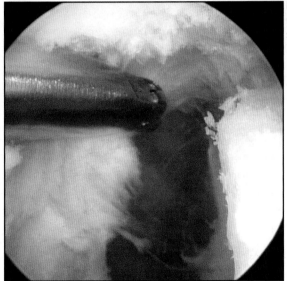

Figure 3-8. Mobilization and release of anterior capsule allows visualization of the subscapularis muscle.

complex is completely mobilized when the subscapularis muscle belly can be clearly visualized (Figure 3-8).

8. The glenoid neck is then carefully prepped with a shaver (burr is rarely needed), attempting to retain as much bone stock as possible, especially in those cases of chronic glenoid erosion. Accurate placement of the double-loaded anchors onto the glenoid face by 1 to 2 mm (Figure 3-9) is critical to re-establishing the depth of the glenoid as well as the concavity-compression phenomenon (see Chapter 3 video). Placement onto the glenoid face also allows for better bone purchase. Approaching the glenoid at a 45-degree angle relative to the articular surface helps ensure anchor purchase in bone. The position of the first anchor is always guided by the pathology and should be at the level of the inferior aspect of the labral tear. If the tear extends beyond the 6 o'clock position, the inferior-most anchor can be inserted through a posterolateral portal and is technically easier than using an anteroinferior portal.

Figure 3-9. Double-loaded glenoid suture anchors are placed along the glenoid rim.

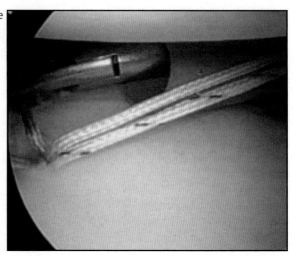

9. Using a #1 absorbable suture loaded into a 60-degree angled suture hook with the correct orientation (eg, right hook for a right shoulder), the inferior glenohumeral ligament is penetrated 1 to 2 cm inferior to the anchor. The inferior glenohumeral ligament is then shifted inferior to superior as well as lateral to medial (Figure 3-10; also see Chapter 3 video). The #1 absorbable suture is then used as a "poor man's suture shuttle," and once the actual suture tail is tied to the absorbable suture, the permanent suture is retrograded through the labrum (Figure 3-11). It should be noted that the suture tail and absorbable shuttle are collected, tied, and then retrograded through the posterior working cannula. For those with associated ligamentous laxity, a plication stitch, in which a portion of the capsule is captured by the hook prior to passage through the labrum, can be used to decrease capsular volume in addition to repairing the Bankart lesion.

10. A minimum of 3 double-loaded suture anchors should be utilized. With each suture passage, tissue should be shifted from an inferior to a superior position while also closing the Bankart lesion. When tying knots, the limb that passes through the labrum should serve as the post so that the knot is prevented from resting adjacent to the articular surface. This also facilitates pushing the labrum onto the glenoid face and recreating labral height. At the completion of the repair, the anterior labral "bumper," which deepens the glenoid, should be visible (Figure 3-12).

11. Once the Bankart repair has been completed, a rotator interval closure can be performed, especially if a patulous rotator interval is present. Through the anteroinferior portal, a straight suture hook loaded with a #1 absorbable suture is passed through the superior aspect of the rotator interval, capturing the superior glenohumeral ligament. A straight or angled tissue penetrator is passed through the anteroinferior portal, grasping the middle glenohumeral ligament. Both limbs of the absorbable suture are retrieved, the arm is positioned in neutral rotation, and the suture tied blindly in an extracapsular fashion (Figure 3-13).

12. At the conclusion of the Bankart repair, while viewing from the anterosuperior portal, the humeral head should be well centered in the glenoid, and the Hill-Sachs lesion, if present, should not engage the anterior glenoid as the shoulder is rotated. Attempts to dislocate the shoulder should reveal robust tension within the inferior glenohumeral ligament, preventing any abnormal excursion.

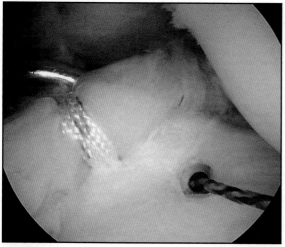

Figure 3-10. Suture hooks are used to introduce a shuttle through the inferior glenohumeral ligament to create a superior shift.

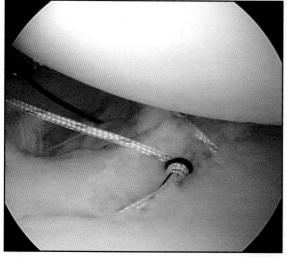

Figure 3-11. A monofilament suture can be used to shuttle braided anchor sutures under labrum and through anterior capsular ligaments.

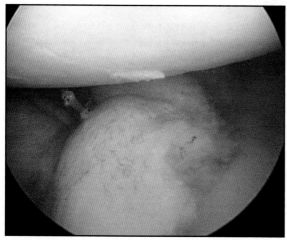

Figure 3-12. Tying the sutures with the knot lateral to the labrum produces a bumper appearance to the repair.

Figure 3-13. Rotator interval closure brings superior margin of middle glenohumeral ligament to superior ligament.

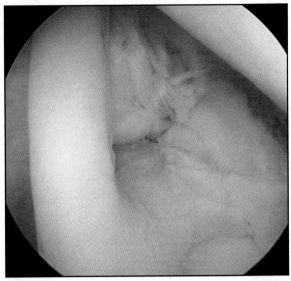

POSTOPERATIVE MANAGEMENT

The goals of an arthroscopic procedure are to identify and repair damaged articular structures. The purpose of early rehabilitation is to allow adequate time to heal, without disturbing the structures that have been injured and repaired. Although the arthroscope has been thought to be a technique that accelerates healing, the biology of healing is unchanged in arthroscopic or open approaches.

Complications can occur during the postoperative period. Early chondrolytic cases were recognized when thermal devices were being used to create capsular changes. Today, the use of sustained analgesia with articular pain pumps has raised concerns. The shoulder has unique characteristics that place it at risk when bathed with anesthetic agents adjacent to the articular surfaces. Chondrolysis is a progressive problem that begins after a "silent" postoperative period. Patients eventually develop increased symptoms of pain and stiffness. At this time, articular pain pumps are not recommended until risk factors can be clearly identified.

The early postoperative course begins by placing a patient in a sling with a small pillow to neutralize the glenohumeral articulation, allowing for the inferior capsular structures to heal. Limited range of motion in abduction, external and internal rotation, and flexion is permitted. Commonly, hands-to-face and external rotation to 20 degrees are allowed to perform activities of daily living. After 4 to 6 weeks, these motions can be increased to forward elevation above the head, external rotation to 45 degrees (60 degrees in throwers), cross-chest, and early internal rotation behind the back.

Strengthening is a process that may start early to improve proprioception, maximize core strength, and reduce recovery time. Isometrics and postural exercises can be started prior to sling removal. After 6 to 8 weeks, gentle therabands and light weights can be added with limited arc exercises permitted. These exercises are increased in resistance and motion arcs at 10 to 12 weeks. Scapular stabilizing exercises are started early.

Sport-specific training can begin after flexibility and basic strength is achieved. Closed arc exercises that combine lower extremity, torso, and upper extremity training is started after 12 to 16 weeks, depending on the patient's goals. Risk of reinjury or new injury is important to a recovering athlete. Proficiency testing may be important to evaluate the recovering worker or athlete. Bracing is of potential assistance in certain athletes. Cutaneous proprioception with taping may be helpful in certain overhead athletes. Ultimately, it is the strength of the repaired structures, protective activities of the surrounding muscles, and the overall condition of the patient protects against recurrence.

The anticipated return to work or sport depends on the degree of healing and the risk factors related to their activity. Generally, 4 months are considered for noncontact or collision activities, and 6 months for the high-velocity collision activities. This time period needs to individualized based on healing parameters, range of motion, strength, and apprehension.

TIPS AND PEARLS

Every effort is made to maximize the success rate of an arthroscopic Bankart repair. That said, proper patient selection is the single most important decision that the surgeon can make. Avoid an arthroscopic approach in those patients who have poor tissue quality, significant bone loss (usually greater than 20% to 25% glenoid loss or in combination with an engaging Hill-Sachs lesion), or an inability to comply with the postoperative protocol. Suspected bone loss should be quantified with a 3-dimensional computed tomography (CT) which can be more reliable than the MRI for assessing bone deficiencies.

During surgery, the lateral decubitus position is the position of choice, as it allows unfettered access to the anterior and posterior aspects of the shoulder while facilitating favorable ergonomics for the surgeon. Use of the anterosuperior portal for viewing is recommended, as visualization of the anteroinferior glenoid and the inferior glenohumeral ligament (IGHL) is unparalleled. Furthermore, liberation of the torn IGHL can be accurately assessed as the subscapularis muscle fibers can be seen through the defect once a satisfactory release has been achieved (see Chapter 3 video).

The anchors should be placed 1 to 2 mm onto the glenoid face. The anchors should be double-loaded to decrease the load to failure, and a minimum of 3 anchors should be deployed. The suture should be passed 1 to 2 cm inferior to the corresponding anchor so that the Bankart lesion is not only closed, but that the IGHL is shifted in an inferior-to-superior direction. Releasing traction on the extremity while the suture is placed can assist in proper retensioning. When knot-tying, the knot should slide down the limb of the suture that has passed through the IGHL (see Chapter 3 video). The knot serves to "push" the labrum onto the glenoid face, deepening the depth of the glenoid and reconstituting the concavity-compression phenomenon.

Adjunctive rotator cuff interval closure may be beneficial in anterior stabilization cases and should be considered especially in those with associated ligamentous laxity. Placing the arm in external rotation while sutures are placed assists in minimizing external rotation loss. Postoperative immobilization is a critical aspect of the procedure and should be utilized for a minimum of 3 weeks. Resistive strengthening should be avoided for 8 weeks, and a return to full contact sports should be avoided for at least 5 months. For overhand throwing athletes, range of motion exercises are initiated earlier with a goal of achieving full range at 2 to 3 months.

COMPLICATIONS

The complications associated with arthroscopic Bankart repair are those that are experienced with most other procedures including infection, stiffness, neurovascular injury, and recurrence. Early recognition is the key to successful management of these complications. A thorough débridement(s) in conjunction with possible hardware and suture removal may be necessary in deep infections while, rarely, persistent stiffness may require a selective release at a later date. Severe restrictions in external rotation should be a cause of concern in the early postoperative phase. Most stiff shoulders following a Bankart repair gain a functional range of motion over time unless a significant nonanatomic repair has been performed such as closure of a normal sublabral recess above the glenoid equator. The axillary nerve passes closest to the glenoid (approximately 12 mm) at the 5 o'clock position (right shoulder). Knowledge of this anatomical relationship is critical in avoiding inadvertent nerve injury. Recurrent instability can occur in up to 5% to 10% of cases according to the recent published literature, and causation must as ascertained in order to treat this complication. Failure to retension the IGHL, medial placement of the anchors on the glenoid neck, an inadequate number of suture anchors, and unrecognized bone loss are the most common causes of recurrence.

REFERENCES

1. Fabbriciani C, Milano G, Demontis A, et al. Arthroscopic versus open treatment of Bankart lesion of the shoulder: a prospective randomized study. *Arthroscopy.* 2004;20:456-462.
2. Kim S-Ho, Ha KI, Kim S-Hyun. Bankart repair in traumatic anterior shoulder instability: open versus arthroscopic technique. *Arthroscopy.* 2002;18:755-763.
3. Ryu RK. Open versus arthroscopic stabilization for traumatic anterior shoulder instability. *Sports Med Arthroc Rev.* 2004;12:90-98.
4. Baker CL. Arthroscopic evaluation of acute initial shoulder dislocations. *Instr Course Lect.* 1996;45:83-89.
5. Taylor DC, Arciero RA. Pathologic changes associated with shoulder dislocations: arthroscopic and physical examination findings in first-time, traumatic anterior dislocations. *Am J Sports Med.* 1997; 25:306-311.
6. Carreira DS. Mazzocca AD, Oryhon J, et al. A prospective outcome evaluation of arthroscopic Bankart repairs. *Am J Sports Med.* 2006;34:771-777.
7. Mishra DK, Fanton GS. Two-year outcome of arthroscopic Bankart repair and electrothermal-assisted capsulorrhaphy for recurrent traumatic anterior shoulder instability. *Arthroscopy.* 2001;17:844-849.
8. Bacilla P, Field LD, Savoie FH. Arthroscopic Bankart repair in a high-demand patient population. *Arthroscopy.* 1997;13:51-60.
9. Burkhart SS, De Beer, JF. Traumatic glenohumeral bone defects and their relationship to failure of arthroscopic Bankart repairs: significance of the inverted-pear glenoid and the humeral engaging Hill-Sachs lesion. *Arthroscopy.* 2000;16:677-694.
10. Itoi E, Lee SB, Amrami KK, et al. Quantitative assessment of classic anteroinferior bony Bankart lesions by radiography and computed tomography. *Am J Sports Med.* 2003;31(1):112-118.
11. Ito H, Takayama A, Shirai Y. Radiographic evaluation of Hill-Sachs lesion in patients with recurrent shoulder instability. *J Shoulder Elbow Surg.* 2000;9:495-497.
12. Bedi A, Ryu RK. Management of the first-time anterior shoulder dislocation. AAOS *Instructional Course Lectures.* 2008; Vol 58.
13. Robinson CM, Kelly M. Wakefield AE. Redislocation of the shoulder during the first six weeks after a primary anterior dislocation: risk factors and results of treatment. *J Bone Joint Surg.* 2002;84A:1552-1559.
14. Kirkley A, Griffin S, Richards C, et al. Prospective randomized clinical trial comparing the effectiveness of immediate arthroscopic stabilization versus immobilization and rehabilitation in first-traumatic anterior dislocations of the shoulder. *Arthroscopy.* 1999;15:507-514.

15. Robinson CM, Howes J, Murdoch H, et al. Functional outcome and risk of recurrent instability after primary traumatic anterior shoulder dislocation in young patients. *J Bone Joint Surg.* 2006;88:2326-2336.

16. Arciero RA, Taylor DC, Snyder RJ, Uhorchak JM. Arthroscopic bioabsorbable tack stabilization of initial anterior shoulder dislocations: a preliminary report. *Arthroscopy.* 1995;11:410-417.

17. Bottoni CR, Wilckens JH, DeBerardino TM, et al. A prospective randomized evaluation of arthroscopic stabilization versus nonoperative treatment of acute, traumatic, first-time shoulder dislocation. *Arthroscopy.* (abs) 2000;16:432.

18. Tesla RL, Brand R, Marti RK. A prospective arthroscopic study of acute first-time anterior shoulder dislocation in the young: a five-year follow-up study. *J Shoulder Elbow Surg.* 2003;12:529-534.

19. Sachs RA, Stone ML, Paxton E, et al. Can the need for future surgery for acute traumatic anterior shoulder dislocation be predicted? *J Bone Joint Surg.* 2007; 89:1665-1674.

20. Hovelius L, Olofsson A, Sandström B, et al. Nonoperative treatment of primary anterior shoulder dislocation in patients forty years of age and younger: a prospective twenty-five year follow-up. *J Bone Joint Surg.* 2008;90:945-952.

21. Sugaya H, Moriishi J, Kanisawa I, Tsuchiya A. Arthroscopic osseous Bankart repair for chronic recurrent traumatic anterior glenohumeral instability. *J Bone Joint Surg (Am).* 2005;87:1752-1760.

22. Abrams JS. Revision instability surgery. In: Angelo RL, Esch JC, Ryu RKN, eds. *AANA Advanced Shoulder Arthroscopy.* Philadelphia, PA: Elsevier; 2010:147-156.

23. Ryu R KN. Arthroscopic approach to traumatic anterior shoulder instability. *Arthroscopy.* 2003;19(suppl):94-101.

24. Gartsman GM, Roddey TS, Hammerman SM. Arthroscopic treatment of anterior-inferior glenohumeral instability: two to five-year follow-up. *J Bone Joint Surg (Am).* 2000;82:991-1003.

**Please see video on the accompanying Web site at
http://www.slackbooks.com/unstableshouldervideos**

4

Knotless Suture Anchor Techniques to Repair the Unstable Shoulder

Raymond Thal, MD

Arthroscopic Bankart repair procedures have been developed in an effort to restore stability to the shoulder while avoiding some of the morbidity associated with the open repair. Several currently used arthroscopic repair techniques provide adequate labral fixation for successful shoulder stabilization. The fixation methods used in early arthroscopic repairs (tacks, staples, transglenoid sutures) were different than commonly described open repair fixation methods (suture anchors, osseous tunnels) and often resulted in higher recurrence rates. More recent arthroscopic repair studies describe the use of suture anchors with arthroscopic knot tying. Arthroscopic suture anchor repair continues to have pitfalls related to the quality, consistency, and technical challenges associated with arthroscopic knots.[1] While many surgeons have become more comfortable with the arthroscopic knot-tying process, the potential for intra-articular knot impingement persists with bulky arthroscopic knot designs.

KNOTLESS SUTURE ANCHOR DESIGNS

In 1998, a knotless suture anchor (Knotless Suture Anchor, DePuy/Mitek, Inc, Norwood, MA) was developed, and a technique was described that eliminated the need for arthroscopic knot tying during arthroscopic instability surgery.[2-5] This knotless suture anchor has a titanium body with an attached suture loop that is captured by the notch at the tip of the anchor (Figure 4-1). The capturing of the suture loop eliminates the knot tying required with standard suture anchors. Bone fixation is achieved by nitinol arcs. In 2001, a wedge-shaped, bioabsorbable, knotless suture anchor (BioKnotless Suture Anchor, DePuy/Mitek) was developed (Figure 4-2). An attached suture loop and notch at the tip of the anchor are similar to the metal knotless anchor. Toggle of the wedge-shaped anchor body provides bone fixation with the BioKnotless Suture Anchor. These knotless suture anchor designs have been shown to provide

Abrams JS. *Management of the Unstable Shoulder: Arthroscopic and Open Repair* (pp. 59-76).
© 2011 SLACK Incorporated

Figure 4-1. Metallic knotless suture anchor design. (Reprinted with permission from Thal R. Knotless suture anchor fixation for shoulder instability. In: Miller MD, Cole BJ, eds. *Textbook of Arthroscopy.* Philadelphia, PA: Elsevier, 2004:115.)

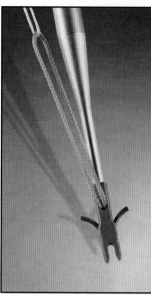

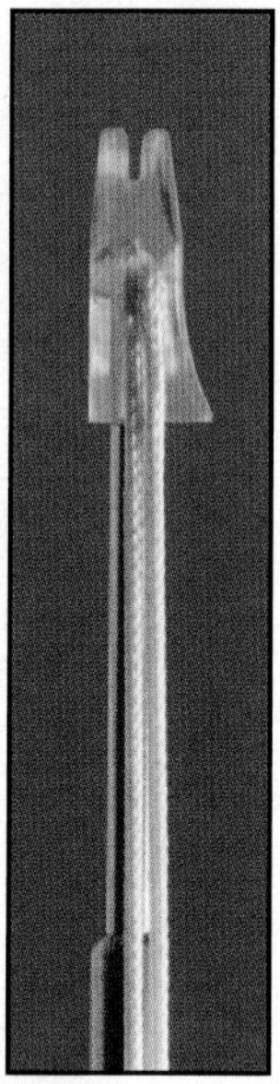

Figure 4-2. BioKnotless suture anchor design. (Reprinted with permission from Thal R. Knotless suture anchor fixation for shoulder instability. In: Miller MD, Cole BJ, eds. *Textbook of Arthroscopy.* Philadelphia, PA: Elsevier, 2004:115.)

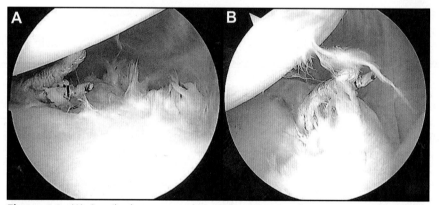

Figure 4-3. (A) Standard suture anchor with prominent knot. (B) Standard suture anchor with abrasion of humeral head from knot impingement.

consistent, strong, low-profile repairs. Increased superior capsular shift can be achieved.[6] The knotless procedure avoids many suture management challenges associated with arthroscopic knot tying. Potential difficulties associated with the use of special knot-tying devices and various knot designs are also eliminated. Additionally, knotless suture anchor fixation eliminates the potential weakness of knot security and knot impingement associated with the use of standard suture anchors (Figure 4-3).

In recent years, several other knotless suture anchor designs have been developed. As with the earlier knotless anchors, these anchors eliminate the need for arthroscopic knot tying. With these devices, knotless fixation is achieved by 1 of 3 methods: 1) compression of the suture within the anchor body (Opus MiniMagnum & Opus LabraLock P, Arthrocare, Sunnyvale, CA), 2) compression of the suture between the anchor and the drill hole (Pushlock, Arthrex, Naples, FL), or 3) sliding a pre-tied knot within the anchor (Kinsa, Smith & Nephew, Andover, MA).

PATIENT SELECTION

Patients with recurrent shoulder instability are indicated for surgical stabilization. Arthroscopic stabilization may be used in most patients with anterior and/or posterior instability. The presence of a significant anterior glenoid bone defect may require an anterior bone graft to address this structural deficiency. The uncommonly encountered humeral avulsion glenohumeral ligament (HAGL) lesion requires repair when present. These lesions are difficult to address arthroscopically and may require an open repair. Capsular redundancy can be addressed arthroscopically by superior capsular shift, capsular plication, or selective capsular resection as indicated.

HIGHLIGHTED SURGICAL TECHNIQUE

Initial arthroscopic visualization is achieved via a standard posterior portal (see Chapter 4 video). Dual anterior portals are established for instrumentation. The antero-inferior portal is placed as close as possible to the superior edge of the subscapularis tendon to allow access to the anterior and inferior aspect of the glenoid rim. The antero-superior portal is placed in the rotator cuff interval just anterior to the biceps tendon.

Thorough arthroscopic evaluation is done with examination of the articular surfaces, labrum, biceps tendon, rotator cuff, and glenohumeral ligaments. If visualization of the anterior labrum and anteroinferior glenohumeral ligament (AIGHL) complex from the posterior portal is inadequate, then visualization can be achieved from the anterior superior portal with instrumentation through the anteroinferior portal.

LIGAMENT PREPARATION AND MOBILIZATION

Preparation of the anteroinferior glenohumeral ligament is determined by the pathologic findings encountered (see Chapter 4 video). The exposed labral edge of a Bankart lesion (Figure 4-4) is débrided with a motorized shaver to promote healing after repair. Care is taken to adequately release and mobilize the anteroinferior glenohumeral ligament from the glenoid and underlying subscapularis tendon. When an anterior labroligamentous periosteal sleeve avulsion (ALPSA) lesion is the cause of instability (Figure 4-5), the periosteum should be incised to release the anteroinferior glenohumeral ligament from the glenoid. This essentially converts an ALPSA lesion to a Bankart lesion (Figure 4-6). The anteroinferior glenohumeral ligament often is scarred to the subscapularis muscle, requiring dissection in this area. Once the ligament is mobilized, a grasper is used to pull the ligament superiorly and to the articular margin while capsular tension, mobility, and capsular laxity are evaluated (Figure 4-7).

Associated capsular stretch can be managed in several ways. Complete capsular mobilization, as described above, allows for superior capsular shift that often corrects associated capsular stretch. Additional capsular plication is rarely needed when the capsule is mobilized and adequately shifted superiorly. A variety of capsular plication techniques have been described as well. Capsular plication can be performed in conjunction with a suture anchor repair by first passing the suture through the ligament, just lateral to the labrum, before passing the suture through the labrum (Figure 4-8). Alternatively, additional capsular plication sutures can be placed after suture anchor repair is completed (Figure 4-9). Capsular stretch can also be addressed by shortening the anteroinferior glenohumeral ligament with a resection of a small section of the capsule (Figure 4-10).[6] Adequate tissue quality must be present to use this method of addressing capsular stretch.

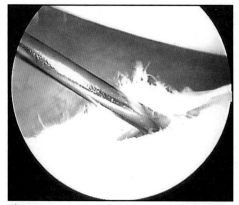

Figure 4-4. Bankart lesion (posterior view).

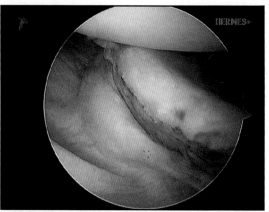

Figure 4-5. ALPSA lesion (anterior view).

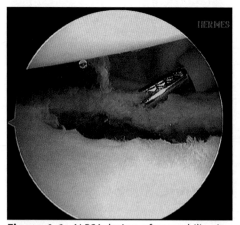

Figure 4-6. ALPSA lesion after mobilization (posterior view).

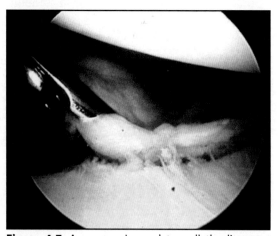

Figure 4-7. A grasper is used to pull the ligament superiorly while capsular tension and mobility are evaluated. The degree of capsular laxity can also be assessed at this time (posterior view).

Figure 4-8. Capsular plication is performed in conjunction with a suture anchor repair by first passing the suture through the ligament, just lateral to the labrum, before passing the suture through the labrum.

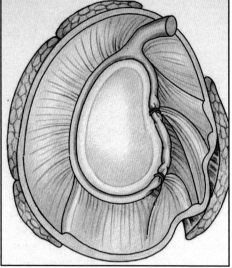

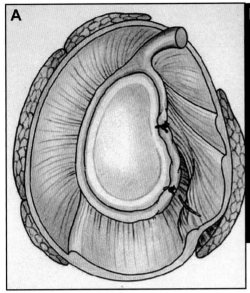

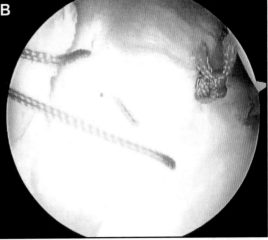

Figure 4-9. (A) An additional capsular plication suture is placed after suture anchor repair. (B) Plication suture prior to arthroscopic knot-tying.

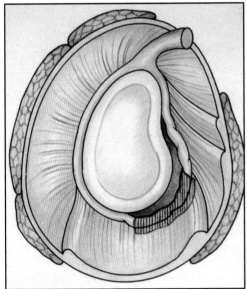

Figure 4-10. A small section of the capsule is resected to shorten the anteroinferior glenohumeral ligament prior to repair.

GLENOID PREPARATION AND DRILL HOLE PLACEMENT

A motorized burr is used to decorticate the anterior glenoid neck from the edge of the articular cartilage medially 1 to 2 cm (see Chapter 4 video).

The anteroinferior cannula then is replaced by a larger 8-mm cannula to accommodate the drill guide, suture passer, and Knotless or BioKnotless Suture Anchors. Three drill holes are made in the anterior glenoid rim using a 2.9-mm arthroscopic drill bit (DePuy/Mitek; Figure 4-11). These drill holes are spaced along the edge of the articular cartilage. It is important to direct the drill bit medially, away from the articular surface of the glenoid, by at least a 15 degree angle, to avoid damage to the articular surface. Furthermore, it is important not to torque the drill when establishing the drill hole

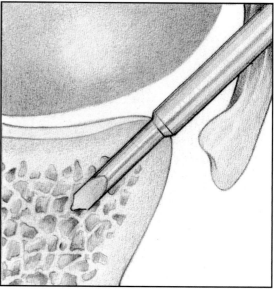

Figure 4-11. Three 2.9-mm drill holes are made in the anterior glenoid rim. (Reprinted with permission from Thal R. Knotless suture anchor fixation for shoulder instability. In: Miller MD, Cole BJ, eds. *Textbook of Arthroscopy.* Philadelphia, PA: Elsevier, 2004:116.)

location, as this can cause difficulty in achieving appropriate alignment for knotless suture anchor insertion. The drill holes are marked with a basket forceps, suction punch, or electrocautery to ease drill hole identification during anchor insertion.

SUTURE PASSAGE

Before implant placement, the utility loop of the knotless suture anchor assembly is passed through the anteroinferior glenohumeral ligament at a selected site via the anteroinferior portal (see Chapter 4 video). This can be achieved using various arthroscopic suture-passing instruments and techniques. Our preferred technique for arthroscopic passage of the utility loop is a suture loop shuttle technique (Figure 4-12).[7] The passage of the utility loop through the ligament at a precise location using this technique allows for proper capsule shift. The location for suture loop placement is determined by grasping the ligament with the suture punch and pulling it superiorly to the drill hole site, while ligament tension is assessed. A 48-inch long, 2-0 Prolene (Ethicon, Inc, Somerville, NJ) suture loop then is passed through the ligament using a Shutt suture punch (Linvatec, Largo, FL). The Prolene suture loop serves as a suture shuttle and is used to pull the utility loop into the anteroinferior portal, through the anteroinferior glenohumeral ligament, and then out the anterosuperior portal.

The utility loop is then used to pull the anchor loop through the anteroinferior glenohumeral ligament. As the utility loop pulls the anchor loop through the anteroinferior glenohumeral ligament, the attached anchor is brought down the anteroinferior cannula while being controlled on the threaded inserter rod (Figure 4-13).

LOOP CAPTURE AND ANCHOR INSERTION

Once the anchor loop has passed through the anteroinferior glenohumeral ligament, one strand of the anchor loop is captured or snagged in the channel at the tip

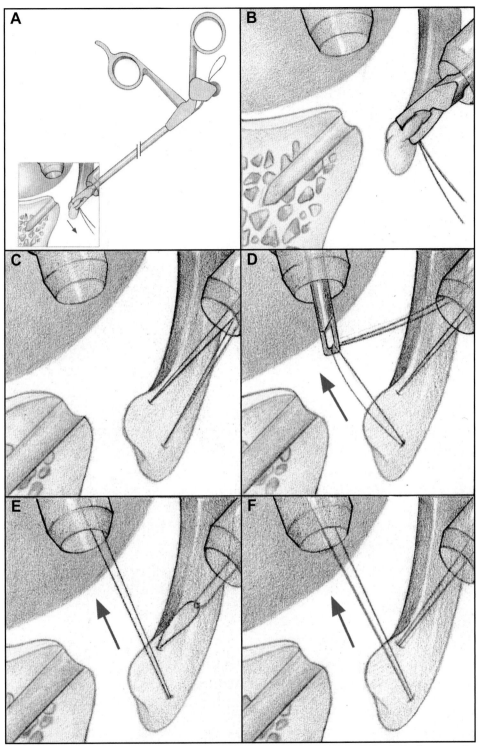

Figure 4-12. (A, B, C) A 48-inch long, 2-0 Prolene suture loop is passed through the ligament by a suture punch. (D) The free ends of the Prolene suture loop are pulled out the anterosuperior portal while the loop remains out the anteroinferior portal. (E, F) The Prolene suture loop is used as a suture shuttle to pull the utility loop through the ligament. (Reprinted with permission from Thal R. Knotless suture anchor fixation for shoulder instability. In: Miller MD, Cole BJ, eds. *Textbook of Arthroscopy*. Philadelphia, PA: Elsevier, 2004:118.)

Figure 4-13. The utility loop is used to pull the anchor loop through the anteroinferior glenohumeral ligament. (Reprinted with permission from Thal R. Knotless suture anchor fixation for shoulder instability. In: Miller MD, Cole BJ, eds. *Textbook of Arthroscopy*. Philadelphia, PA: Elsevier, 2004:117.)

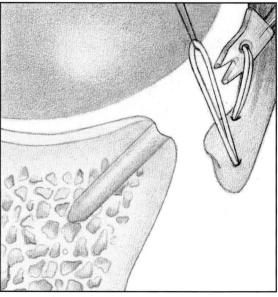

Figure 4-14. One suture strand of the anchor loop is captured or snagged in the channel at the tip of the anchor. (Reprinted with permission from Thal R. Knotless suture anchor fixation for shoulder instability. In: Miller MD, Cole BJ, eds. *Textbook of Arthroscopy*. Philadelphia, PA: Elsevier, 2004:117.)

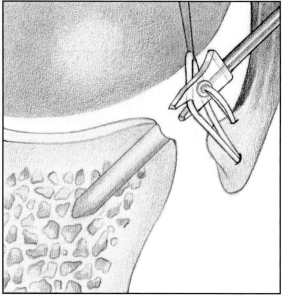

of the anchor (Figure 4-14, and see Chapter 4 video). The anchor then is inserted and tapped into the glenoid drill hole to the desired depth to achieve appropriate tissue tension (Figure 4-15). The anchor should not bottom-out in the drill hole. The depth of anchor insertion is determined by observing the ligament approximation to the glenoid and by intermittently pulling the utility loop to test the tension of the anchor loop during insertion. Once this process has been completed, the anteroinferior glenohumeral ligament is noted to shift superiorly and securely approximate to the glenoid rim in a low-profile manner. The utility loop and inserter rod are then removed (Figure 4-16).

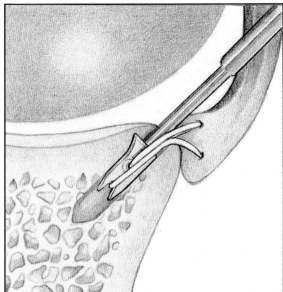

Figure 4-15. The anchor is inserted and tapped into the glenoid drill hole to the desired depth to achieve appropriate tissue tension. (Reprinted with permission from Thal R. Knotless suture anchor fixation for shoulder instability. In: Miller MD, Cole BJ, eds. *Textbook of Arthroscopy.* Philadelphia, PA: Elsevier, 2004:117.)

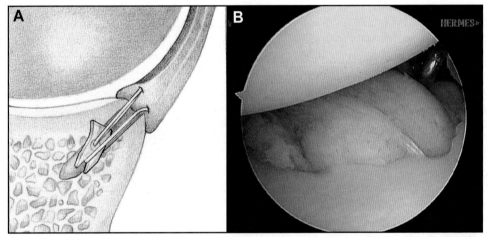

Figure 4-16. (A) The utility loop and inserter rod are removed after the anchor has been inserted to the appropriate depth. (Reprinted with permission from Thal R. Knotless suture anchor fixation for shoulder instability. In: Miller MD, Cole BJ, eds. *Textbook of Arthroscopy.* Philadelphia, PA: Elsevier, 2004:117.) (B) Final knotless suture anchor repair.

ALTERNATIVE KNOTLESS SUTURE ANCHOR DESIGNS AND TECHNIQUES

When alternative knotless suture anchor designs are used, ligament and glenoid preparations are performed as described previously.

When using the Kinsa suture anchor, a loop of suture is passed through the ligament, as described for the Knotless and BioKnotless Suture Anchors. Rather than capturing the suture loop with a notch in the anchor as with the Knotless and BioKnotless Suture Anchors, the Kinsa anchor is passed through the suture loop. Compression fixation of the anchor in the glenoid drill hole is then achieved. Ligament tensioning is then achieved by pulling on a suture strand attached to a pre-tied, sliding knot located within the anchor body. This excess suture strand is then cut with an arthroscopic cutter once the desired ligament tension is achieved.

Opus MiniMagnum and Opus LabraLock P anchors use standard sutures rather than suture loops. Standard sutures are first passed through the ligament to be repaired at the desired location. With the Opus-style anchors, the sutures are then loaded into the anchor body prior to inserting the anchor into the glenoid drill hole. Repair tension is achieved by manually pulling the sutures prior to deploying the anchor's bone-securing mechanism. The suture is secured by compression within the anchor body while bone fixation is achieved.

The PushLock suture anchor also uses a standard suture that is passed through the ligament prior to inserting the anchor into the glenoid drill hole. The suture is passed through an islet portion at the tip of this 2-part anchor. The islet tip is inserted into the glenoid drill hole, and the suture is pulled to tension the repair. The anchor body is then inserted into the drill hole to achieve compression fixation to bone. The suture is compressed between the anchor and the drill hole to provide suture fixation.

TIPS AND PEARLS

The location of passage of the utility loop and anchor loop through the anteroinferior glenohumeral ligament is very important. It should be located inferiorly with respect to the glenoid drill hole so that a superior shift of the anteroinferior glenohumeral ligament is achieved when the anchor is inserted into the drill hole (see Chapter 4 video). The anchors are inserted in the most inferior site first, progressing to the more superior sites. This concept is not unique to the knotless suture anchor technique. This principle is important for all suture anchor repair techniques.

Several techniques have been found to ease capture of the anchor loop when using the knotless suture anchor. For the inferior 2 anchors, pass the Prolene suture loop from the intra-articular side of the ligament to the extra-articular side (Figure 4-17), which positions the utility loop similarly after shuttling. For the superior anchor, pass the suture loop from the extra-articular side of the ligament to the articular side (Figure 4-18). This orients the anchor loop at a better angle and facilitates ease in capturing of the anchor loop. Pull the utility loop through the anterosuperior portal to orient the anchor loop at a better angle with respect to the anchor and ease loop capture (Figure 4-19).

Test the tension of the anchor loop and repair site by intermittently pulling the utility loop during anchor insertion. This is an important step in the appropriate use of the knotless suture anchor as it can help ensure appropriate tension at the repair site.

Special attention must be given to the arcs on the metallic Knotless Suture Anchor to avoid inadvertent cutting of the anchor loop. The anchor loop must pass directly from the base of the anchor into the ligament. If, instead, the anchor loop is allowed to wrap around the body of the anchor, then the anchor loop will be at risk of being cut by the closing anchor arc as the anchor is inserted into bone (Figure 4-20). Additionally, one arc must be passed through the anchor loop before anchor insertion. The utility loop is used to pull the anchor loop over the anchor arc and hold the anchor loop safely away from the arcs during the first stages of anchor insertion. If this is not done, the anchor loop will be cut on insertion into bone. Tension on the anchor loop is relaxed once the arcs have entered the bone. This is not a concern with use of the BioKnotless Suture Anchor because bone fixation is achieved by toggle of the wedge-shaped anchor body rather than by metal arcs.

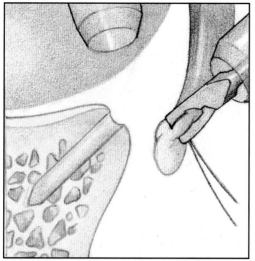

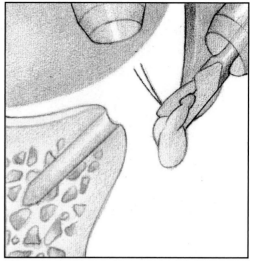

Figure 4-17. The Prolene suture loop is passed from the intra-articular side of the ligament to the extra-articular side for the inferior two anchors. This positions the utility loop similarly after shuttling, which has been found to ease anchor loop capture. (Reprinted with permission from Thal R. Knotless suture anchor fixation for shoulder instability. In: Miller MD, Cole BJ, eds. *Textbook of Arthroscopy*. Philadelphia, PA: Elsevier, 2004:118.)

Figure 4-18. The Prolene suture loop is passed from the extra-articular side of the ligament to the intra-articular side for the superior anchor, which has been found to ease anchor loop capture.

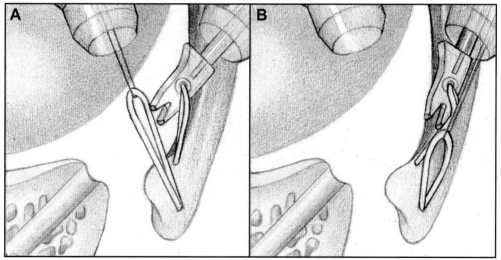

Figure 4-19. (A) The utility loop is pulled out the anterosuperior portal to orient the anchor loop at a better angle with respect to the anchor and thus facilitate loop capture. (B) Loop capture is more difficult when the loop is pulled toward the same portal as the anchor. (Reprinted with permission from Thal R. Knotless suture anchor fixation for shoulder instability. In: Miller MD, Cole BJ, eds. *Textbook of Arthroscopy*. Philadelphia, PA: Elsevier, 2004:119.)

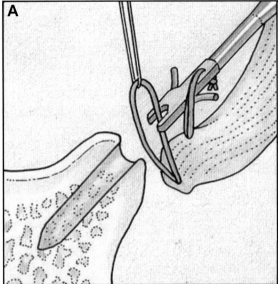

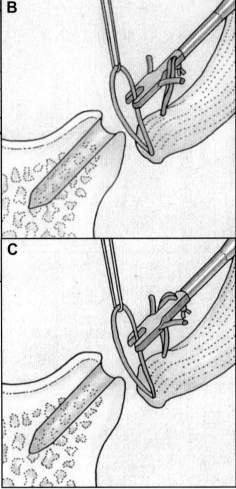

Figure 4-20. (A) One anchor arc has not been passed through the anchor loop and will cut the anchor loop when the anchor is inserted into bone. (B) The anchor loop is incorrectly wrapped around the anchor. (C) The anchor loop is incorrectly wrapped around the anchor. (Reprinted with permission from Thal R. Knotless suture anchor fixation for shoulder instability. In: Miller MD, Cole BJ, eds. *Textbook of Arthroscopy*. Philadelphia, PA: Elsevier, 2004:119-120.)

MANAGING COMPLICATIONS

Fortunately, complications unique to the use of the knotless suture anchor are rare. In fact, knotless suture anchors help avoid several potential intraoperative complications experienced with the use of standard suture anchors. Suture pullout from the anchor, knot-tying difficulties, knot abrasion of the articular surface, and knot interposition between the labrum and the glenoid are eliminated with the use of knotless suture anchors.

The incidence of suture breakage has been significantly decreased with the use of high-strength sutures for both standard and knotless suture anchors. If an anchor loop breaks during insertion of a knotless suture anchor, the repair can be successfully completed by stacking another knotless anchor into the same drill hole.

Inadequate repair tension is a potential complication with both standard suture anchors and knotless suture anchors. Knot-tying deficiencies can cause this complication with standard suture anchors. This complication can occur with knotless suture anchors if the anchor is not inserted to the appropriate depth. Testing the tension of the anchor loop and repair site by intermittently pulling the utility loop during anchor insertion will ensure appropriate repair tension. This is an important step in the proper use of the knotless suture anchor and should be performed before removing the inserter rod. If inadequate repair tension is identified after the inserter rod has been removed, the repair tension can sometimes be adjusted by carefully reattaching the inserter rod to the knotless anchor and advancing the knotless anchor to a more appropriate depth.

POSTOPERATIVE MANAGEMENT

The postoperative rehabilitative protocol involves use of a sling for the first 4 postoperative weeks. During that time, pendulum exercises, range of motion exercises of the shoulder and elbow, and isometric exercises of the forearm are performed. External rotation is limited to neutral. At 4 weeks postoperatively, progressive active and passive range of motion exercises are begun. External rotation is limited to 45 degrees. In addition, isometric exercises of the deltoid and periscapular exercises are begun. At 6 weeks postoperatively, progression to a full active range of motion is allowed. At 8 weeks, resistive training with the use of isotonic and isokinetic modalities is performed in a progressive manner but with no limitation on the patient. Participation in contact and overhead sports was not allowed until 5 months postoperatively.

COMPARISON OF KNOTLESS SUTURE ANCHORS

Several studies have demonstrated comparable clinical results with standard suture anchor and knotless suture anchor repairs.[8,9] Any device that provides adequate ligament fixation would be expected to result in comparable healing rates. Therefore, with appropriate ligament repositioning, comparable results would be expected with these repairs. All of the knotless suture anchor designs discussed in this chapter provide a low-profile repair and eliminate the risk of knot impingement that can occur with suture anchors that require knot tying.

An objective comparison of the merits of the various knotless suture anchor features is difficult. There is a paucity of peer-reviewed literature with direct biomechanical comparisons or clinical outcomes with the use of these devices. Each knotless device has unique functional and technique characteristics. The relative benefits of many of these characteristics are very subjective. In this section, we will discuss the potential benefits and weaknesses of the various anchor designs with regard to specific criteria. When appropriate, we will also describe methods of overcoming the potential weakness with the anchor design feature. For the purpose of this discussion, we will categorize the knotless anchors into 4 separate groups: Knotless (Knotless, BioKnotless, BioKnotless BR), Opus (MiniMagnum, LabraLock P), PushLock, and Kinsa (Table 4-1). Each category of knotless anchor will be assessed based on anchor material, suture strength and material, bone fixation, mechanical considerations, and technique considerations.

Anchor Material

Knotless suture anchors are manufactured with 4 types of implant material: metal (titanium), polyetheretherketone (PEEK), bioabsorbable (poly-L-lactic acid [PLLA]), and biocomposite (tricalcium phosphate [TCP] and polylactic acid [PLA] blend).

Table 4-1

NAME	COMPANY	MATERIAL	TENSION METHOD	BONE FIXATION	SUTURE FIXATION
Knotless	DePuy/Mitek	Titanium	Depth of anchor insertion	Nitinol arcs	Capture closed loop
BioKnotless	DePuy/Mitek	PLLA	Depth of anchor insertion	Toggle of wedge-shaped anchor	Capture closed loop
BioKnotless BR	DePuy/Mitek	Biocryl rapide	Depth of anchor insertion	Toggle of wedge-shaped anchor	Capture closed loop
Opus Mini-Magnum	Arthrocare	Titanium	Suture compression within anchor body at selected position	Anchor expansion	Suture compression within anchor body
Opus LabraLock P	Arthrocare	PEEK	Suture compression within anchor body at selected position	Anchor expansion	Suture compression within anchor body
PushLock	Arthrex	PEEK or PLLA body and PEEK eyelet	Suture compression between anchor and bone at selected position	Compression	Suture compression between anchor and bone
Kinsa	Smith & Nephew	PEEK	Sliding pre-tied knot within the anchor	Compression	Pre-tied knot within the anchor

PLLA = Poly-L-Lactide Acid; PEEK = Polyetheretherketone

PEEK and metal offer strength advantages; however, revision surgery can be more challenging with these nonabsorbable anchor materials. Specific situations (poor bone quality, presence of bone cysts, or revision) and surgeon preference influence the desired anchor material.

The Knotless and Opus suture anchors are available in titanium versions. The Opus, PushLock, and Kinsa anchors are available in PEEK. The BioKnotless and BioKnotless BR anchors are the only fully absorbable or biocomposite anchors. The PushLock anchor is available with a PEEK islet and a bioabsorbable anchor body.

Suture Strength and Material

The Knotless anchor group and the Kinsa anchor use a suture loop, while the Opus and PushLock anchors use standard sutures. A suture loop has been shown to be stronger than the single suture strand when the same suture material is used. The use of high-strength suture material minimizes the strength advantage of a suture loop. Adequate suture strength is likely achieved with a single strand of high-strength suture.

All of the knotless suture anchors described are available with high-strength suture. The Knotless anchor group is available with high-strength suture or absorbable suture material.

Bone Fixation

The metal Knotless Suture Anchor achieves bone fixation by 2 nitinol arcs. The wedge-shaped BioKnotless Suture Anchors toggle within the drill hole to achieve fixation. The Opus anchors have a deployment mechanism whereby deformation of the anchor body occurs within the drill hole after the anchor is inserted. The Kinsa and PushLock anchors achieve bone fixation by compression within the drill hole.

Mechanical Considerations

Knot security and loop security are issues often discussed when evaluating standard suture anchors with arthroscopic knot tying. Knot security is defined as the effectiveness of a knot to resist slippage when load is applied. Knot security depends on 3 factors: friction, internal interference, and slack between throws. Loop security is the ability to maintain a tight secure loop as a knot is tied. It is possible to have an ineffective repair despite good knot security if the suture loop is loose and does not adequately approximate the edges of the tissue to be repaired.

The security of a repair using knotless suture anchors can be evaluated using equivalent terms. Knot tying is eliminated by a variety of mechanisms with the various knotless suture anchors. The security of the particular knot-eliminating mechanism will determine the "knot security equivalent" for a knotless suture anchor. Similarly, the "loop security equivalent" for a knotless suture anchor can be defined as the ability to maintain a tight secure loop as the knotless suture anchor is implanted.

Direct comparisons of the knot security or loop security "equivalents" for the various knotless suture anchors have not been reported. The mechanical differences between the various knotless suture anchors will be described, and the potential effect on repair security will be discussed.

The Knotless anchors all function in a similar fashion. The captured suture loop provides a rigid construct. This construct maximizes knot security equivalent because slippage cannot occur within the closed suture loop as might be experienced with a tied knot. Loop tension is achieved by the depth of anchor insertion with the knotless anchor group. Loop security must be assessed during anchor insertion and adjusted prior to removal of the inserter rod. Similar to a standard suture anchor repair with knot tying, it is possible to have an ineffective repair with the knotless anchor group if the anchor is not inserted to the appropriate depth to achieve the desired repair tension.

The Kinsa anchor achieves repair tension by sliding a pre-tied knot within the anchor body. This pre-tied knot determines the knot security of this anchor. Loop security is determined by the ability to provide the appropriate repair tension while sliding this pre-tied knot. Even with acceptable knot security, an ineffective repair can occur with the Kinsa anchor if the pre-tied knot ceases sliding before adequate repair tension is achieved.

The Opus suture anchors eliminate knot tying by compression of the suture within the anchor body. The knot security equivalent with this system is determined by the ability of this suture compression mechanism to resist suture slippage. Reports indicate that the suture will break before suture slippage occurs with this mechanism. Loop security is determined by the ability to achieve and maintain the appropriate repair tension, while the anchor compression mechanism is deployed. Even with acceptable suture compression security, an ineffective repair can occur with the Opus anchor if adequate repair tension is not achieved prior to anchor deployment.

The PushLock suture anchor eliminates knot tying by compression of the suture between the anchor body and the bone. The knot security equivalent with this system is determined by the ability of this suture compression to resist suture slippage. Bone quality would be expected to affect the resistance to suture slippage. Any suture abrasion during anchor insertion would be expected to have an adverse effect on suture strength. Loop security is determined by the ability to achieve and maintain the appropriate repair tension while the anchor is inserted. Even with acceptable suture compression security, an ineffective repair can occur with the PushLock anchor if adequate repair tension is not achieved prior to and maintained during anchor insertion.

Technique Considerations

Once the suture loop of the Knotless anchor group is captured in the notch at the tip of the anchor, a rigid construct is created. The amount of tissue incorporated into the repair, however, is limited due to the fixed length of the suture loop. This is a potential shortcoming if incorporation of a large capsular plication within the repair is desired. The suture loop is long enough to perform a significant capsular plication; however, the fixed loop length does limit the size of this plication.

Some surgeons might find that intra-articular suture loop capture can be challenging with the Knotless anchor group. The use of the utility loop to manipulate the anchor loop can ease loop capture. The "Tips and Pearls" section on p. 68 of this chapter describes this technique in more detail.

The Knotless anchor group provides a unique method of adjusting ligament repair tension. Ligament tension is assessed as the anchor is inserted. The anchor is gently tapped deeper into the drill hole if additional ligament tension is desired. This allows for fine adjustment in ligament repair tension.

The Kinsa anchor also uses a suture loop; however, the size of this loop can be adjusted by sliding the pre-tied knot located within the anchor body. Therefore, a much larger capsular plication or bite of capsule can be achieved with this anchor.

Because the Kinsa anchor body has been passed through the suture loop, the suture loop tightens and contracts around the ligament as the suture loop is shortened. With the Knotless anchor group, the suture loop is captured in the notch at the tip of the anchor, which prevents the potential tissue strangulation that might occur as the ligament is tensioned with the Kinsa anchor. It is difficult to determine if the tissue compression that occurs with the Kinsa anchor suture loop has an adverse effect on tissue healing.

The Opus and PushLock anchors all use standard suture strands. Therefore, the amount of tissue incorporated into the repair is not limited. Repair tension is adjusted by manually pulling on the suture limbs with both the Opus and PushLock anchors. Anchor deployment is different with these anchors, however. The desired repair tension must be maintained, while the PushLock anchor is tapped into the drill hole. It can be difficult to precisely adjust ligament tension with the PushLock anchor. The anchor body must be advanced past the re-approximated ligament while ligament tension is maintained. Ligament tension cannot be adjusted with the PushLock anchor once the anchor has been inserted into the drill hole. With the Opus anchors, the anchor is inserted into the drill hole before adjusting ligament tension. Once the desired ligament tension has been achieved, the anchor is deployed and the suture compression mechanism is activated. The Opus anchors cannot advance after anchor deployment if additional ligament tension is desired.

REFERENCES

1. Loutzenheiser TD, Harryman DT II, Yung SW, France MP, Sidles JA. Optimizing arthroscopic knots. *Arthroscopy.* 1995;11:199-206.
2. Thal R. A knotless suture anchor: design, function, and biomechanical testing. *American Journal of Sports Medicine.* 2001;29(5):646-649.
3. Thal R. A knotless suture anchor: technique for use in arthroscopic Bankart repair. *Arthroscopy.* 2001;17(2):213-218.
4. Thal R. Knotless suture anchor. Arthroscopic Bankart repair without tying knots. *Clin Ortho Relat Res.* 2001;390:42-51.
5. Thal R, Lizardi J, Reese K. A knotless suture anchor: technique for use in arthroscopic bankart repair and biomechanical testing. Paper presented at: 24th Annual Meeting of the American Orthopaedic Society for Sports Medicine; July 12, 1998; Vancouver, British Columbia, Canada.
6. Berg JH, Thal R, Tamai J. A comparison of capsular shift in medially based repairs for glenohumeral instability: a cadaveric study. Paper presented at: 19th Annual Meeting of the Arthroscopy Association of North America; April 16, 2000; Miami Beach, FL.
7. Thal R. A technique for arthroscopic mattress suture placement. *Arthroscopy.* 1993;9:605-607.
8. Thal R. Arthroscopic anterior stabilization of the shoulder with a knotless suture anchor: technique and results. Paper presented at: 27th Annual Meeting of the American Orthopaedic Society for Sports Medicine; June 30, 2001; Keystone, CO.
9. Thal R, Nofziger M, Bridges M, Kim JJ. Arthroscopic Bankart repair using Knotless or BioKnotless suture anchors: 2- to 7-year results. *Arthroscopy.* 2007;23(4)367-375.

Please see video on the accompanying Web site at http://www.slackbooks.com/unstableshouldervideos

When We Should Consider Posterior Plication Sutures and Interval Plication

Mark T. Wichman, MD

The concepts and techniques in the first section of this book deal with arthroscopic management of the unstable shoulder. They are valuable for determining patient selection and techniques for stabilizing shoulders with anterior, posterior, and multidirectional instability patterns. This chapter will provide a better understanding of how the surgeon may "fine tune" an arthroscopic repair. Like most orthopedic pathology, instability has many degrees of magnitude. The surgeon must have tools to handle not only unidirectional traumatic instability cases, but also complex cases with multidirectional laxity, generalized ligament hyperlaxity, or revision cases alike.

One peculiar aspect of the use of posterior plication sutures and interval plication is that while some well-accomplished surgeons may use them in every case, other equally experienced surgeons may seldom use them, if ever. How can one reconcile these opposite approaches, presuming that both groups of surgeons are obtaining good results? One reasonable theory is that most arthroscopic stabilizations are, in essence, volume-reduction procedures. That is, in addition to anatomical repair of the pathologic anatomy, they involve superior mobilization of the capsule, lateralization of the capsular insertion onto the glenoid face, and reduction of the overall volume of the glenohumeral joint capsule. It is plausible that those who choose to avoid interval closure and posterior plication make up the volume reduction elsewhere. Perhaps they use more aggressive plication sutures or a more vigorous "south to north" repair. By the same argument, those surgeons who currently are seeing favorable outcomes with low recurrence rates should think very carefully before adding interval closure or posterior plication to their current technique without slight modifications of those techniques.

Abrams JS. *Management of the Unstable Shoulder: Arthroscopic and Open Repair* (pp. 77-88).
© 2011 SLACK Incorporated

Figure 5-1. The anatomy of the rotator interval. This is the triangular area bordered by the biceps tendon superiorly, glenoid medially, and the subscapularis inferiorly.

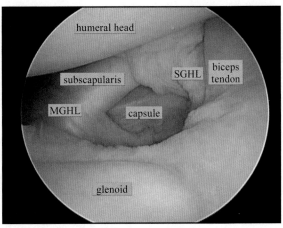

THE ROTATOR INTERVAL

The rotator interval (RI) is defined as the triangular-shaped area between the supraspinatus and subscapularis tendons (Figure 5-1). It includes the coracohumeral ligament (not seen intra-articularly), biceps tendon, superior and middle glenohumeral ligaments, and adjacent capsule. Despite numerous clinical and cadaveric studies during the past few decades, the precise role of the RI in unstable shoulders remains a matter of debate. The classic teaching of an increased sulcus sign as a telltale sign of pathological laxity in the rotator interval led to the concept of RI closure in open instability surgery. However, using knowledge of the RI learned from open approaches to the shoulder to make meaningful statements in arthroscopic shoulder surgery may constitute quite a leap. Not only is the arthroscopic view of the RI vastly different from the open surgical exposure, but one may argue whether current techniques of arthroscopic RI closure truly have a consistent effect on the coracohumeral ligament.

Recent studies by Provencher and colleagues[1,2] and Mologne and coworkers[3] demonstrate significant variations from earlier work by Harryman and colleagues[4] on the function of the rotator interval. The precise effect of RI closure has, therefore, become less clear. Provencher's work focused on differences between open and arthroscopic RI closure. Open RI closure involves a medial-lateral imbrication as demonstrated in Figure 5-2. Therefore, a true shortening of the coracohumeral ligament can only occur in open surgery. However, in arthroscopic surgery, RI closure involves more of an inferior-superior closure. They also found that there was significant improvement in *anterior* stability after both open and arthroscopic closure of the RI, but they found no significant improvement in *posterior* stability in open or arthroscopic RI closure. One potentially problematic finding was that both open and arthroscopic RI closure can potentially cause significant losses of external rotation.[5-9] This loss of external rotation is the most consistent finding between groups who have studied the effects of RI closure. We must remember, however, that most published reports looking at rotator interval closure have been biomechanical studies on cadaveric specimens. There are certainly additional unknown elements encountered when applying these data to in vivo cases.

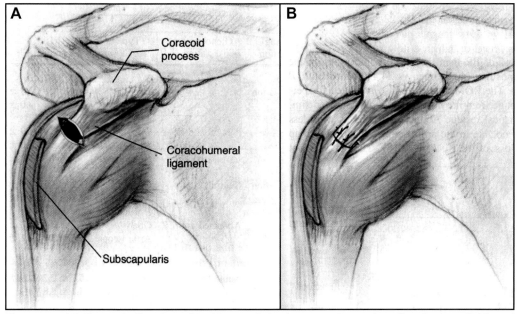

Figure 5-2. (A) The vertically oriented incision made in the rotator interval to allow for a medial-lateral shortening of the coracohumeral ligament. (B) The effect of this type of rotator interval closure as performed by Harryman in open surgery. (Reprinted from Provencher MT, Mologne TS, Hongo M, Zhao K, Tasto JP, An KN. Arthroscopic versus open rotator interval closure: biomechanical evaluation of stability and motion. *Arthroscopy*. 2007;23(6):583-592, with permission from Elsevier.)

INDICATIONS

There are 4 broad categories of patients who could benefit from arthroscopic rotator interval closure combined with instability repair. These include patients with *multidirectional instability* who are also having capsular plication, labral repair, or both. Other patients often seeking treatment for instability are those with *generalized ligament hyperlaxity*. These patients often have hyperextension at the elbows and knees, and can often oppose the thumb to the volar surface of the forearm. In these shoulders, it will take a larger volume reduction in the shoulder capsule to accomplish the same amount of stabilization. They often tend to stretch out the repaired tissue more readily. Often, these shoulders are noted to have hypotrophic glenohumeral ligaments, such as that seen in Figure 5-3. There is often a positive "drive-through" sign as seen in Figure 5-4. The third group of patients who may need additional techniques for capsular reduction are those with *numerous instability episodes*. The patient with a multi-year history of multiple dislocations each year presents a problem with stretched out secondary stabilizers and often thin, hemosiderin-stained capsule from the frequent, chronic instability. These patients may have issues with bone loss as well, which is covered in Sections II and III of this book. The fourth patient population that may benefit from rotator interval closure are those with histories of *failed prior surgical treatment*. The circumstances leading to surgical failure may be different for each of these cases, but additional strategies of capsular volume reduction are often necessary when managing these difficult revisions. Any of the above conditions may coexist with a lesion of the rotator interval. This is seen when a patient with an unstable shoulder and positive sulcus sign has particularly thin, patulous tissue in the

Figure 5-3. This is an arthroscopic photograph demonstrating a thin hypotrophic band of the middle glenohumeral ligament. This anatomic variation is more common in patients with multidirectional instability.

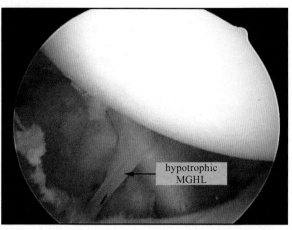

Figure 5-4. This is a drawing depicting the arthroscopic strategy for closure of the rotator interval. It demonstrates the inferior-superior closure that occurs while closing the middle glenohumeral ligament to the superior ligament. (Reprinted from Provencher MT, Mologne TS, Hongo M, Zhao K, Tasto JP, An KN. Arthroscopic versus open rotator interval closure: biomechanical evaluation of stability and motion. *Arthroscopy.* 2007;23(6):583-592, with permission from Elsevier.)

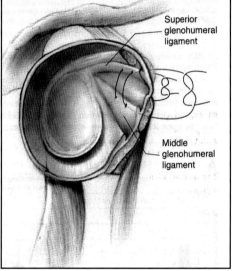

rotator interval. The diagnosis is clinical because no radiographic studies can actually confirm this lesion. The rotator interval lesion combined with one of the clinical presentations above would present an ideal case for adding RI closure to the surgical management of instability.

Contraindications

Though there are no absolute contraindications, closure of the RI may be of greater risk than potential benefit in certain patients. Because there is a risk of loss of external rotation, the dominant shoulder of a throwing athlete is particularly at risk for potential over-tightening. In this particular patient population, the loss of motion may be more difficult to manage than the instability. This principle obviously holds true for other overhand athletes, such as those who play tennis or volleyball. One must even consider these factors in swimmers because they also require full overhead excursion in freestyle competition. Any patient whose shoulder would clearly be worse if there was a mild loss of external rotation can usually be adequately stabilized *without* using RI closure techniques.

Technique

Arthroscopic closure of the rotator interval is often performed near the conclusion of the procedure for 2 reasons. First, the degree of interval plication can be fine-tuned depending on the magnitude of the primary repair. Second, the closure of the RI often obliterates the anterior working portal(s), so it must occur when those portals are no longer needed. There are numerous techniques for RI closure.[10-12] Some surgeons close from the supraspinatus tendon to the subscapularis tendon, and others plicate only capsular structures. Most techniques represent a variation of the capsular plication, though one newer technique includes the use of a suture anchor in the humeral head.[13]

Because the subscapularis and supraspinatus have their own innervations and are 2 distinct musculotendinous structures, it is anatomically undesirable to create a tenodesis. This also could potentially change the force vector of one or both tendons. By arthroscopically placing mattress sutures through the superior extent of the middle glenohumeral ligament (MGHL) and retrieving the suture with a pass through the superior glenohumeral ligament (SGHL), the RI closure may be completed (see Figures 5-4 and 5-5). Two such sutures can be placed using either absorbable monofilament or braided permanent suture material, tying the knots extra-capsular by removing the anterior cannulae. The effect can be documented with the scope remaining in the posterior portal as the knots are tied. It is desirable to have an assistant hold the shoulder in 30 degrees of external rotation during this portion of the procedure. The surgeon must avoid any degree of internal rotation during interval closure to avoid capturing the shoulder. A closed arthroscopic suture cutting device is optimal to avoid cutting out the knot, yet cutting close enough to the knot to avoid excessive suture tails. Many different RI closure techniques have been described. The surgeon should practice these techniques to choose what works best in his or her hands to be prepared for the situation when it is appropriate.

POSTERIOR PLICATION

In addition to rotator interval plication, there are other techniques the surgeon may use to allow for more volume reduction during arthroscopic shoulder stabilization. The addition of posterior-inferior capsular plication sutures is one additional technique. Though it has not been as controversial or vigorously studied, it has a place in the management of shoulder instability. As surgeons tackle multidirectional instability (MDI) using newer arthroscopic techniques, it is important to consider the posterior capsule. The classic open capsular shift addressed this portion of the capsule indirectly as the inferior axillary pouch was shifted superiorly. The arthroscopic surgeon needs to manage this portion of the capsule very specifically and individually, because the anterior plication techniques are not as effective in tightening the posterior band of the inferior glenohumeral ligament.

Posterior-inferior capsular plication is routinely performed in arthroscopic repair of posterior instability. Its use in management of anterior instability and MDI is more variable. Again, we can see a dichotomy of experienced surgeons who use it in every case and others who rarely find it necessary. The relevant anatomical structure is the posterior band of the inferior glenohumeral ligament complex. This structure is highly variable. Plication involves capturing a portion of the posterior-inferior capsule and advancing it superiorly to the posterior labrum. It is usually performed with a curved

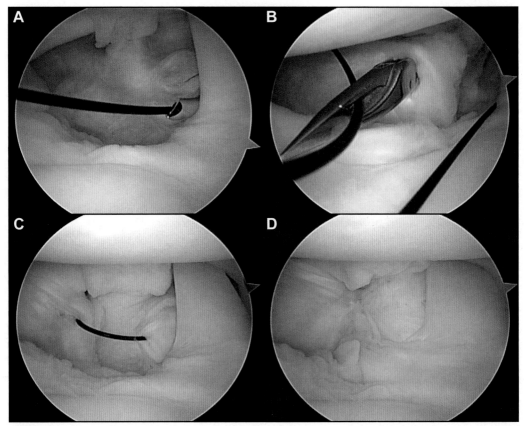

Figure 5-5. The arthroscopic technique for closure of the rotator interval includes (A) placement of sutures using a 30-degree suture hook through the SGHL and (B) retrieving this through a suture retriever passed through the MGHL. This monofilament suture can then be tied or used as a suture shuttle for a nonabsorbable suture. (C, D) Note the reduced distance between the biceps tendon and the MGHL as the suture is placed and tied.

suture hook and can be done with either nonabsorbable braided suture or monofilament suture material.

Indications

The patients who most benefit from the addition of posterior plication sutures fall into the same 4 broad categories as with RI closure. In addition, patients with a very patulous posterior capsule (Figure 5-6) or one that attaches to the glenoid in a very medial position may benefit from continuation of the plication around the 6 o'clock position and up the posterior side. Often, patients with this anatomy will fall into 1 of the previous 4 categories. The rationale for "balancing" the repair with posterior sutures involves the concept of potentially diminishing stress on the anteroinferior corner by placement of posterior sutures. In addition, a robust anterior repair in a shoulder with a relatively deficient posterior band could allow for inadvertent posterior translation of the humeral head. In general, most surgeons use these posterior plication sutures to "fine tune" a repair so that capsular volume reduction is appropriate to balance an unstable shoulder.

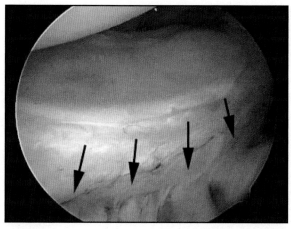

Figure 5-6. Note the patulous posterior capsular insertion pattern seen in this shoulder (arrows). This pattern is also common in multidirectional instability of the shoulder.

Contraindications

This technique does not quite have the potential to overconstrain the shoulder because the posterior band is not so stout of an anatomic structure. These sutures are mandatory in arthroscopic stabilization of a patient with MDI. Controversy exists in the classic traumatic, unidirectional instability case with a Bankart lesion. Many surgeons find it unnecessary in such a case, especially if there have only been 1 or 2 instability episodes. In these cases, anatomy is often restored with the anterior labral and capsular repairs alone. One good strategy is to be proficient at this technique so that it may be employed whenever necessary, but it need not be used routinely in true unidirectional instability cases.

Technique

Posterior capsular plication is performed by viewing from the anterosuperior portal and working from the posterior portal. Seldom are auxiliary portals necessary. The technique is identical to that used for plication on the anterior side. Steps in the technique are demonstrated in Figure 5-7. The portion of the capsule is initially treated with excoriation to encourage healing. A nonaggressive shaver blade is optimal for this. Variable-shaped suture hooks are useful for this step. If the primary procedure was anterior stabilization, a large bore cannula need not be placed posteriorly for this step. It is possible to place the curved suture hook directly through the skin using the tract from the cannula (removed). A 60-degree hook works well near the 6 o'clock position and lesser curvature as the sutures move up the posterior aspect of the glenoid. A suture shuttle may be used when using nonabsorbable suture, and monofilament may be used directly through the suture passer if absorbable suture is preferred. Both tails of suture must be pulled out anteriorly before reinserting the posterior cannula. Both tails can then be withdrawn from the posterior cannula to tie the knot. Range of motion of the shoulder can be assessed after these sutures to verify that it has not been compromised. Performing this procedure in the lateral position is particularly useful because the arm is held near 70 degrees of abduction, which maintains a margin of safety in this regard. One must be aware of the axillary nerve in suture placement in this portion of the capsule. Most studies have shown that it is a safe distance, but one must never plunge deep with the suture hook in this anatomic region of the shoulder.

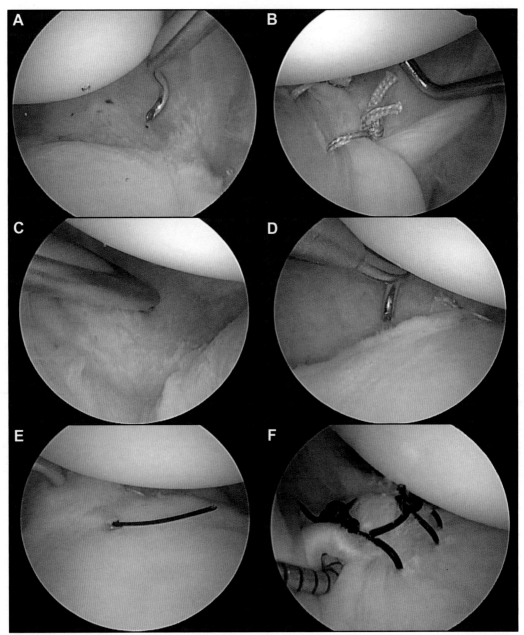

Figure 5-7. (A, B) Anterior capsular plication is seen in this patient with multidirectional instability. The steps of the posterior plication are seen in C through F. Note that the nonaggressive shaver is used to prepare the capsule. The curved suture hook is used to place sutures up the posterior-inferior corner. It is placed directly through the skin to avoid use of a 7- to 8-mm portal through this thin capsule. The opening from the cannula can be closed near the conclusion of the surgery with a very similar technique to the rotator interval closure. Many different suture configurations work well. This demonstrates simple sutures, but mattress or figure-8 sutures are helpful in different circumstances.

Case Studies

Case 1

A 24-year-old female volleyball player has a Bankart tear and mild posterior laxity in her dominant shoulder. This patient needs a stable shoulder for all of her overhead activities. Note the large Hill-Sachs lesion seen in Figure 5-8A and the corresponding Bankart fracture lesion in Figure 5-8B. Figures 5-8C and 5-8D show the anterior repair and the subsequent increased tension on the avulsion of the inferior glenohumeral ligament. This shoulder was treated with the addition of posterior plication sutures to her anterior Bankart repair (Figures 5-8E and F). A rotator interval closure was not added due to good soft tissue balance at the conclusion of the procedure. There was also concern about loss of external rotation in this athlete.

Case 2

A 21-year-old throwing athlete had a partial undersurface rotator cuff tear and anterior instability. He was treated with intra-articular closure of the rotator cuff defect and anterior capsular plication. He actually had a tight posterior capsule as is commonly seen in these patients. He was *not* treated with either posterior plication or RI closure, though the repair began at the 6 o'clock position as seen (Figure 5-9).

Case 3

A 24-year-old professional hockey player has recurrent anterior instability and a Bankart tear. He has a mild degree of multidirectional laxity. Because hockey players require very stable shoulders with the arms down near the body for use of the stick, mild loss of external rotation is well-tolerated. He is treated with Bankart repair and interval closure (photos not shown).

CONCLUSION

Shoulder instability presents in a multitude of ways and has many different variations. Our patients have similar variability in the presentation of these pathological conditions of the shoulder. It is highly desirable that surgeons have many different techniques available to modify the surgical procedures to meet the needs of a patient's pathology, expectations, and needs. The selective use of RI closure and posterior capsular plication can add considerably to our ability to tend to those factors.

REFERENCES

1. Provencher MT, Mologne TS, Hongo M, Zhao K, Tasto JP, An KN. Arthroscopic versus open rotator interval closure: biomechanical evaluation of stability and motion. *Arthroscopy.* 2007;23(6):583-592.
2. Provencher MT, Saldua NS. The rotator interval of the shoulder: anatomy, biomechanics, and repair techniques. *Oper Tech Orthop.* 2007;18:9-22.
3. Mologne TS, Zhao K, Hongo M, Romeo AA. The addition of rotator interval closure after arthroscopic repair of either anterior or posterior shoulder instability: effect on glenohumeral translation and range of motion. *Am J Sports Med.* 2008;36:1123-1131.
4. Harryman DT 2nd, Sidles JA, Harris SL, et al. The role of the rotator interval capsule in passive motion and stability of the shoulder. *J Bone Joint Surg Am.* 1992;74:53-66.
5. Plausinis D, Bravman JT, Heywood C, Kummer JF, Kwon YW, Jazrawi LM. Arthroscopic rotator interval closure: effect of sutures on glenohumeral motion and anterior-posterior translation. *Am J Sports Med.* 2006;34(10):1656-1661.

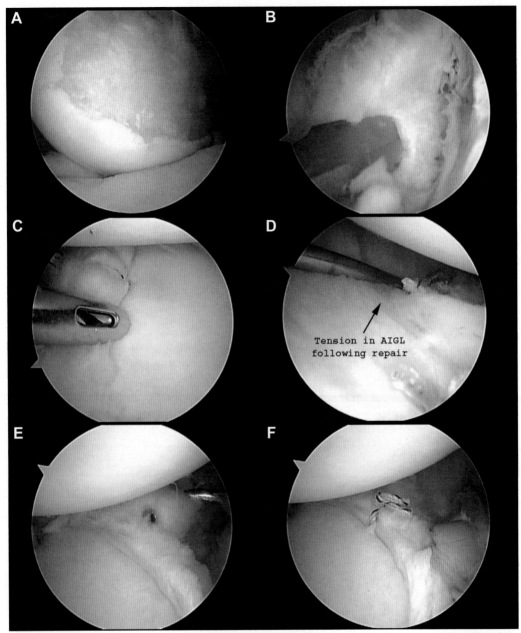

Figure 5-8. Posteroinferior plication is added to this patient along with a Bankart repair. (A, B) The magnitude of instability with a significant Hill-Sachs lesion as well as a Bankart tear. (C) Placement of a pilot hole for subsequent anchor placement. (D) Tension noted in the repaired anterior inferior glenohumeral ligament. (E) Suture hook placed from the posterior portal performing the plication of the posterior-inferior capsule as shown in F.

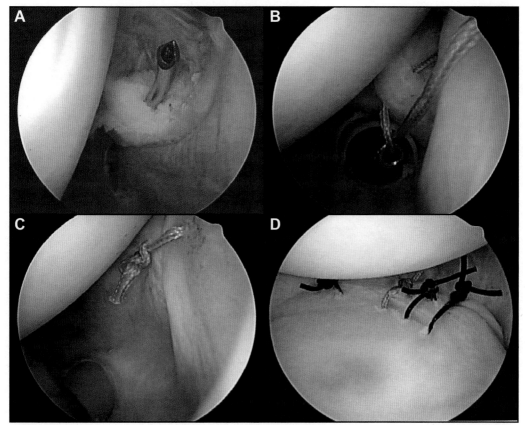

Figure 5-9. Case of recurrent instability leading to a partial articular sided tendon avulsion (PASTA lesion). (A through C) One technique of closure of a fairly shallow infraspinatus tear with 2 side-to-side sutures. (D) The pattern of repair of the instability that led to the PASTA lesion. Note the combination of absorbable and nonabsorbable suture material.

6. Yamamoto N, Itoi E, Tuoheti Y, et al. Effect of rotator interval closure on glenohumeral stability and motion: a cadaveric study. *J Shoulder Elbow Surg.* 2006;15(6):750-758.

7. Almazan A, Ruiz M, Cruz F, Perez FX, Ibarra C. Simple arthroscopic technique for rotator interval closure. *Arthroscopy.* 2006;22(2):230.e1-230.e4.

8. Wolf RS, Zheng N, Iero J, Weichel D. The effects of thermal capsulorrhaphy and rotator interval closure on multidirectional laxity in the glenohumeral joint: a cadaveric biomechanical study. *Arthroscopy.* 2004;20(10):1044-1049.

9. Shafer BL, Mihata T, McGarry MH, Tibone JE, Lee TQ. Effects of capsular plication and rotator interval closure in simulated multidirectional shoulder instability. *J Bone Joint Surg Am.* 2008;90:136-144.

10. Lewicky YM, Lewicky RT. Simplified arthroscopic rotator interval capsule closure: an alternative technique. *Arthroscopy.* 2005;21(10):1276.

11. Calvo A, Martinez AA, Domingo J, Herrera A. Rotator interval closure after arthroscopic capsulolabral repair: a technical variation. *Arthroscopy.* 2005;21(6):765.

12. Creighton RA, Romeo AA, Brown FM, Hayden JK, Verma NN. Revision arthroscopic shoulder instability repair. *Arthroscopy.* 2007;23(7):703-709.

13. Farber AJ, El Attrache NS, Tibone JE, McGarry MH, Lee TQ. Biomechanical analysis comparing a traditional superior-inferior arthroscopic rotator interval closure with a novel medial-lateral technique in a cadaveric multidirectional instability model. Am J Sports Med. 2009;37(6):1178-85.

6

Techniques to Repair the Multidirectionally Unstable Shoulder

Marcus S. Briones, MD; Michael J. Pagnani, MD;
William J. Mallon, MD; and John H. Flint, MD

Multidirectional instability (MDI) was first described by Neer and Foster in 1980.[1] They described 3 groups of patients: 1) anteroinferior dislocation with posterior subluxation, 2) posteroinferior dislocation with anterior subluxation, and 3) global dislocations. They also described the inferior capsular shift, the prototype open surgery used to stabilize such shoulders. It is likely that the entity was seen prior to 1980, but not classified as such.[2]

Neer and Foster considered the hallmark of MDI to be looseness of the inferior capsule.[1] The shoulder capsule is normally large, loose, and redundant to allow for the large range of shoulder motion. The capsule contains discrete capsular ligaments, which are important in understanding shoulder instability. There are 3 main ligaments in the anterior part of the shoulder that help prevent subluxation or dislocation. These ligaments are known as the superior glenohumeral ligament (SGHL), the middle glenohumeral ligament (MGHL), and the inferior glenohumeral ligament complex (IGHLC).

Damage or laxity in the IGHLC, which supports the bottom part of the shoulder capsule like a hammock, is related to most cases of anterior shoulder instability. Defects or injuries in the rotator interval area (which includes the SGHL and MGHL) usually contribute to inferior instability. Both the rotator interval and the posterior capsule are important in preventing posterior instability. Damage or insufficiency to one or both of these areas is usually present with a posterior component of instability.

Most patients with atraumatic MDI have a large inferior capsular pouch that extends both anteriorly and posteriorly. Anterior capsulolabral detachment is generally not associated with this type of capsular redundancy. In contrast, a traumatic type of MDI exists in which both capsular redundancy and a Bankart lesion of varying size may occur. This traumatic type of MDI occurs primarily in the athletic population.

Several studies have looked at muscular control and disturbances of the glenohumeral rhythm in patients with MDI. Kronberg et al[3] and Ozaki[4] studied patients with MDI and noted that the rhythm of scapular abduction was not synchronous during arm elevation. Patients with MDI have also been found to have biochemical abnormalities.

Abrams JS. *Management of the Unstable Shoulder:*
Arthroscopic and Open Repair (pp. 89-100).
© 2011 SLACK Incorporated

Figure 6-1. Examination of a patient with MDI, showing the sulcus sign beneath the lateral border of the acromion.

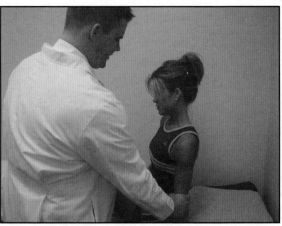

The Japanese have termed this *loose shoulder joint syndrome*, and Tsutsui and colleagues found there was no difference in collagen typing between the shoulder capsule in patients with MDI or normal shoulders, but patients with MDI had significantly reduced numbers of collagen cross-links compared with normal shoulders.[5] Belle and Hawkins also studied the collagen in patients with MDI and compared them to a healthy control group.[6] They also found no differences in collagen typing, but in their study, patients with MDI had a significant increase in the rate of collagen formation.

DIAGNOSIS AND TREATMENT

Shoulder laxity is not synonymous with instability; many individuals with "loose" shoulders function at a high level. It is the presence of recurrent symptoms due to increased laxity that separates patients with instability from those with laxity. It is important to obtain a careful history from the patient complaining of symptoms consistent with MDI. The inciting events and shoulder positions recreating subjective sensations of pain and instability are paramount to diagnosis and formulating a treatment plan. When patients complain of recurrent pain with subluxation or dislocation during sleep, this heralds significant decompensation of shoulder control that may not improve with conservative measures.

A thorough physical examination is also necessary to delineate the primary direction of instability. Shoulders with MDI by definition have increased laxity in multiple directions; however, the instability is likely to be worse in either the anterior or posterior direction. Anterior and posterior laxity are evaluated with load and shift testing as well as apprehension and relocation testing. The predominant direction of instability will guide the surgeon to stabilize the appropriate side of the capsule. A sulcus sign on examination indicates the presence of inferior laxity common to almost all cases of MDI (Figures 6-1 and 6-2). If the sulcus sign remains present with the arm at the side in 45 degrees of external rotation, this suggests a rotator interval deficiency that needs to be addressed operatively.[7,8]

Imaging studies need to be obtained for surgical planning. In most instances, plain radiographs are all that is necessary during the initial evaluation process. CT scans are valuable to further delineate glenoid morphology if plain films are insufficient. Magnetic resonance (MR) arthrograms can be helpful to assess intra-articular

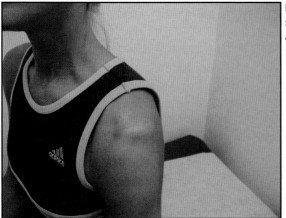

Figure 6-2. A close-up of the sulcus sign, showing the gap between the humeral head and the lateral acromion.

pathology, such as SLAP tears, Bankart lesions, or posterior labral pathology consistent with Kim's lesion.[9,10]

Treatment for MDI can be challenging. Many patients have a predisposition to increased joint laxity, and symptoms of instability can be difficult to treat in this setting; however, with MDI, many patients' chief complaint is pain and not instability. As opposed to traumatic unidirectional instability where pain and instability are experienced at the extremes of range of motion, the patient with MDI often experiences pain at the mid-range of motion. This is particularly disabling for patients because it negatively impacts normal daily activities. Treatment is focused on alleviating pain, reducing instability, and returning patients to their activities.

The mainstay of treatment for MDI is nonoperative and consists of patient education, activity modification, and an aggressive rehabilitation program. Increasing the strength of the dynamic shoulder stabilizing muscles leads to pain reduction and reduced instability. MDI patients should be counseled that the rehabilitation program could take up to 6 months to gain maximum stability and pain reduction, and a maintenance program needs to be continued thereafter. The success rate of therapy for returning patients pain-free to their activities has been reported as 83%.[11]

Surgical intervention is recommended for the patient who remains symptomatic despite compliance with a specific therapy program. Issues of voluntary control over dislocation should be specifically addressed during surgical decision making. The patient with psychological and emotional problems who purposefully dislocates is not a candidate for surgical stabilization until these issues are resolved.[2] Patients with underlying connective tissue disorders, such as Marfan syndrome and Ehlers-Danlos, may often fail a soft tissue reconstruction to reduce joint volume, as they will stretch it out.[12]

Several surgical procedures have been described, including arthroscopic capsular plication, open inferior capsular shift, and thermal capsulorrhaphy. Adding rotator interval closure during arthroscopic capsular plication is based on preoperative clinical examination findings and the predominant direction of instability being posteroinferior. Biomechanical models of arthroscopic closure of the rotator interval have indicated a significant risk of external rotation loss after closure of the interval. This technique should be used with caution in patients in whom restoration of external rotation is especially important for function, specifically the overhead athlete.[13,14] Regardless of the surgical method used, the goal is to symmetrically reduce the overall capsular volume and stabilize the shoulder.

OPEN STABILIZATION

The open capsular shift as originally described by Neer and Foster in 1980 remains the gold standard for surgical treatment of MDI.[1] Additional studies since Neer's paper describe satisfactory results after inferior capsular shift with good to excellent results ranging from 86% to 94%. Recurrence rates range from 4% to 10% with limited loss of motion.[15,16] Bigliani and colleagues' series of inferior capsular shift procedures in overhead athletes with predominantly anteroinferior instability revealed encouraging results.[17] Ninety-four percent of athletes reported good to excellent results, and 92% returned to sports, although only 75% did so at the same competitive level.[17] Several authors have described modifications to the original capsular shift procedure, but the overall goal of capsular imbrication to reduce redundancy and restore capsule-ligamentous tension is common to all.[18,19]

Author's Preferred Open Stabilization Technique

The patient is carefully examined under anesthesia to determine the magnitude and direction of laxity. The patient is placed in the beach chair position, and the arm is draped free. A deltopectoral approach is used. Subcutaneous flaps are mobilized, and the delto-pectoral interval is developed, taking the cephalic vein and deltoid laterally. The subscapularis and the adherent anterior capsule is exposed after dividing the clavipectoral fascia. The subscapularis is then divided either by a vertical release laterally, leaving a cuff of tissue to repair later, or a transverse muscle-splitting approach to the capsule. The subscapularis is divided or peeled from the capsule while leaving the capsule attached at its insertions at the humerus and glenoid. This requires patient and careful dissection to identify and follow the plane of transition from the tendinous subscapularis to the capsular tissue. The capsule is then released from lateral with a vertical incision off of bone, followed by a lateral to medial horizontal incision creating a T-type incision. After release and division of the 2 limbs, the inferior capsule limb is fully mobilized to its posteroinferior border to allow maximum excursion of the limb and freedom to tension the inferior limb as clinically needed. The inferior capsular limb is then taken superiorly as much as clinically needed to decrease the volume in the axillary pouch and attached to the subscapularis stump laterally or with a suture anchor if desired. The superior limb of the capsule is then brought inferiorly and likewise attached to the stump of the subscapularis tendon or via a suture anchor. This effectively decreases capsular volume, provides a double capsular layer in the anterior capsule, tightens up the IGHLC, and reduces the redundancy found in the posterior capsule. One must attend to the position of the arm when shifting the flaps so as to not over-tighten the shoulder. The arm should be held in slight flexion and 10 degrees of external rotation. Others have recommended more abduction and more external rotation, especially in overhead athletes or throwers. The subscapularis tendon is then repaired back to its stump laterally. Standard closure of the delto-pectoral interval and skin is performed (see Chapter 6 video).

ARTHROSCOPIC STABILIZATION

There has been increasing interest in arthroscopic stabilization procedures for MDI in recent years. Multiple techniques have evolved over time in an effort to treat this difficult problem. Current arthroscopic techniques emphasize capsular plication with or without a rotator interval closure.

The advantages of arthroscopic capsular plication are improved intra-articular diagnostic visualization and less perioperative morbidity. Several studies looking specifically at arthroscopic treatment of MDI exist. The findings are encouraging, with results that are comparable to open techniques. McIntyre et al[20] and Treacy et al[21] both describe an older technique with a trans-glenoid approach for capsular plication with 95% and 88% satisfactory results, respectively, with recurrent instability in the other 5% and 12%. Gartsman and colleagues prospectively evaluated 47 patients treated with arthroscopic capsular plication and rotator interval closure in select patients.[22] Ninety-four percent of patients obtained good to excellent results, with 85% returning to sports at their desired level. Kim and coworkers stressed the importance of evaluating and recognizing hidden posterior labral pathology in the patient with symptomatic posteroinferior MDI.[9] When posterior labral lesions were identified in the setting of MDI, they were successfully stabilized with arthroscopic labral repair, capsulolabroplasty consisting of posteroinferior labroplasty, superior shift of the posteroinferior and anteroinferior capsule, and rotator interval closure. Alpert and colleagues[23] analyzed the results of arthroscopic treatment of MDI with concomitant frank labral tear in 13 patients. A 270-degree labral repair and capsulorrhaphy was performed in all patients and rotator interval closure in select cases. Good to excellent results were obtained in 85%, with 2 patients experiencing recurrent dislocation. Overall, the short- to mid-term results of arthroscopically stabilized MDI appear to approach and even match open repair results.

Electrothermal arthroscopic shoulder capsulorrhaphy has fallen out of favor in recent years. There was initial enthusiasm for its application in MDI by reducing capsular volume through denaturing and shrinking the collagen triple helix through heat application. Several studies looking at 2- to 5-year follow-up showed a high failure rate with this technique.[11,24] Hawkins and colleagues showed a nearly 60% failure rate for electrothermal capsulorrhaphy in the MDI patient.[24] The current recommendation is to not use this modality alone. It may be used with caution to augment capsular interval repairs. One potential complication of this procedure is significant chondrolysis, resulting in an early osteoarthritic joint. If it is used to augment a repair, the period of immobilization needs to be increased prior to starting rehabilitation.

Author's Preferred Arthroscopic Surgical Technique

After the administration of anesthesia, examination under anesthesia (EUA) is performed in the supine position to determine the predominant direction and magnitude of laxity. The position for the procedure may be either lateral decubitus or beach chair, depending on the surgeon's preference. The senior author (WJM) prefers the beach chair position as this allows adequate visualization and the ability to address associated pathology, such as a rotator cuff tear. In this position, the arm can easily be held in 30 degrees of external rotation and 30 degrees of abduction during capsular plication to prevent over-tightening.

The shoulder joint is entered through a posterior portal, often slightly lateral to the standard posterior portal. Lateral portal placement allows better visualization of the posterior labrum and its pathology. An anteroinferior portal is placed at the superior edge of the subscapularis tendon in line with the joint using a spinal needle to guide placement. An additional anterosuperior portal may be placed through the rotator interval. This portal should be lateral and superior to the previously placed portal to avoid crowding during repair. An accessory posterior portal can be added either laterally or inferiorly to aid in anchor placement of suture shuttling.

Diagnostic arthroscopy is performed, and the joint is systematically examined. Associated pathology is addressed, such as débriding partial thickness rotator cuff tears and chondral lesions. The capsule and labrum are examined, taking note of all pathology. It is common to find a drive-through sign upon entering the joint, widening of the rotator interval, capsular redundancy, and associated anterior or posterior labral tears. The humeral head can be translated anteriorly, posteriorly, and inferiorly to assess the level of laxity.

The repair process is initiated by gently abrading the redundant capsule with a rasp or shaver on reverse to create a surface receptive to healing. Deficient areas of the labrum are identified and are elevated from the medial glenoid neck. If there are deficient areas of labrum present, this indicates that labral repair and capsular plication should be performed with the addition of suture anchors. Suture anchors should be positioned at the edge of the articular margin of the glenoid face, not on the neck of the glenoid. If the labrum is intact, the capsular plication can be performed without the use of anchors by placing the plication suture beneath the labrum into the adjacent edge of articular cartilage. We prefer to work beginning anteroinferiorly with plication in a superior direction to reduce the redundant inferior capsule. Plication is then performed posteriorly followed by rotator interval closure. The suture of choice is a #2 nonabsorbable suture.

The first plication suture is important for reducing inferior redundancy. Using a curved suture passing hook (Figures 6-3 and 6-4), the inferior capsule is penetrated at approximately the 6 o'clock position in the mid-portion of the valley created by the capsule below the glenoid. The capsular tissue is advanced superiorly to the 5:30 position and secured. The suture is cut prior to passing subsequent stitches. The next suture is placed in the capsule adjacent to the one prior and is advanced to the 4:30 position (Figures 6-5 and 6-6). Three to 4 sutures are placed in this manner until the capsule is imbricated to approximately the 2:30 position. A reduction in the anteroinferior capsular volume should be apparent, and the head of the humerus should be more centered on the glenoid.

The arthroscope is repositioned in the anterosuperior portal to visualize the posterior imbrication. The amount of plication necessary is based on the amount of posterior capsular redundancy, clinical laxity, and instability pattern. Starting inferiorly, the capsule is elevated and plicated until the capsular redundancy is decreased and the humeral head is centered. This may require 1 to 4 sutures depending on the amount of posterior instability present.

The rotator interval may be a substantial contributor to MDI, although there is some controversy concerning this. For this reason, the senior author performs a rotator interval closure on nearly all instability patients with the exception of high-level overhead athletes. The interval closure is performed by advancing the superior edge of the subscapularis tendon to the anterior edge of the supraspinatus tendon. The arm is held in 30 degrees of external rotation during interval closure. The suture is passed medial to the biceps sling to prevent entrapment of the biceps tendon. Passage through the subscapularis tendon is directly visualized from the posterior portal. A penetrating suture grasper is advanced through the anterosuperior portal into the supraspinatus, and the free end of the suture is shuttled through the supraspinatus. The suture is tied through the anterior portal while visualizing the amount of interval closure arthroscopically. The knot is not visualized and is tied down by feel. One suture is typically sufficient to adequately close the interval. Additional sutures can be added if needed, but care should be taken not to over-tighten the interval and restrict external rotation.

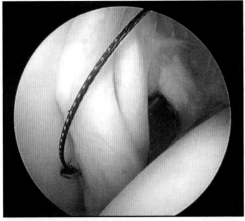

Figure 6-3. A shuttle relay suture bringing the anteroinferior glenohumeral pouch up to an intact labrum.

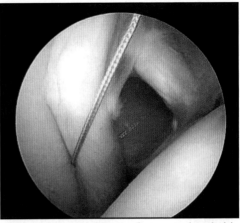

Figure 6-4. Shuttling of a nonabsorbable #2 suture through the anteroinferior glenohumeral pouch and intact labrum.

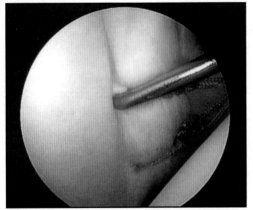

Figure 6-5. After tying 2 sutures to the labrum to tighten the anteroinferior glenohumeral pouch, checking the tightness of the construct with a probe.

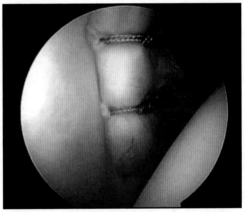

Figure 6-6. The final appearance of 2 sutures imbricating the anteroinferior glenohumeral pouch to the anteroinferior labrum.

TIPS AND PEARLS—ARTHROSCOPIC AND OPEN ANTERIOR INSTABILITY REPAIR

When surgical stabilization of an unstable shoulder is indicated and can be performed arthroscopically, patients can have excellent outcomes and return to function. However, there are several critical tenets that must be considered and followed for the operation and postoperative rehabilitation to be successful. These include adequate history and physical examination, appropriate patient selection, patient positioning, EUA, portal placement, soft tissue mobilization, suture anchor placement, suture management, capsular plication and rotator interval closure, avoiding neural damage during open repair, and diagnosis of other shoulder pathologies, such as concomitant rotator cuff tears, especially in patients older than 40 years.[25,26]

The most important tip/pearl regarding surgical stabilization of an unstable shoulder is the appropriate preoperative evaluation and diagnosis. The patient's pattern of instability must be identified, as this dictates the operative indication and plan. Arthroscopic findings can be correlated with the preoperative history and examination. Equally important is the postoperative rehabilitation protocol. The surgeon must be astute in judging the patient's ability to comply with the postoperative therapy protocol in offering the patient surgical stabilization.

Patient positioning is also critical to successful arthroscopic stabilization. Either the beach chair position or lateral decubitus position can be used. Arguments can be made for either position. Some surgeons feel that the lateral decubitus position is the preferred position due to increased ability to access the entire capsule and labrum, and it allows the opportunity to place a bolster in the axilla to increase access and visualization to the anteroinferior capsulolabrum complex.

Correctly placing portals is critical to success in arthroscopic stabilization. One must be able to access the inferior glenoid to appropriately place sutures and suture anchors. This can be accomplished by establishing portals using the outside-in technique and if necessary placing suture anchors percutaneously through the subscapularis tendon. The posterior portal must be placed so that the arthroscope can assume a position parallel to the glenoid surface.

Rotator interval closure should be used judiciously in the high-level overhead athlete. Excessive interval closure may limit external rotation for the patient, especially if more medial sutures are placed to close the interval.[27] Swimmers, pitchers, and volleyball and tennis players do not tolerate this loss of external rotation. Thus, in this patient population, conventional wisdom is that it is better to leave this group of athletes too loose rather than too tight.[27] During knot tying, placing the shoulder in 30 to 40 degrees of external rotation for nonthrowing athletes or patients and 60 to 70 degrees of external rotation and abduction for throwing or overhead athletes will prevent patients from being over-tightened by rotator interval closure.[27] Additionally, sutures should not be placed in the most medial aspect of the rotator interval to limit the risk of loss of external rotation.

During open capsular repair, the axillary nerve is at considerable risk given its close intimate relationship with and the need to mobilize the inferior capsule. Neural injury can be avoided by fully understanding the neural anatomy and the 3-dimensional relationships around the shoulder. Additionally, placing the arm in a flexed, adducted, and externally rotated position places the nerve at the lowest risk for injury. Nerve injury is rare in arthroscopic stabilization procedures.

MANAGING COMPLICATIONS— ARTHROSCOPIC AND OPEN

The first step in managing complications is to avoid them in the first place. However, they do occur, and it is important to determine the cause of failure. Recurrent instability is devastating for the patient after months of restrictions and rehabilitation. Causes for recurrent instability include failed initial repair of any Bankart lesions (eg, capsulolabral tissue not mobilized and lateralized sufficiently), excessive capsular laxity that was not addressed at the time of surgery, incorrect diagnosis of anterior instability when the patient had either posterior or multidirectional instability, and unrecognized and untreated humeral avulsion of the glenohumeral ligament lesions. Other complications unrelated to recurrent instability include superficial or deep infection, migration of or articular cartilage penetration by anchors, excessive tightness or loss of external rotation, and failure to diagnose and treat a rotator cuff tear.[26,28]

After the cause of failure has been correctly established by careful examination of the preoperative history and physical examination, imaging, surgical report, findings and photographs, and by ordering additional tests as warranted, the appropriate management plan can be put into action. If the patient is found to have excessive capsular laxity, then repeat capsulorrhaphy, either open or arthroscopically, can be performed with rotator interval closure if not performed previously. If anchors are found to have migrated or to have penetrated the articular surface, they must be removed.

Excessive tightness after arthroscopic stabilization for MDI is very rare. Appropriate rehabilitation and physical therapy will usually resolve this problem. In nonthrowing athletes, a slight loss of motion may be well tolerated and not require any further treatment. But if loss of motion is a problem and does not resolve with therapy, consideration should be given for either manipulation under anesthesia or arthroscopic lysis of adhesions. While manipulation under anesthesia works well for idiopathic adhesive capsulitis, postoperative stiffness usually requires an arthroscopic lysis of adhesions to fully resolve the problem.

POSTOPERATIVE MANAGEMENT

Although the debate over arthroscopic versus open repair of anterior shoulder instability continues, the healing time and return to full activity is no different, regardless of the technique, and patients must be equally compliant with postoperative restrictions.[29] However, the immediate postoperative course does differ between the 2 techniques. For the arthroscopic technique, the operation is typically done on an outpatient basis. The patient wears a sling in neutral rotation with a 10-degree abduction pillow continuously for 5 to 6 weeks after capsular plication. The patient is instructed to perform elbow, wrist, and hand range of motion exercises. The patient begins physical therapy after his or her first postoperative visit at 1 to 2 weeks, which includes pendulums, passive abduction in the plane of the scapula to 90 degrees, passive external rotation to 0 degrees with the shoulder adducted, and internal rotation to the chest.[30] Patients discontinue the sling at 5 to 6 weeks and begin active assisted range of motion exercises with the intention of having the patient achieve full motion at 3 months. Terminal passive stretching exercises are avoided in this patient population. Full range of motion is restored in nearly all patients without the use of stretching. Patients start strengthening exercises for the rotator cuff and scapular stabilizing muscles when full motion is obtained, typically at 8 to 10 weeks. Collision sports and manual labor are not allowed until 6 months postoperatively.

For open capsular repair of MDI, the postoperative regimen consists of immobilization of the affected extremity in a shoulder immobilizer with the arm in internal rotation for 4 weeks. The immobilizer may be removed to dress and shower but with rigid restrictions on avoiding external rotation past neutral. Elbow, wrist, and hand motions are encouraged multiple times a day. Immobilization is discontinued 4 weeks after surgery, and a passive shoulder stretching program is initiated. External rotation is limited to 30 degrees for 6 weeks after starting the stretching program, and forward elevation is limited to 160 degrees. During the third postoperative month, external rotation is increased to 60 degrees and elevation to 170 degrees. At 12 weeks after surgery, a strengthening program of the rotator cuff and deltoid muscles is instituted. During the next 6 weeks, periscapular muscles are added to the strengthening program. Patients are not allowed to return to collision sports or manual labor for 4 to 6 months.[29]

REFERENCES

1. Neer CS, Foster CR. Inferior capsular shift for involuntary inferior and multidirectional instability of the shoulder. *J Bone Joint Surg.* 1980;62:897-908.
2. Rowe CR, Pierce DS, Clark JG. Voluntary dislocation of the shoulder: a preliminary report on a clinical, electromyographic, and psychiatric study of twenty-six patients. *J Bone Joint Surg.* 1973;55-A:445-460.
3. Kronberg M, Broström L-Å, Németh G. Differences in shoulder muscle activity between patients with generalized joint laxity and normal control. *Clin Orthop.* 1990;257:76-85.
4. Ozaki J. Gleno-humeral movements of the involuntary inferior and multidirectional instability. *Clin Orthop.* 1989;238:107-111.
5. Tsutsui H, Yamamoto R, Kuroki Y, et al. Biochemical study on collagen from the loose shoulder joint capsules. In: Post M, Morrey BF, Hawkins RJ, eds. *Surgery of the Shoulder.* St. Louis, MO: Mosby; 1991:108-111.
6. Belle RM, Hawkins RJ. Collagen typing and production in multi-directional instability of the shoulder. *Orthop Trans.* 1991;15:188.
7. Levy AS, Lintner S, Kenter K, Speer KP. Intra- and interobserver reproducibility of the shoulder laxity examination. *Am J Sports Med.* 1999;27:460-463.
8. Linter SA, Levy AS, Kenter K, Speer KP. Gleno-humeral translation in the asymptomatic athlete's shoulder and its relationship to other clinically measurable anthropometric variables. *Am J Sports Med.* 1996;24:716-720.
9. Kim SH, Ha KI, Yoo JC, Noh KC. Kim's lesion: an incomplete and concealed avulsion of the posteroinferior labrum in posterior or multidirectional posteroinferior instability of the shoulder. *Arthroscopy.* 2004;20:712-720.
10. Kim SH, Kim HK, Sun JI, Park JS, Oh I. Arthroscopic capsulolabroplasty for posteroinferior multidirectional instability of the shoulder. *Am J Sports Med.* 2004;32:594-607.
11. Burkhead WZ, Rockwood CA. Treatment of instability of the shoulder with an exercise program. *J Bone Joint Surg.* 1992;74-A:890-896.
12. Jerosch J, Castro WHM. Shoulder instability in Ehlers-Danlos syndrome. An indication for surgical treatment? *Acta Orthop Belg.* 1990;56:451-453.
13. Mologne TS, Zhao K, Hongo M, Romeo AA, An K-N, Provencher MT. The addition of rotator interval closure after arthroscopic repair of either anterior or posterior shoulder instability: effect on gleno-humeral translation and range of motion. *Am J Sports Med.* 2008;36:1123-1131.
14. Plausinis D, Bravman JT, Heywood C, Kummer FJ, Kwon YW, Jazrawi LM. Arthroscopic rotator interval closure: effect of sutures on gleno-humeral motion and anterior-posterior translation. *Am J Sports Med.* 2006;34:1656-1661.
15. Cooper RA, Brems JJ. The inferior capsular-shift procedure for multidirectional instability of the shoulder. *J Bone Joint Surg.* 1992;74-A:1516-1521.
16. Pollock RG, Owens JM, Flatow EL, Bigliani LU. Operative results of the inferior capsular shift procedure for multidirectional instability of the shoulder. *J Bone Joint Surg.* 2000;82:919-928.
17. Bigliani LU, Kurzweil PR, Schwartzbach CC, Wolfe IN, Flatow EL. Inferior capsular shift procedure for anterior-inferior shoulder instability in athletes. *Am J Sports Med.* 1994;22:578-584.
18. Altchek DW, Warren RF, Skyhar MJ, Ortiz G. T-plasty modification of the Bankart procedure for multidirectional instability of the anterior and inferior types. *J Bone Joint Surg.* 1991;73-A:105-111.
19. Bak K, Spring BJ, Henderson JP. Inferior capsular shift procedure in athletes with multidirectional instability based on isolated capsular and ligamentous redundancy. *Am J Sports Med.* 2000;28:466-471.
20. McIntyre LF, Caspari RB, Savoie FH III. The arthroscopic treatment of multidirectional shoulder instability: two-year results of a multiple suture technique. *Arthroscopy.* 1997;13:418-425.
21. Treacy SH, Savoie FH III, Field LD. Arthroscopic treatment of multidirectional instability. *J Shoulder Elbow Surg.* 1998;8:345-350.
22. Gartsman GM, Roddey TS, Hammerman SM. Arthroscopic treatment of multidirectional gleno-humeral instability: 2- to 5-year follow-up. *Arthroscopy.* 2001;17:236-243.
23. Alpert JM, Verma N, Wysocki R, Yanke AB, Romeo AA. Arthroscopic treatment of multidirectional shoulder instability with minimum 270-degree labral repair: minimum 2-year follow-up. *Arthroscopy.* 2008;24:704-711.
24. Hawkins RJ, Krishnan SG, Karas SG, Noonan TJ, Horan MP. Electrothermal arthroscopic shoulder capsulorrhaphy: a minimum 2-year follow-up. *Am J Sports Med.* 2007;35:1484-1488.

25. Carter C, Ahmad CS, Levine WN. Arthroscopic anterior instability repair: technical pearls, pitfalls, and complications. In: Duwelius PJ, ed. *Instructional Course Lectures.* Rosemont, IL: American Academy of Orthopaedic Surgeons; 2008:773.
26. Neviaser RJ, Neviaser TJ, Neviaser JS. Concurrent rupture of the rotator cuff and anterior dislocation of the shoulder in the older patient. *J Bone Joint Surg Am.* 1988;70(9):1308-1311.
27. Conway JE. Arthroscopic rotator interval repair and placation in the management of shoulder instability. In: Zuckerman JD, ed. *Advanced Reconstruction Shoulder.* Rosemont, IL: American Academy of Orthopaedic Surgeons; 2007:21-27.
28. Rhee YG, Lee DH, Chun IH, Bae SC. Gleno-humeral arthropathy after arthroscopic anterior shoulder stabilization. *Arthroscopy.* 2004;20(4):402-406.
29. Brems JJ. Open capsular repair for anterior instability. In: Zuckerman JD, ed. *Advanced Reconstruction Shoulder.* Rosemont, IL: American Academy of Orthopaedic Surgeons; 2007:47-56.
30. Rokito AS, Khajavi K. Arthroscopic anterior shoulder repair. In: Zuckerman JD, ed. *Advanced Reconstruction Shoulder.* Rosemont, IL: American Academy of Orthopaedic Surgeons; 2007:3-9.

SUGGESTED READING

Arciero RAS, Jeffrey T. Complications in arthroscopic shoulder stabilization: pearls and pitfalls. In: Duwelius PJ, ed. *Instructional Course Lectures.* Rosemont, IL: American Academy of Orthopaedic Surgeons; 2008:773.

Basmajian JV, Bazant FJ. Factors preventing downward dislocation of the adducted shoulder joint. *J Bone Joint Surg.* 1959;41-A:1182-1186.

Bigliani LU, Newton PM, Steinmann SP, Connor PM, McLlveen SJ. Glenoid rim lesions associated with recurrent anterior dislocation of the shoulder. *Am J Sports Med.* 1998;26(1):41-45.

Boileau P, Villalba M, Hery JY, Balg F, Ahrens P, Neyton L. Risk factors for recurrence of shoulder instability after arthroscopic Bankart repair. *J Bone Joint Surg Am.* 2006;88(8):1755-1763.

Burkhart SS, De Beer JF. Traumatic gleno-humeral bone defects and their relationship to failure of arthroscopic Bankart repairs: significance of the inverted-pear glenoid and the humeral engaging Hill-Sachs lesion. *Arthroscopy.* 2000;16(7):677-694.

D'Alessandro DF, Bradley JP, Fleischli JE, Connor PM. Prospective evaluation of thermal capsulorrhaphy for shoulder instability: indications and results, two to five year follow-up. *Am J Sports Med.* 2004;32:21-33.

Kaar TK, Schenck RC Jr, Wirth MA, Rockwood CA Jr. Complications of metallic suture anchors in shoulder surgery: a report of 8 cases. *Arthroscopy.* 2001;17(1):31-37.

O'Brien SJ, Neves M, Arnowski S, Warren RF. The anatomy and histology of the inferior gleno-humeral ligament complex of the shoulder. *Am J Sports Med.* 1990;18:449-456.

Pagnani MJ, Warren RF. Stabilizers of the gleno-humeral joint. *J Shoulder Elbow Surg.* 1994;3:173-190.

Rook RT, Savoie FH, Field LD. Arthroscopic treatment of instability attributable to capsular injury or laxity. *Clin Orthop.* 2001;390:52-58.

Tauber M, Resch H, Forstner R, Raffl M, Schauer J. Reasons for failure after surgical repair of anterior shoulder instability. *J Shoulder Elbow Surg.* 2004;13(3):279-285.

> **Please see video on the accompanying Web site at**
> **http://www.slackbooks.com/unstableshouldervideos**

Posterior Shoulder Instability
Recognition and Arthroscopic Treatment

Richard L. Angelo, MD

Posterior shoulder instability may be responsible for significant disability. The symptoms related to posterior instability tend to be less specific and physical examination tests less sensitive than those related to anterior instability. In addition, when compared to anterior instability, a much greater range of asymptomatic translational laxity exists in the posterior direction, often making the accurate use of the term *posterior instability* elusive. The absence of an identified "essential lesion" has often contributed to ill-conceived or incomplete surgical solutions. Relatively high rates of failure and complications have been reported with the various open methods previously described.[1] During the past decade, the evolution in the arthroscopic management of posterior shoulder instability has led to successful outcomes comparable to open procedures with substantially less morbidity.[2-4]

PATHOANATOMY

A thickening of the capsule, the posterior band of the inferior glenohumeral ligament, is the most effective structure for providing stability in flexion, internal rotation, and adduction,[5] the jeopardy position for posterior shoulder instability. The posterior labrum, which has been shown to contribute approximately 20% of the concavity-compression component of stabilization for the glenohumeral joint in the posteroinferior direction,[6] may become circumferentially fissured, abraded, or deformed in the unstable shoulder. A reverse Bankart, or frank posterior labral detachment[7] from the glenoid neck, is often the result of a specific traumatic episode. Occasionally, a loss of labral height and deep labral fissure adjacent to the articular cartilage serve as the only hint that a more substantial, hidden underlying Bankart (Kim's lesion) is present.[5,8]

A patulous or redundant posterior capsule[9,10] and associated incompetent glenohumeral ligament are often the primary pathology responsible for posterior shoulder instability. An excessively lax capsule may be physiologic for a particular individual

Abrams JS. *Management of the Unstable Shoulder: Arthroscopic and Open Repair* (pp. 101-110).

or may be secondary to plastic deformation[11,12] due to repetitive microtrauma. Occasionally, an actual midsubstance tear or rent in the capsule may occur following a traumatic event. Rarely, an avulsion of the glenohumeral ligaments from the humeral neck is responsible for posterior instability.

In the past, correction of a "deficiency" of the rotator interval was believed to be a key component of successfully treating posterior instability, particularly when a frank posterior capsulolabral detachment from the glenoid was not present. Recent biomechanical research has shed doubt on this concept with cadaveric studies demonstrating no significant impact on posterior translation with current methods of arthroscopic rotator interval plication.[13,14]

PATIENT SELECTION

In selecting appropriate patients with posterior instability for surgical treatment, 3 criteria must be met: pain and dysfunction is disabling, the pathology responsible must be identified as clearly as possible, and the proposed surgical treatment must have an acceptable success rate for meeting the patient's expected or anticipated shoulder demands. Laxity is the magnitude of glenohumeral translation in a particular direction and, even if greater than the population norm, may or may not be symptomatic. Posterior instability is defined as symptomatic and/or dysfunctional glenohumeral translation in the posterior or posteroinferior direction. Many patients are diagnosed with MDI when unidirectional "instability" with multidirectional "laxity" may be a more accurate term. Regardless, it is essential that all of the pathology responsible for posterior instability be recognized and appropriately addressed.

History

Injury to the posterior shoulder can occur from an acute traumatic event or can be due to repetitive posterior stress. Traumatic posteroinferior instability typically occurs with the shoulder in a position of flexion, adduction, and internal rotation (ie, an offensive football lineman with his arms in the blocking position). Overhead sports can predispose the shoulder to posterior subluxation (ie, the follow-through phase of throwing, the backhand stroke for racquet sports, and the pull-through phase of swimming), but the symptoms may be more gradual in onset. Pain is variable and is often poorly localized. Weakness or intermittent mechanical symptoms are sometimes present. A sensation of the shoulder "slipping out" is occasionally noted, but apprehension is rare. The patient who is very willing to demonstrate his or her posterior laxity should make the clinician concerned that symptoms may not be great enough to warrant surgical treatment.[1,15,16]

PHYSICAL EXAMINATION

Several tests are useful when examining the shoulder for posterior instability. A positive jerk test is often the most reliable sign, but by itself is not diagnostic, as it may be present in both shoulders. After stabilizing the scapula, the humerus is flexed, adducted, and axially loaded to produce a posterior glenohumeral subluxation. As the patient's shoulder is then slowly extended in the horizontal plane, a palpable clunk or jerk is appreciated as the humeral head reduces.

The load and shift test is employed to determine the magnitude of posterior gleno-humeral translation.[17] Up to 50% displacement of the humeral head up onto the glenoid rim is considered the upper limit of normal. It is not unusual to find symmetrical posterior translation despite only one shoulder being symptomatic.[18] The humeral head is loaded with a direct lateral force to center it in the glenoid. A posteriorly directed force is then applied, and a determination of the extent of subluxation made. A sensation of pain and/or a click during the maneuver may be elicited. The Kim's test is a specific variant wherein the shoulder is flexed to approximately 160 degrees and an attempt made to generate a posteroinferior subluxation.[19] The test is considered positive if pain accompanies the posteroinferior subluxation and indicates a poor prognosis for nonoperative treatment.[20]

A diagnosis of posterior predominant multidirectional instability is supported by pain on posterior translation, global glenohumeral laxity, and a positive sulcus sign. Other tests of ligamentous laxity, such as recurvatum of the knee and elbow, hyperextensibility of the thumb and finger at the metacarpophalangeal joint, and hypermobility of the patella, are also often present.

Imaging

An MRI scan provides the best noninvasive study of the posterior soft tissues of the shoulder. The accuracy in identifying subtle posterior labral pathology is improved with the addition of gadolinium contrast dye. Excessive retroversion, hypoplasia, and rim fractures are evaluated best with a CT. Glenoid retroversion in excess of 10 degrees will likely necessitate consideration of a posterior glenoid osteotomy.[21,22]

SURGICAL TECHNIQUES

Efforts to rehabilitate the shoulder with posterior instability have included infraspinatus, teres minor, periscapular, and deltoid strengthening exercises along with biofeedback and activity modification and are successful in 65% to 80% of cases.[15,22,23] Only when those measures fail and the patient remains significantly symptomatic does surgical treatment become an option.

In the absence of an "essential lesion" responsible for posterior shoulder instability, each component of the pathology that may contribute to the abnormal posterior glenohumeral translation must be corrected. Three regions of the posterior shoulder must be evaluated and, if pathologic, addressed. First, if a reverse Bankart lesion is present, the capsulolabral tissue must be secured back to the glenoid rim.[24,25] Second, appropriate tension must be restored to the posterior capsule if lax or attenuated.[26] Third, if the capsule is detached from the humeral neck, it must be reduced and fixed securely back to its anatomic insertion.[27]

Diagnostic Arthroscopy

Shoulder arthroscopy with the patient in the lateral decubitus position offers somewhat easier access to the posterior pathology, although some surgeons prefer to have the patient in the seated or beach chair orientation. The posterior portal is adjusted 1 cm further lateral than the standard portal to permit the proper 45-degree angle approach to the posterior glenoid rim with drill bits and anchors (Figure 7-1). In addition, it should be placed as superior as possible, approximately 5-mm inferior to the posterolateral acromion. The conical blunt tip of the arthroscopic sheath trocar

Figure 7-1. Posterior view of a right shoulder in the lateral decubitus orientation. The posterior (Post) portal is adjusted 1 cm further lateral than the routine posterior portal. The posteroinferior (Post-Inf) portal is 2-cm inferior and 1-cm lateral to the posterior portal.

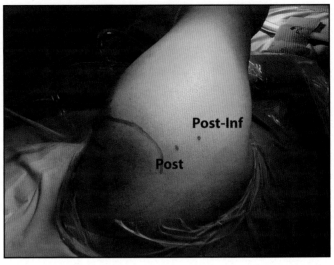

facilitates a superior and lateral entry through the capsule. Next, a mid-anterior portal is created with an obturated cannula introduced 1.5 cm lateral and 1.5 cm inferior to the inferolateral tip of the coracoid and enters the joint just superior to the subscapularis tendon. An anterosuperior portal is established 1 cm lateral and slightly anterior to the anterolateral corner of the acromion and enters the joint immediately anterior to the supraspinatus and posterior to the biceps tendon. This portal path is created with a switching stick. A second switching stick is introduced into the posterior portal, and the arthroscopic sheath is removed and reinserted over the anterosuperior rod. An obturated cannula is then placed at the posterior portal using a metal introducer. When access to the axillary recess is necessary, an accessory posteroinferior portal can be created. Under direct vision with the arthroscope in the anterosuperior portal, a spinal needle and subsequent cannula are introduced 2 cm inferior and 1 cm further lateral to the modified posterior portal described above (see Figure 7-1).[28]

A thorough diagnostic survey is conducted from both the posterior and then anterosuperior portals. A careful evaluation of the entire labrum, the posterior and anterior capsule including its insertion onto the humeral neck, the corresponding glenohumeral ligaments, and the articular surfaces of the glenoid and humeral head is performed.

Posterior Bankart Repair (See Chapter 7 Video)

When the capsulolabral tissues are detached posteriorly (Figure 7-2), they must be secured back to the glenoid rim. A suture anchor technique is preferred when a frank posterior Bankart lesion is present. While viewing from the anterosuperior portal, a full-radius synovial resector is introduced through the posterior portal, and the labrum and marginal articular cartilage are débrided of any ragged or unstable tissue. Using a liberator elevator, the scar tissue tethering the capsulolabral tissue is released at least to the 6 o'clock position, exposing the underlying infraspinatus muscle. A drill is introduced to create a hole at the 7 o'clock position, 2 to 3 mm onto the articular surface of the glenoid. The corresponding anchor is inserted and tested for security (Figure 7-3). The sutures are then retrieved out the anterior cannula. A cannulated suture hook is introduced through the posterior portal and enters the capsulolabral tissue 1 cm inferior and 1 cm lateral to the anchor site so as to superiorly advance and medially plicate the posterior capsule. A #1 monofilament suture is delivered through the suture hook and retrieved out the mid-anterior cannula. A shuttle is created by tying a simple overhand throw in the monofilament suture around the inferior limb of

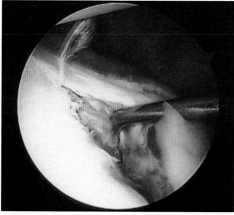

Figure 7-2. Right shoulder in the lateral decubitus orientation. Arthroscopic view (30 degrees) from the anterosuperior portal; hook probe at site of a posterior Bankart lesion.

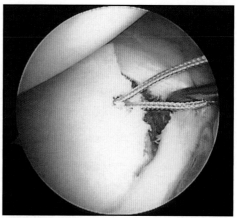

Figure 7-3. Right shoulder in the lateral decubitus orientation. A suture anchor has been implanted along the posterior glenoid rim, 2 mm onto the articular surface.

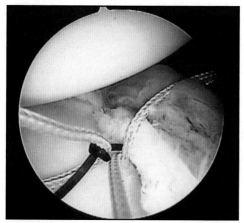

Figure 7-4. Right shoulder in the lateral decubitus orientation. One limb of the anchor suture is being shuttled from anterior to posterior through the capsulolabral tissue with a monofilament suture that had been passed previously.

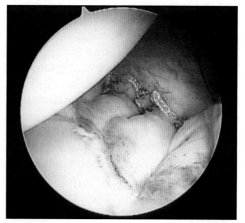

Figure 7-5. Right shoulder in the lateral decubitus orientation. Completed suture anchor posterior Bankart repair with secure refixation of the capsulolabral tissue to the posterior glenoid rim.

the braided anchor suture, which exits the mid-anterior portal. Traction is applied to the limb of monofilament suture exiting the posterior cannula to deliver the inferior limb of braided suture from anterior to posterior through the capsulolabral tissue (Figure 7-4). This becomes the post limb for the sliding knot of choice, which is backed up with 3 or 4 half hitches. Many other devices and methods of suture delivery are available, but the placement of the sutures in the capsule should remain the same. Additional anchors are placed at 8:30 and 10 o'clock on the posterior glenoid, and the sutures are delivered as described above (Figure 7-5).

Posterior Capsular Plication (See Chapter 7 Video)

When posterior capsular laxity is present along with a substantially intact labrum, a posterior capsular plication is undertaken. If a disrupted/deficient labrum is detected, suture anchors will be necessary. A superior shift of the capsule at the time of the medial-lateral plication is also performed.

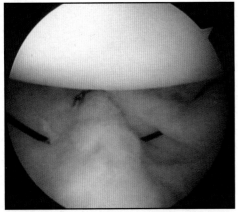

Figure 7-6. A monofilament suture has been passed in a "pinch-tuck" configuration to create a capsular plication when the suture is tied.

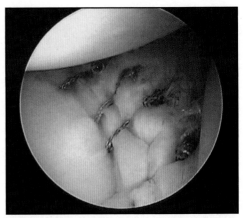

Figure 7-7. Completed posterior capsular plication with creation of a "pseudolabrum." The durability of this "bumper" effect is uncertain.

While viewing from the anterosuperior portal, a rasp or full-radius shaver with the suction turned off is introduced through one of the posterior portals to excoriate the posterior and inferior capsule and adjacent labrum to stimulate a healing response. Care must be exercised to avoid creating rents in the thin capsular tissue. A 45-degree cannulated suture hook is introduced through a posterior portal to create a "pinch-tuck" plication of the capsule. Beginning at the 6 o'clock position, the hook tip is used to penetrate the capsule approximately 12-mm lateral to the labral rim. It is then passed parallel to the capsule to avoid encircling tissue subjacent to the capsule, especially the axillary nerve, and then exits the capsule 7 mm from the glenoid rim. The hook tip is then brought toward the glenoid and passed beneath the annular fibers of the entire labrum to exit adjacent to the articular surface. A #1 PDS suture is delivered and retrieved out the mid-anterior cannula (Figure 7-6). A #2 permanent braided suture is shuttled back through and out the posterior cannula, but the PDS may be employed as the definitive suture. The posterior limb, which exits the capsule laterally, is identified as the post, and a sliding knot is delivered and backed up with 3.5 hitches. As the knot is tightened, it will advance the tissue superiorly as well as create a pseudolabrum, increasing the glenoid concavity (Figure 7-7). A total of 3 to 5 sutures are placed in a similar manner. A hook probe is then used to verify the security of the suture loops and restoration of appropriate capsular tension.

Repair of Posterior Humeral Avulsion of the Glenohumeral Ligaments (See Chapter 7 Video)

The arthroscope is maintained in the anterosuperior portal. Although the 30-degree lens generally provides an adequate view (Figure 7-8), the 70-degree scope is occasionally helpful. The repair is begun by introducing a burr through the posterior portal and lightly excoriating the posterior humeral neck (Figure 7-9). A double-loaded suture anchor appropriate for the cancellous bone of the humeral head is selected, and, if nonmetallic, a hole is punched and tapped. Generally, 2 anchors along the humeral neck are sufficient, and spacing is planned accordingly. Once the anchor is implanted and security tested, the inserter is partially withdrawn and then used to "hand-off" all sutures to a loop grasper, which has been introduced through the anterior portal. Numerous methods exist for delivering sutures through the capsular margin. A loop grasper is used to select the most inferior limb of anchor suture and position it near the capsular margin for ease of grasping. With the capsule reduced with the previously placed superior traction suture, a sharp-tipped penetrator/retriever is introduced through the

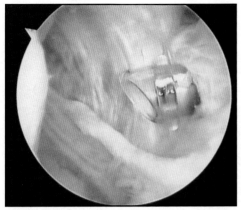

Figure 7-8. Humeral avulsion of the posterior glenohumeral ligaments with exposed infraspinatus muscle. Cannula is posterior and lateral to the free capsular margin.

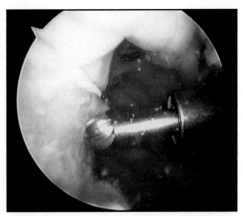

Figure 7-9. Burr introduced through the posterior portal and used to lightly excoriate the posterior humeral neck.

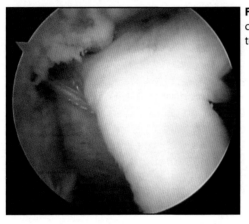

Figure 7-10. Anchor sutures after passage through the capsule; when tension is applied, the capsule is reduced to the posterior humeral neck.

capsule and used to grasp the previously positioned inferior anchor suture. The suture is retrieved in retrograde fashion through the capsule. The remaining anchor limbs are delivered in a similar manner either as 2 horizontal mattresses or as 1 mattress with a simple overlocking suture. In the latter case, it is easiest to work from inferior to superior and pass one mattress limb followed by the simple limb 3 mm to 4 mm more superior and slightly more medial followed by the second mattress limb.

Once all of the sutures are passed, the posterior cannula is removed and reinserted to place the passed sutures outside the cannula. The steps are repeated for the more superior anchor. Once all of the sutures are placed, matched pairs are tied from the posterior approach. As the sutures are tied and the repair progresses superiorly (Figure 7-10), it becomes somewhat more difficult as the posterior cannula becomes "extra-articular." For the final posterosuperior closure, the arthroscope is changed to the mid-anterior portal. From the posterior skin opening, a penetrator loaded with the end of either a #2 permanent braided or a resorbable monofilament suture penetrates the capsule in antegrade fashion. The delivered suture is retrieved out the anterosuperior cannula. The second limb of the free suture is also passed through the same skin opening and through the capsule on the opposite side of the remaining defect and again retrieved. The repair is completed by tying the sutures intra-articularly via the anterosuperior portal.

TIPS AND PEARLS

- Suture anchors must be placed onto the glenoid rim for 2 to 3 mm to obtain an intact posterior wall and prevent anchor suture cut-out.

- Once the suture-delivery device has penetrated the capsule, superior tension is applied to verify that the suture hook remains inferior to the anchor site and will effectively advance the capsule superiorly.

- As plication sutures progress superiorly, care must be taken to avoid increasing the magnitude of the plication with each suture, which can overconstrain the joint.

- During repair of the capsule from the humeral neck, avoid excessive traction on the arm during placement of sutures to prevent inadequate capsular tension once traction is released.

- On completion of the repair, the arm should be removed from suspension and tested for adequate range of motion and acceptable restoration of stability.

POSTOPERATIVE REHABILITATION

The shoulder is immobilized in a sling and loose swath for 4 weeks, during which time rotator cuff and periscapular isometrics are performed. Patients are permitted to use the affected extremity out in front of the body from the waist to the face for light activities. At 4 weeks, gentle passive range of motion exercises are begun, avoiding internal rotation. Full motion is expected at 12 weeks with the exception of internal rotation. Postoperatively, active and passive internal rotation is avoided and just allowed to gradually return unless significant restriction is present at 10 weeks, at which time gentle passive motion efforts are initiated. At 10 to 12 weeks, progressive resistive cuff, periscapular, and deltoid strengthening is begun. Return to sport activities is permitted at 6 months provided shoulder strength is sufficient.

CONCLUSION

The management of posterior shoulder instability remains challenging. Arthroscopic treatment methods are clearly less morbid than open approaches. The early results of a posterior Bankart repair, capsulolabral plication, and repair of a capsular avulsion from the posterior humeral neck appear promising and suggest that a success rate similar to or better than available open procedures is achievable. Refinements in the arthroscopic techniques, instrumentation, and implants will undoubtedly further improve patient outcomes.

REFERENCES

1. Hawkins RJ, Koppert G, Johnston G. Recurrent posterior instability (subluxation) of the shoulder. *J Bone Joint Surg Am.* 1984;66:169-174.
2. Magit DP, Tibone JE, Lee TQ. In vivo comparison of changes in glenohumeral translation after arthroscopic capsulolabral reconstruction. *Am J Sports Med.* 2008;36:1389-1396.

3. Savoie FH 3rd, Holt MS, Field LD, Ramsey JR. Arthroscopic management of posterior instability: evolution of technique and results. *Arthroscopy.* 2008;24:389-396.

4. Kakar S, Voloshin I, Kaye EK, et al. Posterior shoulder instability: comprehensive analysis of open and arthroscopic approaches. *Am J Orthop.* 2007;36:655-659.

5. O'Brien SJ, Schwartz RS, Warren RF, et al. Capsular restraints to anterior-posterior motion of the abducted shoulder: a biomechanical study. *J Bone Joint Surg Am.* 1995;4:298-308.

6. Lippitt SB, Vanderhooft E, Harris SL, et al. Glenohumeral stability from concavity-compression: a quantitative analysis. *J Shoulder and Elbow Surg.* 1993;2:27-35.

7. Mair SD, Zarzour R, Speer KP. Posterior labral injury in contact athletes. *Am J Sports Med.* 1998;26:753-758.

8. Kim SH, Ha KI, Yoo JC, Noh KC. Kim's lesion: an incomplete and concealed avulsion of the posteroinferior labrum in posterior or multidirectional posteroinferior instability of the shoulder. *Arthroscopy.* 2004;20:712-720.

9. Fronek J, Warren RF, Bowen M. Posterior subluxation of the glenohumeral joint. *J Bone Joint Surg Am.* 1989;71:205-216.

10. Rockwood CA Jr, Matsen FA. Glenohumeral instability. In: Rockwood CA Jr, Matsen FA, eds. *The Shoulder.* Philadelphia, PA: WB Saunders; 1990:526-622.

11. Pagnani MJ, Warren RF. Stabilizers of the glenohumeral joint. *J Shoulder Elbow Surg.* 1994;3:173-190.

12. Weber SC, Caspari RB. A biomechanical evaluation of the restraints to posterior shoulder dislocation. *Arthroscopy.* 1989;5:115-121.

13. Provencher MT, Dewing CB, Bell SJ, et al. An analysis of the rotator interval in patients with anterior, posterior and multidirectional shoulder instability. *Arthroscopy.* 2008;24:921-929.

14. Mologne TS, Zhao K, Hongo M, et al. The addition of rotator interval closure after arthroscopic repair of either anterior or posterior shoulder instability: effect on glenohumeral translation and range of motion. *Am J Sports Med.* 2008;36:1123-1131.

15. Burkhead WZ Jr, Rockwood CA Jr. Treatment of instability of the shoulder with an exercise program. *J Bone Joint Surg Am.* 1992;74:890-896.

16. Rowe CR, Pierce DS, Clarke JG. Voluntary dislocation of the shoulder. A preliminary report on a clinical, electromyographic, and psychiatric study of twenty six patients. *J Bone Joint Surg Am.* 1973;55:455-460.

17. Yoldas EA, Faber KJ, Hawkins RJ. Translation of the glenohumeral joint in patients with multidirectional and posterior instability: awake examination versus examination under anesthesia. *J Shoulder Elbow Surg.* 2001;10:416-420.

18. Williams RJ III, Strickland S, Cohen M, et al. Arthroscopic repair for traumatic posterior shoulder instability. *Am J Sports Med.* 2003;31:203-209.

19. Kim SH, Park JS, Jeong WK, Shin SK. The Kim test: a novel test for posteroinferior labral lesion of the shoulder—a comparison to the jerk test. *Am J Sports Med.* 2005;33:1188-1192.

20. Kim SH, Park JC, Park JS, Oh I. Painful jerk test: a predictor of success in nonoperative treatment of posteroinferior instability of the shoulder. *Am J Sports Med.* 2004;32:1849-1855.

21. Fuchs B, Jost B, Gerber C. Posterior-inferior capsular shift for the treatment of recurrent, voluntary posterior subluxation of the shoulder. *J Bone Joint Surg Am.* 2000;82:16-25.

22. Hurley JA, Anderson TE, Dear W, et al. Posterior shoulder instability. Surgical versus conservative results with evaluation of glenoid version. *Am J Sports Med.* 1992;20:396-400.

23. Beall MS Jr, Diefenbach G, Allen A. Electromyographic biofeedback in the treatment of voluntary posterior instability of the shoulder. *Am J Sports Med.* 1987;15:175-178.

24. Bradley JP, Baker CL 3rd, Kline AJ, et al. Arthroscopic capsulolabral reconstruction for posterior instability of the shoulder: a prospective study of 100 shoulders. *Am J Sports Med.* 2006;34:1061-1071.

25. Bottoni CR, Franks BR, Moore JH, et al. Operative stabilization of posterior instability. *Am J Sports Med.* 2005;33:996-1002.

26. Sekiya JK, Willobee JA, Miller MD, et al. Arthroscopic multi-pleated capsular plication compared with open inferior capsular shift for reduction of shoulder volume in a cadaveric model. *Arthroscopy.* 2007;23:1145-1151.

27. Castagna A, Snyder SJ, Conti M, et al. Posterior humeral avulsion of the glenohumeral ligament: a clinical review of 9 cases. *Arthroscopy.* 2007;23:809-815.

28. DiFelice GS, Williams RJ, Cohen MS, et al. The accessory posterior portal for shoulder arthroscopy: Description of technique and cadaveric study. *Arthroscopy.* 2001;17:888-891.

**Please see video on the accompanying Web site at
http://www.slackbooks.com/unstableshouldervideos**

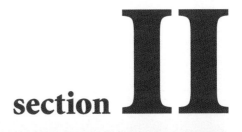

Special Situations in Shoulder Instability

8

The Best Treatment for the First-Time Dislocator

Drew Fehsenfeld, MD, PhD and Robert A. Arciero, MD

The management of the first-time dislocator has been the subject of considerable controversy, especially in patients younger than 25 years old. A thorough understanding of the pathology, natural history, and recent results of outcomes for treatment of this problem serve to assist in appropriate management decisions.

The shoulder is one of the most commonly dislocated joints, with an incidence of 1.7% in people aged 18 to 70 years old.[1] The 1-year incidence is actually higher in young, healthy athletes with a rate of 2.8%.[2] The majority of dislocations (96%) occur anteriorly and are associated with avulsion of the labrum and inferior glenohumeral ligament (IGHL) from the glenoid. This capsulolabral complex is known as a Bankart lesion. The failure of the anterior structures may also occur through intrasubstance tearing of the capsule or avulsion from the humeral insertion but is much less common in the primary dislocation in younger patients. Injury to the capsulolabral complex has been reported in 85% to 100% of young patients with acute shoulder dislocation.[3,4] The avulsion of the capsuloligamentous structures has been a very consistent pathoanatomical lesion in the first-time dislocator at arthroscopy.[5] MRI studies have shown avulsion of the glenohumeral ligaments (66%), tearing of the labrum (73%), and combined injuries (53%).[6]

In the current modern era, the management of the first-time dislocator should not only focus on recurrent instability as a primary goal but should also include quality of life, return to work, return to sports, and a true outcomes assessment. The natural history of the first-time dislocator has been investigated in multiple studies and forms part of the basis for a treatment approach. The traditional literature suggests high recurrence rates of more than 90% in young patients (younger than 20 years; Table 8-1). This high recurrence rate has been challenged by several more recent studies. At 4 years follow-up, Sachs and colleagues found a 56% redislocation rate in young athletic patients, but only 50% of these patients ultimately requested surgical stabilization.[7] A similar lower recurrence rate has been reported in a 25-year follow-up study by Hovelius and colleagues, who showed that patients younger than 22 years either were stable (33%) or became stable (12%).[8] However, the outcomes in patients

Abrams JS. *Management of the Unstable Shoulder:*
Arthroscopic and Open Repair (pp. 113-126).
© 2011 SLACK Incorporated

Table 8-1

DEMOGRAPHICS AND RECURRENCE RATE

Historically, a high recurrence rate has been reported for young patients.

REFERENCE	DEMOGRAPHICS	RECURRENCE RATE
Rowe et al. *JBJS.* 1956.	<20 years old	94%
McLaughlin et al. *Am J Surg.* 1950.	<20 years old	95%
Henry et al. *AJSM.* 1982.	17 to 23 years old	90%
Simonet et al. *AJSM.* 1984.	Athletes <30 years old	82%
West Point	17 to 24 years old	85%
Marans et al. *JBJS.* 1992.	Open physes	100%
Postacchini et al. *JSES.* 2000.	Adolescents	92%

with recurrent dislocation have been found to be significantly worse than patients treated with initial stabilization. In a prospective randomized trial, Kirkley reported improved Western Ontario Shoulder Instability (WOSI) scores and a reduced redislocation rate in surgical (15.9%) versus nonoperative (47%) groups.[9] In a more recent, prospective, randomized trial, patients with an average age of 25 years were found to have improved WOSI and Disabilities of the Arm, Shoulder, and Hand (DASH) scores at 2 years with arthroscopic Bankart repair compared to lavage alone.[10]

This chapter will examine the natural history, pathoanatomy, and results of nonoperative and operative intervention to provide a basis for "the best treatment" of the first-time anterior dislocation.

PATIENT EVALUATION

The key to successful management of instability is patient selection. The history will often describe an episode of forced abduction and external rotation resulting in a "pop," pain, and loss of shoulder function. Most patients require reduction in the emergency room. Initially, because of the acute injury, a complete exam may not be possible, but a positive apprehension/relocation test with laxity on anterior load shift supports the diagnosis of an acute dislocation. A complete neurovascular exam is paramount, as nerve injury, especially the axillary nerve, is observed in up to 8.6% of cases.[10] In older patients, injuries to the brachial plexus and axillary artery have been described after the initial dislocation.

Initial imaging studies should include a true anteroposterior and axillary lateral to evaluate for reduction of the glenohumeral joint. A Stryker notch can be used to assess for humeral head defect, and a West Point axillary view is useful to evaluate the anterior inferior glenoid for fracture. MRI will provide valuable information regarding the presence or absence of a Bankart lesion (Figure 8-1), as well as possible concurrent pathology, such as a humeral avulsion of the glenohumeral ligament, rotator cuff tear, or fracture. If an anterior rim fracture is identified, it may be important to obtain a computed tomography (CT) scan, especially with 3-dimensional reconstructions to fully evaluate the extent of the injury (Figure 8-2).[11]

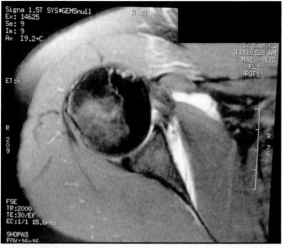

Figure 8-1. Axial T2 MRI view of shoulder showing disruption of the capsulolabral complex from the anterior glenoid rim.

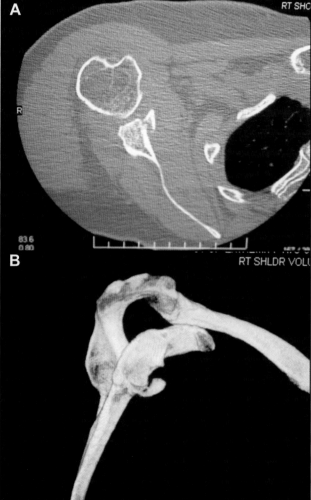

Figure 8-2. Glenoid rim fractures can be better characterized and quantified using CT imaging as shown in this (A) axial and (B) 3-dimensional reconstruction.

Rationale for Nonoperative Treatment

Initial nonoperative management of the primary dislocator is preferred in select patients. Clearly, older patients (older than 30 years) with primary dislocation have lower recurrence rates (15%) but may have associated injuries, such as rim fractures, greater tuberosity fractures, and rotator cuff tears. Patients can be immobilized briefly for pain control and then mobilized. Re-examination for rotator cuff injury is warranted after 4 weeks. MRI should be obtained if no active abduction is present.

In young patients, recent literature has begun to suggest that recurrence alone is not an indication for persistent instability. According to the work of Hovelius in a 25-year follow-up study, patients younger than 40 years of age had an overall recurrence rate of only 57%.[8] Despite a 70% recurrence rate in patients younger than 20 years of age, surgical stabilization was required in only 44%. The authors believe that these findings suggest that primary surgical stabilization is not indicated. In addition, Sachs and colleagues reported a similarly low recurrence rate of 43% in 90 patients younger than 40 years of age.[7] The authors were unable to predict who would need surgical stabilization. As earlier studies have shown, patients younger than 20 years of age and those involved in contact and overhead sports had a higher rate of recurrence.

The nonoperative management in the young patient immobilized in internal rotation has never been shown to alter the natural history.[8] However, Itoi and colleagues have demonstrated apposition of the Bankart lesion on MRI with the arm immobilized in external rotation.[12] They have also shown a reduction in recurrence rates (26% versus 42%) in patients treated with immobilization in external rotation compared to internal immobilization after primary dislocation.[13] However, this treatment has not been compared to primary arthroscopic stabilization.

Management of the in-season athlete presents a challenging problem and represents another subset of patients who could be managed nonoperatively. Buss and colleagues showed that 26 of 30 athletes were able to return to sport at an average of 10 days and complete the season.[14] Approximately half of these patients went on to require surgical intervention in the off season.

Rationale for Primary Surgical Stabilization

There are now multiple studies to support primary surgical stabilization on the basis of reduced recurrence rates *and* improved outcomes. Surgical stabilization is recommended for treating young patients (younger than 30 years) with primary traumatic dislocations. Multiple studies have shown early repair to have improved outcome with a 10% to 15% recurrence rate (Table 8-2). In a prospective study comparing nonoperative and arthroscopic repair in US Military Academy cadets, 80% of nonsurgical patients had recurrent instability compared to only 14% of the surgical group.[15] In a prospective, randomized clinical trial of 40 patients, Kirkley and colleagues showed improved quality-of-life outcome as well as decreased risk of recurrence.[16] These results were confirmed by Bottoni and colleagues in a direct comparison of operative and nonoperative management with an 11% and 75% recurrence rate, respectively.[17] These results have been consistent even at long-term follow-up using a biodegradable tack.[2] In a study by Jakobsen and colleagues, patients treated nonoperatively who had recurrence that required stabilization did not have as good of an outcome as those primarily stabilized both by outcome score and recurrence rate.[18] Patients with persistent instability who chose to "cope" had lower American Shoulder and Elbow Society (ASES), Constant-Murley, and WOSI scores compared to primary dislocators with stable shoulders.[7]

Table 8-2

Recent studies have shown reduced recurrence and improved outcomes in patients treated with surgical stabilization versus nonoperative management.

REFERENCE	TREATMENT	F/U	STUDY DESIGN	RECURRENCE	OUTCOMES
Wheeler. Arthroscopy. 1989.	35 Nonop 9 Repair	26 mo	Retro	Nonop: 92% Repair: 22%	
Arciero. AJSM. 1994.	15 Nonop 21 Repair	33 mo	Retro	Nonop: 80% Repair: 14%	Repair: Rowe 95
Kirkley. Arthroscopy. 1999.	20 Nonop 20 Repair	24 mo	PRCT	Nonop: 47% Repair: 16%	WOSI Nonop: 634 Repair: 287
DeBeradino. AJSM. 2001.	49 Repair	2 to 5 yrs	Retro	Repair: 12%	Repair: Rowe: 92 SF-36: 99
Bottoni. AJSM. 2002.	14 Nonop 10 Repair	36 mo	PRCT	Nonop: 75% Repair: 11%	Sane / L'Insalata Nonop: 57 / 73 Repair: 88 / 94

(continued)

Table 8-2 (continued)

Recent studies have shown reduced recurrence and improved outcomes in patients treated with surgical stabilization versus nonoperative management.

REFERENCE	TREATMENT	F/U	STUDY DESIGN	RECURRENCE	OUTCOMES
Jakobsen. Arthroscopy. 2007.	39 Nonop 36 Repair	10 yrs	PRCT	Nonop: 56% Repair: 3%	Oxford (good/excellent) Nonop: 25% Repair: 72% Fail Nonop Repaired: 63%
Owens. AJSM. 2007.	40 Repair	13 yrs	Pro	Repair: 12.5%	WOSI Rowe SST SANE SF-36 371 25 11.1 92 95
Sachs. JBJS. 2007.	102 Nonop 20 Bankart 9 RTCR	5 yrs	Pro	Age Nonop 12 to 19 56% 20 to 29 38% 30 to 39 27%	ASES Constant WOSI Stable 87 92 84 Unstable 72 84 60 Repair 86 93 78
Robinson. JBJS. 2008.	38 lavage 42 Repair	2 yrs	PRCT	Lavage: 38% Repair: 7%	Decreased WOSI and DASH in lavage versus repair

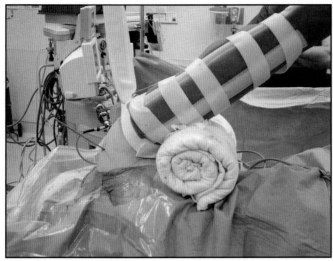

Figure 8-3. Patient positioned in the lateral decubitus position with 7 lbs of distal traction and 5 lbs of lateral traction. A large bump placed in the axilla improves inferior joint exposure.

In a prospective, randomized, 2-year study, patients with recurrent instability had lower WOSI and DASH scores compared to surgically stabilized shoulders.[18] In addition, surgical stabilization resulted in outcomes similar to patients who stabilized after initial dislocation.

Recurrence is not benign and can result in repetitive capsular injury. Repetitive subfailure strains to injured IGHL can decrease the peak load response and result in capsular and ligament elongation.[19,20] Habermeyer and colleagues reported progressive labral-ligamentous injury with repeated instability episodes.[21] A recent study by Hovelius and Seboe reported the rate of moderate to severe arthropathy in patients with multiple recurrence (40%), a single recurrence (35%), surgical repair (26%), and no recurrence (18%),[22] suggesting that persistent instability has long-term consequences.

In summary, a rationale for surgical stabilization of primary dislocation can be strongly made for the young, active patient. This is based on the pathoanatomy, improved outcomes and reduced recurrence rates in prospective randomized studies, avoiding increased capsular and bony injury, and potential decreased post-traumatic osteoarthritis.

Highlighted Surgical Technique

The authors' preferred surgical technique is arthroscopic. Contraindications to an arthroscopic approach include a large HAGL or glenoid rim fracture of greater than 20%. The surgical goals are to re-establish labral anatomy, retension the IGHL, and treat associated pathology. Arthroscopic stabilization may be performed in either the beach chair or lateral decubitus position. The author's preferred position is lateral decubitus due to improved distraction and glenohumeral exposure. The patient is placed lateral on a bean bag with an axillary bump in place (Figure 8-3). An examination under anesthesia should always be performed prior to stabilization. The arm is placed in 7 lbs of distal traction and 5 lbs of lateral traction to provide joint distraction. Additional exposure of the inferior joint may be provided with a towel roll placed in the axilla (see Chapter 8 video).

Portal placement for instability is extremely important to provide good access to the anterior glenoid for anchor placement and suture management (Figure 8-4).

Figure 8-4. Image of portal positions for performing arthroscopic Bankart repair. Three primary portals are used: anteriosuperior, anterioinferior, and posterior.

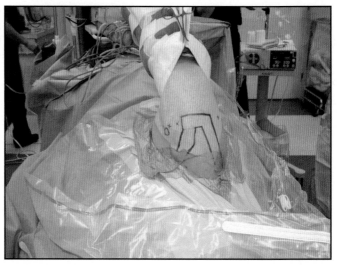

The joint line is palpated posteriorly, and an incision is made approximately 1-cm inferior and 1-cm medial to the posterior corner of the acromion. A hemostat is used to bluntly spread to the joint capsule. The gap between the humeral head and the glenoid is palpated with the tip of the hemostat. The scope is then introduced into the glenohumeral joint. A diagnostic arthroscopy is performed, examining the biceps tendon, rotator cuff, articular cartilage, labrum, and capsule. The Bankart lesion is visualized (Figure 8-5). Special attention should be given to assessing the entire capsule to rule out possible capsular tear or humeral avulsion of the glenohumeral ligament.

Using an outside-in technique, an 18-gauge spinal needle is placed anterior to the anterolateral acromion, entering the joint behind the biceps tendon and at the superior edge of the rotator interval (Figure 8-6). An incision is made in Langer's lines, and a switching stick is placed. The 18-gauge spinal needle is used to create the anteroinferior portal (AIP) just lateral to the coracoid and superior to the subscapularis tendon. The distance between the anterosuperior portal (ASP) and AIP needs to be maximized to prevent interference between the cannulas (Figure 8-7). The angle of entry should allow access to the inferior capsule as well as placement of anchors at the edge of the inferior glenoid. An 8.25 cannula is placed into the AIP for anchor placement and suture management. The scope is then shifted to the ASP over the previously placed switching stick, and an 8.25 cannula is placed posteriorly for suture management (Figure 8-8 and see Chapter 8 video). The majority of the procedure may be performed through these portals; however, placement of an anchor at the 6 o'clock position may require a more inferior approach. A percutaneous trans-subscapular portal can be created using the drill cannula and a small skin incision.

The labrum is typically scarred to the anterior glenoid neck and must be mobilized using an elevator (Figure 8-9). Adequate release of the labrum is important to allow a tensionless repair to the edge of the glenoid. The labrum and capsule should float to the edge of the glenoid, and the subscapularis muscle be visible once adequate release is complete. A 3.5 shaver without suction is introduced into the interval between the capsule and glenoid to débride any scar tissue. The glenoid rim is decorticated with a slap burr to create a bleeding surface (Figure 8-10). A rasp is then used to prepare the capsule.

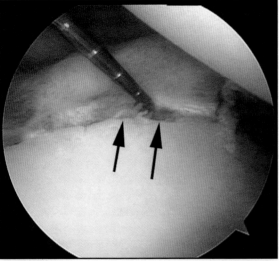

Figure 8-5. A probe is introduced through the AIP to probe the gap between the disrupted labrum and glenoid.

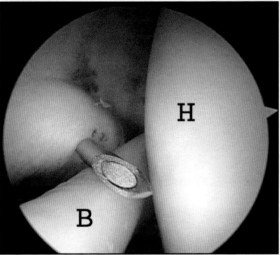

Figure 8-6. The ASP is established under direct visualization using a spinal needle placed through the rotator interval and adjacent to or behind the biceps tendon.

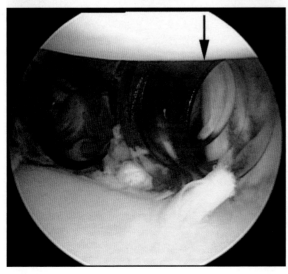

Figure 8-7. The AIP is placed just above the subscapularis tendon. The 2 anterior portals should be separated if possible to avoid interference with each other during repair.

Figure 8-8. Using the ASP, the Bankart is often seen scarred and medialized on the glenoid neck.

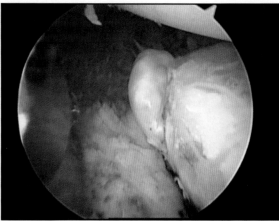

Figure 8-9. The Bankart lesion is mobilized from the anterior glenoid neck using an angled elevator until the muscle of the subscapularis is visualized and the labrum floats to the edge of the glenoid.

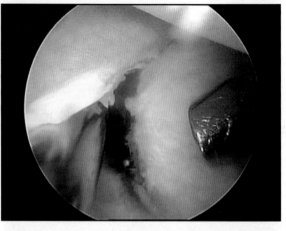

Figure 8-10. The glenoid rim is prepared either with an arthroscopic burr or rasp to create a bleeding surface.

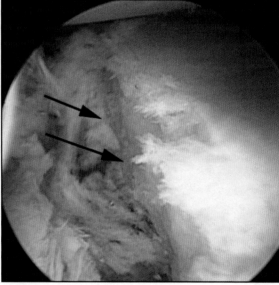

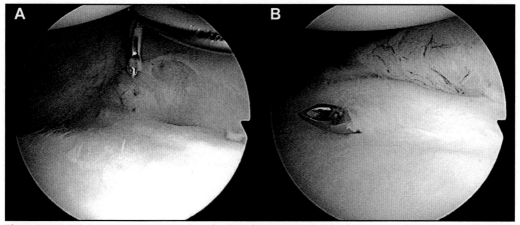

Figure 8-11. (A) A passing suture is placed using the combi stitch technique in which the capsule is plicated and then (B) the suture is passed around the labrum.

The placement of the inferior sutures is critical and can be the most challenging. Several techniques can be used to tension the inferior capsule. One option is to translate the capsule superiorly to the glenoid edge using a 0 polydioxanone suture (PDS) placed inferiorly or using a grasper from the ASP. A second option is to place a PDS through the capsule from the AIP, using the posterior portal for shuttling the PDS. A final alternative is to place the PDS from the posterior portal as viewed from the ASP and shuttle using the AIP (Figure 8-11). The suture can be passed as a "combi" stitch, which plicates the capsule and stabilizes the labrum (see Chapter 8 video). Once the PDS is in place, the inferior anchor is placed 1 to 2 mm on the articular surface and 5 to 7 mm cephalad to the shuttling suture (Figure 8-12). The lateral edge of the cartilage can be removed using a looped curette to allow more stable placement of the drill cannula. As discussed earlier, the AIP may not provide a good trajectory for anchor placement at the inferior glenoid. If this is the case, a percutaneous trans-subscapular portal can be used to place the anchor. One end of the suture is retrieved through the posterior portal, and the PDS is tied to the suture and used to shuttle it around the capsule and labrum. The suture is then tied, repairing the labrum and retensioning the capsule. The next anchor is placed through the AIP slightly more superior (5 to 8 mm) on the glenoid rim. The suture is retrieved through the posterior portal in preparation for shuttling. The crescent hook is used to place a "combi" stitch 5 to 7 mm inferior to the anchor. The shuttling suture is retrieved through the posterior portal, tied to the anchor suture, and used to pass the suture around the capsule and labrum. This process is repeated until the labrum is completely repaired to the glenoid rim (Figure 8-13). A minimum of 3 to 4 suture anchors should be used to provide adequate strength to the repair.

Tips and Pearls

In the event of a small (less than 20%) bony avulsion fracture, an arthroscopic technique may be used to reduce and stabilize the fragment arthroscopically.[23] The initial suture anchor is placed as described above. The fragment is mobilized with the capsulolabral complex attached. The fragment should be easily reducible to the anterior glenoid. An anchor is placed through the AIP just inferior to the fracture. The suture-passing device is then used to palpate the bony fragment and pass the suture

Figure 8-12. The anchor is placed slightly superior to the stitch, allowing superior translation of the capsule and labrum retensioning of the inferior glenohumeral ligament.

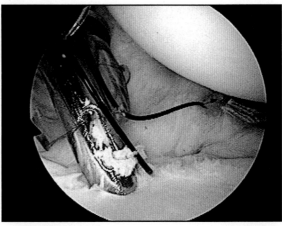

Figure 8-13. The completed Bankart repair reestablishing the labrum to the anterior glenoid and retensioning the inferior glenohumeral ligament.

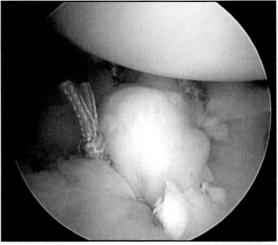

just inferior to the bony fragment. The anchor is then tied, which reduces the inferior portion of the fragment and creates a hinge to reduce the fracture fragment. A second anchor is placed on the glenoid at the midpoint of the glenoid defect and on the anterior edge of the fracture. The suture passing device is used to pass a suture either around or through the fracture fragment. The suture is then tied, stabilizing the fragment. The final anchor is placed just superior to the fracture fragment.

Recently, an alternative technique was described by Millet and Braun.[24] An anchor is placed medial to the fracture on the glenoid neck. The sutures are then shuttled through the capsule medial to the fracture fragment. These sutures are then parked through the AIP. An anchor is placed at the inferior aspect of the fracture as described previously to create a hinge. The bone fragment is now fixed using a bridging technique. The sutures to the medial anchor are retrieved and loaded into a Bio-PushLock anchor (Arthrex, Naples, FL). A drill hole is created on the glenoid face at the junction between the glenoid face and fracture. The suture limbs are tensioned, and the PushLock is inserted, providing reduction and compression of the fracture fragment. At least one further anchor should be placed superior to lock the fragment in place.

Managing Complications

The most common complication with surgical management of shoulder instability is recurrent subluxation or dislocation. The primary reason for failure of arthroscopic stabilization is failure to recognize bone defects. A clinically significant Hill-Sachs or insufficient glenoid has been reported to increase recurrence. Inadequate initial repair may also result in recurrent instability. A good repair requires mobilization of the Bankart, retensioning of the IGHL, placement of anchors at the 6 o'clock position, and adequate fixation points (at least 3 to 4 anchors). The arthroscopic repair should mirror the open method, which is still considered the gold standard for instability repair.

Postoperative Management

The arm is held in neutral or slight internal rotation in a shoulder immobilizer for 3 to 4 weeks. For the first 4 weeks, the patient is allowed supine well-arm assisted forward elevation to 90 degrees, and external rotation to 10 degrees. Range of motion is progressed at 4 weeks to develop full motion. Isometric strengthening of all rotator cuff muscles and scapular stabilization exercises are initiated at 6 weeks after surgery. Resistance training can be started at 8 weeks with bands, cords, or weights. At 6 months, the patient may return to all activities, including contact sports.

REFERENCES

1. Hovelius L. Incidence of shoulder dislocation in Sweden. *Clin Orthop Relat Res.* 1982;166:127-131.
2. Owens BD, DeBerardino TM, Nelson BJ, et al. Long-term follow-up of acute arthroscopic Bankart repair for initial anterior shoulder dislocation in young athletes. *Am J Sports Med.* 2009;37(4):669-673.
3. Baker CL, Uribe JW, Whitman C. Arthroscopic evaluation of acute initial anterior shoulder dislocations. *Am J Sports Med.* 1990;18(1):25-28.
4. Norlin R. Intraarticular pathology in acute, first-time anterior shoulder dislocation: an arthroscopic study. *Arthroscopy.* 1993;9(5):546-549.
5. Taylor DC, Arciero RA. Pathologic changes associated with shoulder dislocations. Arthroscopic and physical examination findings in first-time, traumatic anterior dislocations. *Am J Sports Med.* 1997;25(3):306-311.
6. Wintzell G, Haglund-Akerlind Y, Tengvar M, Johansson L, Eriksson E. MRI examination of the glenohumeral joint after traumatic primary anterior dislocation. A descriptive evaluation of the acute lesion and at 6-month follow-up. *Knee Surg Sports Traumatol Arthrosc.* 1996;4(4):232-236.
7. Sachs RA, Stone ML, Paxton E, Kuney M, Lin D. Can the need for future surgery for acute traumatic anterior shoulder dislocation be predicted? *J Bone Joint Surg Am.* 2007;89:1665-1674.
8. Hovelius L, Olofsson A, Sandstrom B, et al. Nonoperative treatment of primary anterior shoulder dislocation in patients forty years of age and younger. A prospective twenty-five-year follow-up. *J Bone Joint Surg Am.* 2008;90:945-952.
9. Kirkley S. Primary anterior dislocation of the shoulder in young patients. A ten-year prospective study. *J Bone Joint Surg Am.* 1998;80(2):300-301.
10. Robinson CM, Jenkins PJ, White TO, Ker A, Will E. Primary arthroscopic stabilization for a first-time anterior dislocation of the shoulder. A randomized, double-blind trial. *J Bone Joint Surg Am.* 2008;90:708-721.
11. Sugaya H, Moriishi, Dohi M, Kon Y, Tsuchiya A. Glenoid rim morphology in recurrent anterior glenohumeral instability. *J Bone Joint Surg Am.* 2003;85-A(5):878-884.
12. Itoi E, Hatakeyama Y, Kido T, et al. A new method of immobilization after traumatic anterior dislocation of the shoulder: a preliminary study. *J Shoulder Elbow Surg.* 2003;12(5):413-415.
13. Itoi E, Hatakeyama Y, Sato T, et al. Immobilization in external rotation after shoulder dislocation reduces the risk of recurrence. A randomized controlled trial. *J Bone Joint Surg Am.* 2007;89(10):2124-2131.

14. Buss DD, Lynch GP, Meyer CP, Huber SM, Freehill MQ. Nonoperative management for in-season athletes with anterior shoulder instability. *Am J Sports Med.* 2004;32(6):1430-1433.
15. DeBerardino TM, Arciero RA, Taylor DC. Arthroscopic stabilization of acute initial anterior shoulder dislocation: the West Point experience. *J South Orthop Assoc.* 1996;5(4):263-271.
16. Kirkley A, Griffin S, Richards C, Miniaci A, Mohtadi N. Prospective randomized clinical trial comparing the effectiveness of immediate arthroscopic stabilization versus immobilization and rehabilitation in first traumatic anterior dislocations of the shoulder. *Arthroscopy.* 1999;15(5):507-514.
17. Bottoni CR, Wilckens JH, DeBerardino TM, et al. A prospective, randomized evaluation of arthroscopic stabilization versus nonoperative treatment in patients with acute traumatic, first-time shoulder dislocations. *Am J Sports Med.* 2002;30(4):576-580.
18. Jakobsen BW, Johannsen HV, Suder P, Sojbjerg JO. Traumatic anterior dislocation of the shoulder: a randomized study with 10-year follow-up. *Arthroscopy.* 2007;23(2):118-123.
19. Pollock RG, Wang VM, Bucchieri JS, et al. Effects of repetitive subfailure strains on the mechanical behavior of the inferior glenohumeral ligament. *J Shoulder Elbow Surg.* 2000;9(5):427-435.
20. Urayama M, Itoi E, Sashi R, Minagawa H, Sato K. Capsular elongation in shoulders with recurrent anterior dislocation. Quantitative assessment with magnetic resonance arthrography. *Am J Sports Med.* 2003;31(1):64-67.
21. Habermeyer P, Gleyze P, Rickert M. Evolution of lesions of the labrum-ligament complex in posttraumatic anterior shoulder instability: a prospective study. *J Shoulder Elbow Surg.* 1999;8:66-74.
22. Hovelius L, Seboe M. Neer Award 2008: arthropathy after primary anterior shoulder dislocation—223 shoulders prospectively followed up for twenty-five years. *J Shoulder Elbow Surg.* 2009;18:229-247.
23. Sugaya H, Kon Y, Tsuchiya A. Arthroscopic repair of glenoid fractures using suture anchors. *J Arthroscopy.* 2005;21(5):635e1-5.
24. Millett PJ, Braun S. The "Bony Bankart Bridge" procedure: a new arthroscopic technique for reduction and internal fixation of a bony Bankart lesion. *J Arthroscopy.* 2009;25(1):102-105.

Please see video on the accompanying Web site at
http://www.slackbooks.com/unstableshouldervideos

9

Treatment Decisions in the Elite Athlete

Todd C. Moen, MD and Gordon W. Nuber, MD

Traumatic anterior shoulder dislocations occur commonly in young, athletic patients, particularly those involved in contact or collision sports. The age of this subset of patients and the nature of the sports in which these athletes participate puts this group at high risk for recurrent instability. Because of the tremendous demands placed on the shoulder, the expectation of a return to a high level of performance, and the implications of potential failure to return to prior function, the therapeutic decision making in treating these patients can be complex, often with a large number of individuals other than the patient involved in the process. The treating surgeon must discern whether to treat the patient's instability surgically, when is the best time to operate, and the specific procedure that is most appropriate. When surgery is indicated, the choice of technique—open or arthroscopic—is controversial. Regardless of the type of procedure chosen, the surgical goal is the same: to successfully perform the procedure that most accurately restores the injured anatomy and allows optimum return to function.

PATIENT SELECTION

In assessing the high school and/or elite collision athlete with recurrent shoulder instability, the treating surgeon is faced with 3 inter-related decisions. First of all, does the patient require surgery? Second, if the patient requires surgery, when should the surgery be performed? Finally, if the decision to operate has been made, what is the most appropriate procedure? The young and/or elite athlete with shoulder instability presents many challenges, medical and otherwise, which complicates these 3 decisions.

The first decision that must be made is whether to address the patient's instability surgically. In general, a traumatic shoulder dislocation is treated nonoperatively with

Abrams JS. *Management of the Unstable Shoulder: Arthroscopic and Open Repair* (pp. 127-134). © 2011 SLACK Incorporated

a regimen of physical therapy and strengthening of the dynamic shoulder stabilizers; surgery to stabilize the shoulder is indicated with recurrent dislocation and/or symptomatic instability intolerable to the patient. However, the young, elite athlete's age and the nature of their activity mandates that they be approached differently than the general population. The natural history following traumatic anterior shoulder dislocation is well known. The risk of recurrent instability is inversely related to age and is directly proportional to activity level.[1-3] The high-energy collisions and contact in sports such as football, rugby, hockey, and wrestling predispose the participants to recurrent dislocation and subluxation and lowers the threshold to address the instability surgically.

Besides putting the patient at risk for recurrent injury, the patient's involvement in athletics adds additional factors that affect the decision of whether to operate. The patient will have a desire to return to his or her prior level of function, and surgery presents the best opportunity to do so. Following this, the injury itself and a return to prior function, or lack thereof, will have implications on the patient's future athletic career. In the case of a high school athlete, opportunities in higher education and potential participation in collegiate athletics could be at stake. In the case of the professional athlete, an individual's surgical outcome could have a significant effect on future financial income potential. Given these additional issues, the surgeon treating a high-level athlete will often be put in the position of having to interact with parents, coaches, agents, general managers, and even the media, in addition to the actual patient. Regardless of the number of individuals involved in the decision making, it is imperative to keep the individual patient's needs and desires foremost in importance when discerning between operative and nonoperative treatment.

If surgery is chosen, the next decision that must be made is when the surgery should be performed. The specific time during the season when the injury occurs will have an impact on the timing of surgery. If the injury occurs early in the season, the patient may wish to attempt a course of conservative management and play through to the conclusion of the season, with plans for early surgical stabilization immediately following the season. If the injury occurs near the end of the season, the patient may wish to forego playing in the remaining games and have immediate surgery to maximize rehabilitation time prior to the coming season. Again, it is imperative to keep the individual patient's needs at the forefront when planning the timing for surgery.

Regardless of whether a patient wishes to ultimately have surgery, conservative measures can figure significantly into a patient's treatment plan. If a patient decides against surgery, it can serve as definitive treatment. Nonoperative treatment begins with the use of a sling as needed for the patient's comfort following the initial injury, coupled with almost immediate addition of Codman and pendulum exercises. This is followed by isometric exercises to strengthen the dynamic stabilizers of the shoulder, namely the rotator cuff muscles, the deltoid, and the scapular stabilizers. Eventually, isokinetic exercises are added to condition the patient for a return to play. In evaluating when it is safe to return to sport, the main criteria is the patient's ability to protect himself or herself. The patient must have regained sufficient strength, a full range of motion, and an acceptable degree of comfort. Upon returning to contact activities, the patient may wear any number of commercially available shoulder braces that limit abduction and external rotation. Despite widespread use, there is a paucity of literature regarding these protective braces.

SURGICAL TECHNIQUE

Once surgery has been chosen, the final decision that must be made for a young, athletic patient with shoulder instability is the choice of stabilizing procedure. Regardless of what operation is chosen, the ultimate goal is the same, namely to repair the injured structures as anatomically as possible and allow for the best return to function. The main choice is between open and arthroscopic techniques, with each technique having inherent advantages and disadvantages. Historically, there has been a debate in the literature between open and arthroscopic techniques as to the superior method to stabilize the shoulder, with open techniques generally being more favored, given superior results. However, as the understanding of the pathoanatomy of shoulder instability and arthroscopic surgical techniques have improved, the number of absolute indications for open instability surgery are decreasing, and the indications for arthroscopic surgery are increasing.[4]

Given the principle of restoring the pathoanatomy as anatomically as possible, it is useful to review the relevant injuries in an unstable shoulder. Not all unstable shoulders are created equal, and a wide spectrum of pathology can exist following a traumatic dislocation or subluxation. The most common lesion is the Bankart lesion, a detachment of the anteroinferior labrum from the glenoid rim. Depending on the amount of energy and the direction of force vectors involved in the initial injury, a host of other soft-tissue lesions will be present, such as damage to the joint capsule, an associated labral injury (such as a SLAP[5] lesion), tears of the rotator cuff, or, in the case of an old injury, a labrum healed in a medialized position, the so-called anterior labroligamentous periosteal sleeve avulsion (ALPSA) lesion.[6] In more severe injuries, the bony structures of the shoulder may also be damaged, with resultant defects in the humeral head (the Hill-Sachs lesion), the glenoid, or a HAGL lesion. These injuries are superimposed on any other preexisting shoulder conditions, such as an abnormally lax capsule, which predisposes one to instability. Given this diverse potential pathology, it is crucial to completely and accurately identify—through the patient's history, physical examination, imaging studies, and arthroscopic examination—all lesions leading to the patient's instability.[7]

A debate has raged in the literature over how to best repair the injured anatomy in the unstable shoulder; this debate has centered on the choice of open versus arthroscopic techniques, with each technique having distinct advantages and disadvantages. The main advantage of open stabilization surgery is that it allows for a more precise restoration of capsular tension by allowing the surgeon to separate the damaged capsule from the subscapularis tendon and to repair the capsule with the shoulder in an optimal position. Another advantage is that the damaged capsule can be more easily overlapped and reinforced than with arthroscopic techniques.[8] Finally, open repair has been regarded as stronger[9] and allows a superior rotator interval closure.[10] The main disadvantage of open stabilization is the morbidity of the procedure itself. As with all open procedures compared with arthroscopic procedures, open shoulder stabilization causes increased pain, increased trauma to local tissues creating scarring and adhesions, decreased range of motion, and inferior cosmesis. The other main disadvantage of open surgery is the potential to miss associated pathology; if a diagnostic arthroscopy is not performed prior to opening the shoulder, a contributing lesion may be overlooked.

The advantages and disadvantages of arthroscopic stabilization are the virtual opposite of open stabilization. The smaller exposure and incisions are less damaging to surrounding tissues, allowing for improved range of motion, less pain, an easier rehabilitation process, and improved cosmesis. Most importantly, the arthroscope allows the surgeon to fully visualize the entire shoulder and thus completely identify associated pathology. The main disadvantages involve the ability of arthroscopic techniques to repair the damaged structures. Arthroscopic techniques have traditionally been viewed as less secure,[9] although this view is changing.[11-14] It is more difficult to mobilize and repair the damaged capsule using arthroscopic techniques, and an arthroscopic repair of the rotator interval has been shown to be inferior.[10] Finally, although early series suggest otherwise,[15] arthroscopic techniques have historically been inadequate to address major bone defects, which are a significant cause of failed stabilization procedures.[16]

Although the literature regarding the open versus arthroscopic debate has been plagued by heterogeneous study populations, wide varieties of repair techniques and technologies used in studies, varying outcome measures, differing definitions of success and failure, and selection bias, certain trends have emerged. First, the consensus has been that open stabilization procedures are superior to their arthroscopic counterparts for elite collision athletes. Second, bony defects—in either the glenoid or humerus—predispose a patient to failure, regardless of technique. These 2 trends have historically delineated the indications for open and arthroscopic stabilization procedures; however, new literature is blurring these lines.

Historically, open stabilization techniques have shown superior results when compared with arthroscopic techniques. Most of the reports on shoulder stabilization are retrospective case series and come with the usual criticisms inherent to these types of studies. Nevertheless, open stabilization procedures have consistently shown failure rates in the single digits,[8,17,18] while arthroscopic series have shown failure rates in the 10% to 25% range.[11-14,19] The more rigorous studies, primarily meta-analysis but also a small number of controlled trials, have also shown open techniques to have lower failure rates than arthroscopic ones.[20-24] It is important to note, however, that much of this literature was written when arthroscopic stabilization procedures primarily used transglenoid sutures and bioabsorbable tacks for soft tissue fixation. These methods of fixation have been proven to be inferior to, and have subsequently been replaced by, suture anchor techniques,[9] and thus this literature must be interpreted accordingly. Complete long-term results for modern suture anchor techniques is forthcoming and will likely show different results from these studies of inferior techniques.

The other significant trend that has emerged from the literature on shoulder instability is that bone defects, either in the glenoid or in the humerus, put a patient at high risk for recurrent instability. Burkhart and De Beer[25] described an "inverted pear"-shaped glenoid, in which a post-traumatic anterior bony defect causes the glenoid to appear the opposite of normal, like an upside-down piece of fruit. For patients with humeral or glenoid bone defects, such as an "inverted pear," that were not addressed at the time of surgery, the authors cite recurrence rates of 67% for the general population and 89% for the collision athlete.[25] Boileau and colleagues[19] and Warner and coworkers[26] have reported similar results.These authors recommend various procedures—among them the Latarjet procedure and augmentation with autogenous tricortical bone graft—to address the bony deficiencies or else be faced with high percentages of dislocations.

Despite the above trends, new literature suggests a paradigm shift in that many patients with unstable shoulders, even collision athletes and those with significant bony defects, can be successfully treated arthroscopically. Bacilla and colleagues[11] and Owens and coworkers[27] reported that arthroscopic procedures, using modern techniques, can produce acceptable rates of recurrence, while Carreira and colleagues[12] and Mazzocca and coworkers[13] have argued that arthroscopic techniques, even when used to stabilize collision athletes, can have recurrence rates approaching historic controls. Pagnani[17] has argued that bony defects do not increase the risk of recurrence and do not need to be addressed surgically, while Mologne et al[14] has argued that glenoid bone deficiency can be successfully treated arthroscopically. As understanding of the pathoanatomy of shoulder instability and arthroscopic techniques evolves, so does the rationale behind shoulder stabilization.

The debate of open versus arthroscopic techniques is far from being settled and promises to continue for the foreseeable future. However, the debate itself is actually missing the most important principle. Burkhart and De Beer succinctly wrote that "a bad operation is a bad operation, whether it is performed open or arthroscopic."[25] Put another way, a good operation is a good operation—so long as it is the *appropriate* operation—whether it is performed open or arthroscopic. The *appropriate* operation is determined by the patient's injury, the patient's needs, and the abilities of the surgeon.

TIPS AND PEARLS/MANAGING COMPLICATIONS

- The decision whether to proceed to surgery is always in the patient's hands, after being advised and counseled of the relevant information.
- All pathology must be completely identified and addressed for a successful outcome.
- Even if an open stabilization procedure is planned, always perform a diagnostic arthroscopy prior to opening to completely identify all pathology.
- If the patient's capsular tissue is of poor quality, err toward open stabilization.
- Both the labral and capsular tissue must be repaired at the time of stabilization.
- When repairing the labrum, take care to repair the labrum to the face of the glenoid—avoid medialization of the labrum.
- When tensioning the capsule in an open repair, position the shoulder in 40 degrees of abduction and 40 degrees of external rotation. The exception to this rule is the throwing athlete.
- It is important to start range of motion exercises early, particularly in patients who had an open stabilization, to avoid postoperative stiffness. Trend toward more aggressive rehabilitation in patients who underwent open procedures.

POSTOPERATIVE MANAGEMENT

0 to 4 weeks: A sling is to be used when sleeping and when out in public. It may also be used as needed for comfort. Codman, pendulum, saw, and tummy-rub exercises are used to preserve/improve range of motion. No passive external rotation or abduction is allowed past the point at which the capsule was tensioned intraoperatively. No forced external rotation is permitted.

4 to 8 weeks: Begin formal physical therapy and active assisted range of motion exercises. If the subscapularis was violated, no resistive exercises are permitted. Again, no forced external rotation is permitted.

2 to 4 months: Work toward achieving full range of motion, and regain strength by resistive exercises.

4 months: Return to function, contact activities.

CONCLUSION

Post-traumatic instability is a common problem in young elite athletes. This subset of patients presents numerous challenges unique from the general population, and the decision-making process in treating these patients is complex. Although many issues regarding their management remain, certain principles are well established. By reconstructing the injured anatomy as anatomically as possible, one can help maximize a patient's return to function.

REFERENCES

1. Arciero RA, Wheeler JH, Ryan JB, McBride JT. Arthroscopic Bankart repair versus nonoperative treatment for acute, initial anterior shoulder dislocations. *Am J Sports Med.* 1994;22(5):589-594.
2. Tsai L, Wredmark T, Johansson C, Gibo K, Engstrom B, Tornqvist H. Shoulder function in patients with unoperated anterior shoulder instability. *Am J Sports Med.* 1991;19(5):469-473.
3. Warme WJ, Arciero RA, Taylor DC. Anterior shoulder instability in sport: current management recommendations. *Sports Medicine.* 1999;28(3):209-220.
4. Kropf EJ, Tjoumakaris FP, Sekiya JK. Arthroscopic shoulder stabilization: is there ever a need to open? *Arthroscopy.* 2007;23(7):779-784.
5. Snyder SJ, Karzel RP, Del Pizzo W, Ferkel RD, Friedman MJ. SLAP lesions of the shoulder. *Arthroscopy.* 1990;6(4):274-279.
6. Neviaser TJ. The anterior labroligamentous periosteal sleeve avulsion lesion: a cause of anterior instability of the shoulder. *Arthroscopy.* 1993;9(1):17-21.
7. Cole BJ, L'Insalata J, Irrgang J, Warner JJ. Comparison of arthroscopic and open anterior shoulder stabilization. A two- to six-year follow-up study. *J Bone Joint Surg.* 2000;82-A(8):1108-1114.
8. Pagnani MJ, Dome DC. Surgical treatment of traumatic anterior shoulder instability in American football players. *J Bone Joint Surg.* 2002;84-A(5):711-715.
9. Freedman KB, Smith AP, Romeo AA, Cole BJ, Bach BR Jr. Open Bankart repair versus arthroscopic repair with transglenoid sutures or bioabsorbable tacks for recurrent anterior instability of the shoulder: a meta-analysis. *Am J Sports Med.* 2004;32(6):1520-1527.
10. Provencher MT, Mologne TS, Hongo M, Zhao K, Tasto JP, An KN. Arthroscopic versus open rotator interval closure: biomechanical evaluation of stability and motion. *Arthroscopy.* 2007;23(6):583-592.
11. Bacilla P, Field LD, Savoie FH III. Arthroscopic Bankart repair in a high demand patient population. *Arthroscopy.* 1997;13(1):51-60.
12. Carreira DS, Mazzocca AD, Oryhon J, Brown FM, Hayden JK, Romeo AA. A prospective outcome evaluation of arthroscopic Bankart repairs: minimum 2-year follow-up. *Am J Sports Med.* 2006;34(5):771-777.
13. Mazzocca AD, Brown FM Jr, Carreira DS, Hayden J, Romeo AA. Arthroscopic anterior shoulder stabilization of collision and contact athletes. *Am J Sports Med.* 2005;33(1):52-60.
14. Mologne TS, Provencher MT, Menzel KA, Vachon TA, Dewing CB. Arthroscopic stabilization in patients with an inverted pear glenoid: results in patients with bone loss of the anterior glenoid. *Am J Sports Med.* 2007;35(8):1276-1283.
15. Lafosse L, Lejeune E, Bouchard A, Kakuda C, Gobezie R, Kochhar T. The arthroscopic Latarjet procedure for the treatment of anterior shoulder instability. *Arthroscopy.* 2007;23(11):1242 e1241-1245.
16. Burkhart SS, De Beer JF, Tehrany AM, Parten PM. Quantifying glenoid bone loss arthroscopically in shoulder instability. *Arthroscopy.* 2002;18(5):488-491.

17. Pagnani MJ. Open capsular repair without bone block for recurrent anterior shoulder instability in patients with and without bony defects of the glenoid and/or humeral head. *Am J Sports Med.* 2008;36(9):1805-1812.
18. Uhorchak JM, Arciero RA, Huggard D, Taylor DC. Recurrent shoulder instability after open reconstruction in athletes involved in collision and contact sports. *Am J Sports Med.* 2000;28(6):794-799.
19. Boileau P, Villalba M, Hery JY, Balg F, Ahrens P, Neyton L. Risk factors for recurrence of shoulder instability after arthroscopic Bankart repair. *J Bone Joint Surg.* 2006;88(8):1755-1763.
20. Bottoni CR, Smith EL, Berkowitz MJ, Towle RB, Moore JH. Arthroscopic versus open shoulder stabilization for recurrent anterior instability: a prospective randomized clinical trial. *Am J Sports Med.* 2006;34(11):1730-1737.
21. Bottoni CR, Wilckens JH, DeBerardino TM, et al. A prospective, randomized evaluation of arthroscopic stabilization versus nonoperative treatment in patients with acute, traumatic, first-time shoulder dislocations. *Am J Sports Med.* 2002;30(4):576-580.
22. Lenters TR, Franta AK, Wolf FM, Leopold SS, Matsen FA 3rd. Arthroscopic compared with open repairs for recurrent anterior shoulder instability. A systematic review and meta-analysis of the literature. *J Bone Joint Surg.* 2007;89(2):244-254.
23. Mohtadi NG, Bitar IJ, Sasyniuk TM, Hollinshead RM, Harper WP. Arthroscopic versus open repair for traumatic anterior shoulder instability: a meta-analysis. *Arthroscopy.* 2005;21(6):652-658.
24. Rhee YG, Ha JH, Cho NS. Anterior shoulder stabilization in collision athletes: arthroscopic versus open Bankart repair. *Am J Sports Med.* 2006;34(6):979-985.
25. Burkhart SS, De Beer JF. Traumatic glenohumeral bone defects and their relationship to failure of arthroscopic Bankart repairs: significance of the inverted-pear glenoid and the humeral engaging Hill-Sachs lesion. *Arthroscopy.* 2000;16(7):677-694.
26. Warner JJ, Gill TJ, O'Hollerhan JD, Pathare N, Millett PJ. Anatomical glenoid reconstruction for recurrent anterior glenohumeral instability with glenoid deficiency using an autogenous tricortical iliac crest bone graft. *Am J Sports Med.* 2006;34(2):205-212.
27. Owens BD, Deberardino TM, Nelson BJ, et al. Long-term follow-up of acute arthroscopic Bankart repair for initial anterior shoulder dislocations in young athletes. *Am J Sports Med.* 2009;37(4):669-673..

10

Assessment of Bone Loss in the Chronic, Recurrent, Unstable Shoulder

Anshu Singh, MD; Travis G. O'Brien, BA; Jianhua Wang, MD; and Jon J. P. Warner, MD

Assessment of acquired and congenital shoulder pathology is a critical step in treating patients with shoulder instability. Bony lesions, typically of the glenoid rim or humeral head, are predictive of recurrence after nonoperative or arthroscopic management. Accurate assessment allows for proper risk stratification, preoperative planning, and management of patient expectations.

While the surgeon should have the ability to diagnose and treat other pathology as it presents intraoperatively, it is optimal to have a thorough understanding of the lesions that are to be addressed before making an incision. This allows for planning in which implants, graft sources, and surgical approaches are needed to optimize results. In addition, the patient will have a better idea of what to expect postoperatively while obviating the time, expense, and morbidity of a secondary operation.

Multiple authors have reported that the presence and extent of bony lesions are predictive of poor outcome.[1,2] In 2006, Boileau and colleagues reviewed 3-year results of 91 consecutive patients after arthroscopic Bankart repair.[3] They found that anterior glenoid bone loss and large Hill-Sachs lesions were associated with recurrence of subluxation and instability. The destabilizing effect was more pronounced in the setting of ligamentous laxity. This study and others underscore the importance of preoperative risk stratification in this patient population.

This chapter presents the up-to-the-date literature regarding the assessment of bone loss associated with shoulder instability. Radiographic (x-ray), computed tomography (CT), nuclear MRI, and arthroscopic modalities are presented with the goal of cost-effective and timely risk stratification. Finally, we present our current best-practice recommendations.

GLENOID BONE LOSS

In 1923, Bankart described an anterior capsulolabral injury that was the critical lesion in recurrent anterior instability in his classic paper, "Recurrent or Habitual

Abrams JS. *Management of the Unstable Shoulder: Arthroscopic and Open Repair* (pp. 135-148).
© 2011 SLACK Incorporated

Figure 10-1. Anterior glenoid bone loss results in recurrent anterior instability despite soft tissue fixation. (Reprinted with permission from Clavert PH, Millet PJ, Warner JJP. Traumatic anterior instability: open options. In: Warner JJP, Iannotti JP, Flatow EL, eds. *Complex and Revision Problems in Shoulder Surgery*. 2nd ed. Philadelphia, PA: Lippincott, Williams and Wilkins; 2005:23-52.)

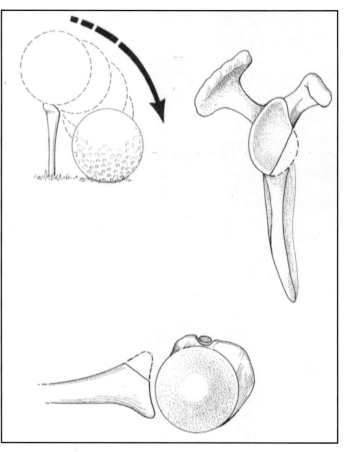

Dislocation of the Shoulder-Joint."[4] We have now come to understand that "Bankart" lesions are present in nearly 100% of first-time traumatic anterior shoulder dislocations. In recurrent cases, the importance of anterior glenoid bone loss has been elucidated in recent years.

The relationship between bone loss and failure of open Bankart repair was first noted in a 1978 report by Rowe and colleagues.[5] Burkhart and De Beer demonstrated that isolated arthroscopic Bankart repair has a significantly higher failure rate in the setting of anterior bone loss in contact athletes.[2] This has been confirmed by several subsequent investigators (Figure 10-1).[6] Therefore, preoperative evaluation of glenoid bone loss has critical implications regarding the type of surgical approach and must be understood by both the surgeon and patient preoperatively.

There are essentially 2 categories of anterior glenoid bone loss patterns in recurrent anterior shoulder dislocation. Most commonly, there is an abrasive erosion of the glenoid by the humeral head during multiple dislocation episodes. This results in anterior bone loss in the scapular plane, which clinically appears anteroinferior, given the flexed posture of the joint in the sagittal plane. The second type of loss is traumatic fracture. This may be a smaller "Bony Bankart" fragment or a larger glenoid fracture. The implication is that fracture results in an osseous fragment that may be anatomically repaired, as opposed to an abrasive lesion that necessitates bony reconstruction if it is of significant size and orientation.

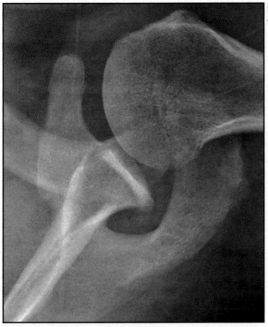

Figure 10-2. An axillary radiograph in the plane of the scapula demonstrates attritional bone loss.

X-ray

After dislocation, the standard of care is to obtain orthogonal anteroposterior and axillary views of the shoulder. This is a very accurate way to determine the adequacy of reduction, but typically underestimates anteroinferior bone loss.[7] This is because standard axillary films are taken in reference to the anatomic plane, not the scapular plane. To provide an orthogonal view of the anteroinferior glenoid, several views have been described, including the apical oblique,[8] West Point,[9] and Bernageau views.[10]

The West Point, or "modified axillary view," was first described by Rokous and colleagues in 1972.[9] The patient is prone with the film placed under the shoulder (Figure 10-2). The arm is adducted 90 degrees, and the elbow is flexed 90 degrees. The central beam projects 25 degrees below horizontal and 25 degrees medially to parallel the anteroinferior glenoid.

The Bernageau view is performed by maximally abducting the shoulder and flexing the elbow over the patient's head.[11] The beam is directed from the opposite side of the patient in the plane of the scapula and 30 degrees inferiorly tangent to the glenoid. This produces a sharp triangular outline of the glenoid. The "cliff sign" is apparent with attritional bone loss at the rim (Figure 10-3).

Most experts generally use radiography as a screening tool. For preoperative planning, advanced axial and parasagittal imaging is recommended.

Computed Tomography

CT is the gold standard for elucidating glenoid bone loss because it offers unparalleled delineation of complex bony pathology. When possible, we recommend 3-dimensional CT reconstruction. Some surgeons worry that the algorithm will "average" out fine detail, but with modern technology, this problem is not clinically relevant. Taken with the traditional axial and para-sagittal imaging, 3-dimensional reconstruction offers a complete understanding of traumatic bone loss.

Figure 10-3. (A) The Bernageau view is taken with the shoulder maximally abducted and results in a sharp outline of the osseous glenoid vault. (B) Bone loss is evident by a positive "cliff sign" versus the contralateral side. (Reprinted with permission from Gilles Walch, MD.)

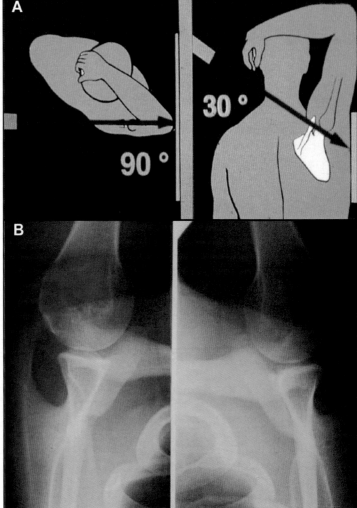

The literature is nearly universal that bony insufficiency will lead to an increased failure rate of isolated soft tissue procedures, but there is no agreement on a standard method of quantifying bone loss. Most authors agree, however, that 20% to 30% of glenoid bone loss leads to increased failure rates of soft tissue reconstruction.[12] We present 2 methods of measuring bone loss: one based on axial imaging and the other based on parasagittal imaging.

Axial CT is performed in the anatomic plane, 45 degrees retroverted from the scapular plane. Thus, the location of the bony deficit appears anteroinferior in the anatomic plane, when this finding is located anterior referenced to the shoulder. In 2005, Saito and colleagues demonstrated the finding that the defect is anterior with reference to the glenoid, or at the 3-o'clock position on a right shoulder, if the base of the coracoid is considered 12 o'clock.[13]

Saito and colleagues and Sugaya and coworkers have studied the anatomy and imaging of the glenoid extensively.[13,14] Given the orientation of the defect, they found that axial imaging below the coracoid tends to overestimate the defect size. Therefore,

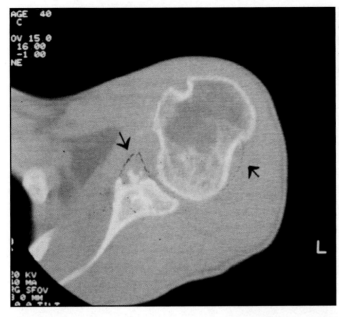

Figure 10-4. Axial CT accurately depicts the bony anatomy, but it may be difficult to judge precisely where the normal glenoid should be to quantitate the amount of bone loss.

a true 25% defect of the glenoid will appear on an axial image as a 50% defect if the cut corresponds to the bottom quarter of the glenoid.[7] However, it may be difficult to estimate where the intact anatomic edge of the glenoid should be in the absence of contralateral imaging (Figure 10-4).

Therefore, we prefer the "circle method" on CT scan. It allows for simple, reproducible measurement of readily-available para-sagittal or 3-dimensional unilateral CT scans and accounts for different orientations and magnitudes of bone loss (Figure 10-5). In the parasagittal view, the bottom of the intact glenoid makes a circle where the humeral head is centered and typically located. Sugaya et al use simple geometry to calculate the surface area of lost glenoid on computer-generated 3-dimensional reconstruction.[14]

We find the method published by Gerber and Nyffeler simple and reproducible.[15] The distance between the anatomic center of the glenoid and the edge of this circle (the radius) is measured (Figures 10-6 and 10-7). Then, a measurement is made of the length of the bony defect. If the length of the defect is equal to or larger than the radius, then the force required for dislocation after isolated Bankart repair is 70% less than the intact shoulder. This, in our opinion, is an indication for restoring bony anatomy by an autograft procedure.

Magnetic Resonance Imaging

MRI has several advantages in the setting of instability, including added sensitivity evaluating soft tissues, such as the ligaments, inferior capsule, rotator cuff, and labrum. In a recent cadaveric study, Huijsmans and colleagues demonstrated that 3-dimensional CT and sagittal MRI had identical rates of diagnosing glenoid bone loss and very high inter- and intraobserver reliability.[16] This validates the use of MRI in a controlled cadaveric model of bone loss.

Figure 10-5. Using the "circle method" on para-sagittal imaging allows for a more accurate estimation of bone loss without the need for contralateral images.

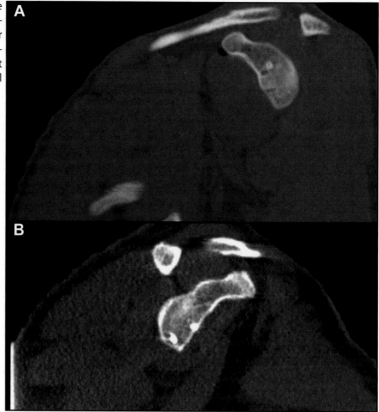

Figure 10-6. The method popularized by Gerber allows for rapid determination of the clinical relevance of bone loss. If the length of the defect (x) is greater than the radius (w/2), then we recommend allograft reconstruction. The 3-dimensional image in Figure 10-7 demonstrates such a case.

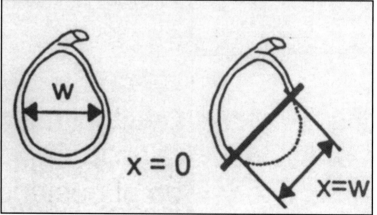

Diagnostic Arthroscopy

Direct arthroscopic visualization of the glenoid bone defect has been encouraged by Burkhart and colleagues,[17] Lo and coworkers,[18] and others. They recommend using the bare spot to approximate the center of the glenoid as a reference to measure the radius. Recently, authors have shown in a cadaver model that the bare spot is not a reliable estimate of the center of the joint.[19] Other investigators, in a larger cadaver study, have confirmed that the bare spot accurately approximates the center of the glenoid.[20] We agree with Provencher and colleagues that arthroscopy is an accurate method to

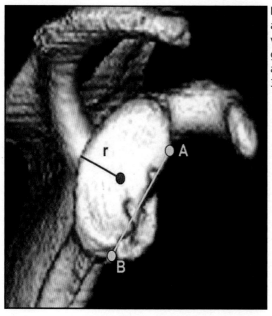

Figure 10-7. The method popularized by Gerber allows for rapid determination of the clinical relevance of bone loss. If the length of the defect (x) is greater than the radius (w/2), then we recommend allograft reconstruction (refer to Figure 10-6). The 3-dimensional image demonstrates such a case.

measure clinically relevant bone loss,[21] but we rarely use it in practice (Figure 10-8). There are no outcomes data that justify the added time, expense, and distortion of tissue planes that is caused by routine arthroscopy before open surgery. To the contrary, proponents of the open Latarjet coracoid transfer have demonstrated excellent results without diagnostic arthroscopy in thousands of cases.

Determining Glenoid Version

Version should be measured on an axial image at the midpoint of the glenoid (generally just below the coracoid root). Glenoid version is the angle subtended by a line drawn across the face of the glenoid and a line perpendicular to the scapular spine. In rare cases, excessive congenital or acquired glenoid version may play a role in instability.[22,23] The only reliable way to evaluate this is with axial CT or MRI, as axillary x-ray has been shown to overestimate retroversion and have poor correlation with CT measurements (Figure 10-9).[24]

HUMERAL HEAD

In the late 1800s, case reports described a "typical defect" consisting of a groove on the posterior aspect of the humeral head noted after humeral head resection as treatment for recurrent shoulder dislocation. In the early 1900s, investigators confirmed its presence using radiographic technology. Hill and Sachs reported this finding in their classic 1940 article, "The Grooved Defect of the Humeral Head: A Frequently Unrecognized Complication of Dislocations of the Shoulder Joint."[25] While other authors had previously described this pathology, Hill and Sachs correctly described it as a compression fracture produced by the relatively osteopenic humeral head resting on the dense anterior glenoid. Thus, their name is now associated with this pathologic lesion (Figure 10-10).

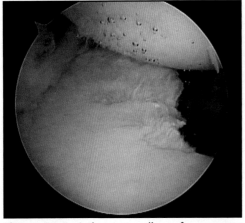

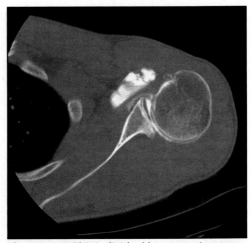

Figure 10-8. Arthroscopy allows for accurate determination of glenoid bone loss, but routine arthroscopy has not improved clinical outcomes in the literature.

Figure 10-9. This individual has excessive posterior glenoid version contributing to symptomatic posterior glenoid subluxation that was successfully treated with opening wedge osteotomy.

Figure 10-10. The Hill-Sachs lesion is an acquired compression fracture on the posterior humeral head.

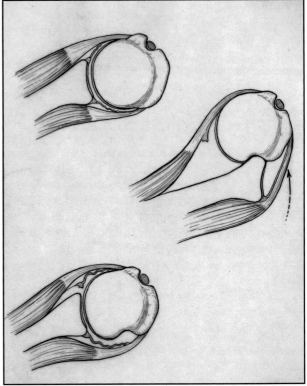

The reported incidence of Hill-Sachs lesion is approximately 50% in first-time dislocators[26] and more than 90% in patients with recurrent anterior shoulder instability. Small lesions have a trivial effect on shoulder stability, but larger lesions may contribute to symptomatic subluxation, crepitus, and frank dislocation. Therefore, it is important to evaluate this in both the first-time and multiple dislocator.

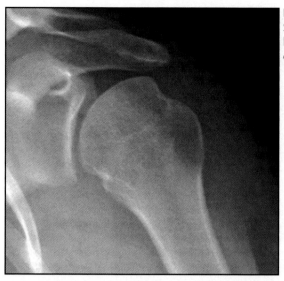

Figure 10-11. Internal rotation brings the Hill-Sachs lesion into profile and away from the bony metaphysis, which may obscure it on standard AP radiographs.

Unlike glenoid bone loss, the literature varies widely on what constitutes a "significant" Hill-Sachs defect, with values ranging from 20% to 40%.[12] We believe this is because both the magnitude of bone loss and the orientation of the deficit are clinically relevant. Hill-Sachs lesions are evaluated by x-ray, CT, MRI, and direct open or arthroscopic visualization.

X-ray

Radiography has been shown to be less accurate than axial imaging or arthroscopy for visualizing humeral head impaction fractures. However, only large Hill-Sachs lesions are likely to be symptomatic. Thus, plain radiography is a good screening tool for large Hill-Sachs lesions.

In the anatomic position, the compressive lesion is generally located on the posterior humeral head, oriented from superior-lateral to inferior-medial, although this varies depending on the position of the arm at the time of dislocation. The optimal screening radiograph is an anteroposterior view with the arm in internal rotation. Internal rotation brings the defect perpendicular to the beam x-ray, so it is outlined and not obscured by the bony humeral metaphysis (Figure 10-11).

Computed Tomography

Computerized tomography is considered the gold standard for noninvasive evaluation of Hill-Sachs lesions. On an axial image, the size of the wedge-shaped lesion is determined as a percentage of the circular intact humeral head. The precise size and shape of the defect may be appreciated as a planning tool for bony reconstruction (Figures 10-12 and 10-13).

Magnetic Resonance Imaging

MRI has been shown to have 100% sensitivity for Hill-Sachs lesions with arthroscopy as a gold standard. The correlation of defect size with CT and arthroscopy is poor, so we use CT for preoperative planning in our practice.

Figure 10-12. This patient had symptoms despite reduction of a fixed posterior dislocation. We used this CT scan to template open osteochondral allograft reconstruction of the defect (refer also to Figure 10-13).

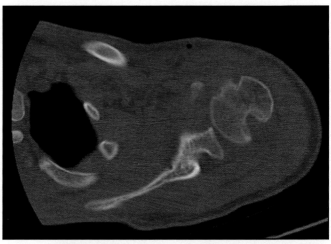

Figure 10-13. This patient had symptoms despite reduction of a fixed posterior dislocation. We used this CT scan to template open osteochondral allograft reconstruction of the defect (refer also to Figure 10-12).

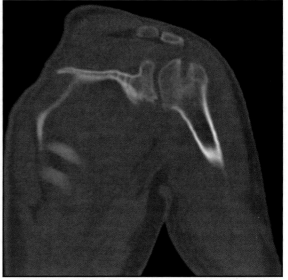

Arthroscopy

Dynamic arthroscopy allows the surgeon to accurately determine the clinical relevance of a humeral head compression fracture. Viewing from a standard posterior portal, the humerus is manually abducted and externally rotated while visualizing the glenohumeral articulation. This establishes whether the Hill-Sachs lesion is of adequate size and orientation to "engage" the glenoid (Figure 10-14). Engaging lesions require intervention to ensure that the patient does not have symptomatic crepitus, locking, or subluxation.[2] This can be achieved by increasing the anteroposterior dimension of the glenoid, filling the defect, or performing capsular plication.

PHYSICAL EXAMINATION

A detailed history and physical examination are critical for planning purposes and stratifying recurrence risk after repair. Boileau and colleagues elegantly presented

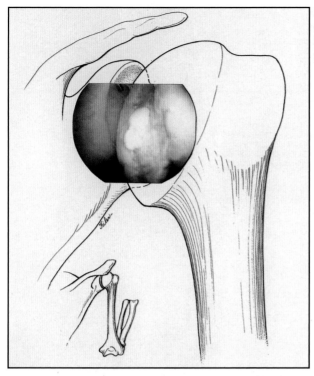

Figure 10-14. Arthroscopy allows for dynamic testing to determine if the Hill-Sachs lesion "engages" the anterior glenoid.

these factors in a 2006 *JBJS* study.[3] Patients with more than 90 degrees of external rotation with the elbow at the side may have anterior capsular hyperlaxity, requiring interval closure or capsular placation. The Gagey test evaluates plastic deformation of the inferior capsule and inferior glenohumeral ligament. A positive test is an independent risk factor for failure of arthroscopic Bankart repair.[3] A positive Gagey test is defined as more than 10 degrees difference in hyperabduction between the affected and contralateral side (Figures 10-15).[27]

In a pilot study, the "bony apprehension test" has been shown to predict large osseous anterior glenoid lesions. Apprehension, not pain, at 45 degrees of abduction and 45 degrees of external rotation should prompt the surgeon to order axial imaging in order to evaluate the glenoid. This has not been confirmed by other examiners or a larger study.

Neurovascular examination of the affected extremity must also be documented, as transient neuropraxia is common following shoulder dislocation.

AUTHOR'S PREFERRED METHOD

All patients with a history of instability are screened with standard anteroposterior radiographs in internal and external rotation, as well as an axillary radiograph. A detailed physical examination is mandatory. Advanced imaging is ordered in the following cases:

- History of recurrent instability
- Instability with minimal force (eg, sleep)
- Planned operative management

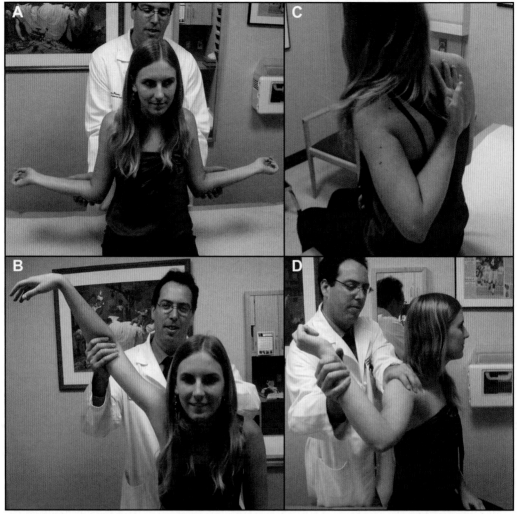

Figure 10-15. This individual has laxity in the rotator interval, noted by more than 90 degrees of external rotation with the elbow at the side. Her inferior capsule is also relaxed, noted by abduction over 90 degrees with the scapula stabilized. She also has evidence of general ligamentous laxity.

In individuals younger than 40 years old, CT arthrogram is ordered as it is economical, expedient, and provides information about the bony architecture, labrum, cartilage, and full-thickness rotator cuff tears. In patients older than 40 years, rotator cuff tears often coincide with instability. Therefore, MR arthrogram is our study of choice for this age group.

REFERENCES

1. Bigliani LU, Newton PM, Steinmann SP, Connor PM, McLlveen SJ. Glenoid rim lesions associated with recurrent anterior dislocation of the shoulder. *Am J Sports Med.* 1998;26(1):41-45.
2. Burkhart SS, De Beer JF. Traumatic glenohumeral bone defects and their relationship to failure of arthroscopic Bankart repairs: significance of the inverted-pear glenoid and the humeral engaging Hill-Sachs lesion. *Arthroscopy.* 2000;16(7):677-694.

3. Boileau P, Villalba M, Hery JY, Balg F, Ahrens P, Neyton L. Risk factors for recurrence of shoulder instability after arthroscopic Bankart repair. *J Bone Joint Surg Am.* 2006;88(8):1755-1763.
4. Bankart A. Recurrent or habitual dislocation of the shoulder joint. *Br Med J.* 1923;2:1132-1133.
5. Rowe CR, Patel D, Southmayd WW. The Bankart procedure: a long-term end-result study. *J Bone Joint Surg Am.* 1978;60(1):1-16.
6. Mologne TS, Provencher MT, Menzel KA, Vachon TA, Dewing CB. Arthroscopic stabilization in patients with an inverted pear glenoid: results in patients with bone loss of the anterior glenoid. *Am J Sports Med.* 2007;35(8):1276-1283.
7. Itoi E, Lee SB, Amrami KK, Wenger DE, An KN. Quantitative assessment of classic anteroinferior bony Bankart lesions by radiography and computed tomography. *Am J Sports Med.* 2003;31(1):112-118.
8. Garth WP Jr, Slappey CE, Ochs CW. Roentgenographic demonstration of instability of the shoulder: the apical oblique projection. A technical note. *J Bone Joint Surg Am.* 1984;66(9):1450-1453.
9. Rokous JR, Feagin JA, Abbott HG. Modified axillary roentgenogram. A useful adjunct in the diagnosis of recurrent instability of the shoulder. *Clin Orthop Relat Res.* 1972;82:84-86.
10. Bernageau J, Patte D, Debeyre J, Ferrane J. Value of the glenoid profile in recurrent luxations of the shoulder. *Rev Chir Orthop Reparatrice Appar Mot.* 1976;62(2 suppl):142-147.
11. Edwards TB, Boulahia A, Walch G. Radiographic analysis of bone defects in chronic anterior shoulder instability. *Arthroscopy.* 2003;19(7):732-739.
12. Bushnell BD, Creighton RA, Herring MM. Bony instability of the shoulder. *Arthroscopy.* 2008;24(9):1061-1073.
13. Saito H, Itoi E, Sugaya H, Minagawa H, Yamamoto N, Tuoheti Y. Location of the glenoid defect in shoulders with recurrent anterior dislocation. *Am J Sports Med.* 2005;33(6):889-893.
14. Sugaya H, Moriishi J, Dohi M, Kon Y, Tsuchiya A. Glenoid rim morphology in recurrent anterior glenohumeral instability. *J Bone Joint Surg Am.* 2003;85-A(5):878-884.
15. Gerber C, Nyffeler RW. Classification of glenohumeral joint instability. *Clin Orthop Relat Res.* 2002;400:65-76.
16. Huijsmans PE, Haen PS, Kidd M, Dhert WJ, van der Hulst VP, Willems WJ. Quantification of a glenoid defect with three-dimensional computed tomography and magnetic resonance imaging: a cadaveric study. *J Shoulder Elbow Surg.* 2007;16(6):803-809.
17. Burkhart SS, De Beer JF, Tehrany AM, Parten PM. Quantifying glenoid bone loss arthroscopically in shoulder instability. *Arthroscopy.* 2002;18(5):488-491.
18. Lo IK, Parten PM, Burkhart SS. The inverted pear glenoid: an indicator of significant glenoid bone loss. *Arthroscopy.* 2004;20(2):169-174.
19. Kralinger F, Aigner F, Longato S, Rieger M, Wambacher M. Is the bare spot a consistent landmark for shoulder arthroscopy? A study of 20 embalmed glenoids with 3-dimensional computed tomographic reconstruction. *Arthroscopy.* 2006;22(4):428-432.
20. Huysmans PE, Haen PS, Kidd M, Dhert WJ, Willems JW. The shape of the inferior part of the glenoid: a cadaveric study. *J Shoulder Elbow Surg.* 2006;15(6):759-763.
21. Provencher MT, Detterline AJ, Ghodadra N, et al. Measurement of glenoid bone loss: a comparison of measurement error between 45 degrees and 0 degrees bone loss models and with different posterior arthroscopy portal locations. *Am J Sports Med.* 2008;36(6):1132-1138.
22. Brewer BJ, Wubben RC, Carrera GF. Excessive retroversion of the glenoid cavity. A cause of non-traumatic posterior instability of the shoulder. *J Bone Joint Surg Am.* 1986;68(5):724-731.
23. Weishaupt D, Zanetti M, Nyffeler RW, Gerber C, Hodler J. Posterior glenoid rim deficiency in recurrent (atraumatic) posterior shoulder instability. *Skeletal Radiol.* 2000;29(4):204-210.
24. Nyffeler RW, Jost B, Pfirrmann CW, Gerber C. Measurement of glenoid version: conventional radiographs versus computed tomography scans. *J Shoulder Elbow Surg.* 2003;12(5):493-496.
25. Hill HA, Sachs MD. The grooved defect of the humeral head: a frequently unrecognized complication of dislocations of the shoulder joint. *Radiology.* 1940;35:690-700.
26. Calandra JJ, Baker CL, Uribe J. The incidence of Hill-Sachs lesions in initial anterior shoulder dislocations. *Arthroscopy.* 1989;5(4):254-257.
27. Gagey OJ, Gagey N. The hyperabduction test. *J Bone Joint Surg Br.* 2001;83(1):69-74.

11

Applying a Soft Tissue Repair in a Chronic Unstable Shoulder With Bone Loss

Robert T. Burks, MD

The effects of bone loss in shoulder stability have become a topic of significant interest in the past few years. A quick review of the literature shows only one article on bone loss from 1990 to 2000,[1] but since 2000, more than 12 articles on bone loss and shoulder stability have been published.[2-5] These articles have recognized that an important reason for failure in some stability surgeries is inadequate bone on the glenoid and/or humeral side of the joint (Figure 11-1). Although it is clearly a true statement to say that there are levels of bone loss that are simply too great for soft tissue procedures to successfully stabilize, the issues are 1) how significant does bone loss need to be, 2) how often is bone loss really an issue, and 3) can soft tissue surgery solve some of these bone loss problems?

In determining how much glenoid bone loss is important, Burkhart and De Beer and Lo and colleagues described the inverted pear as seen on arthroscopy.[6,7] This represents the inferior aspect of the glenoid appearing somewhat narrower than the superior aspect of the glenoid and would represent an approximate 25% loss of glenoid width inferiorly (Figure 11-2). The authors use the bare area of the glenoid as a marker for the center of the glenoid. Because a glenoid could be estimated to average 26 mm from anterior to posterior in the inferior aspect, the authors felt the inverted pear would imply a bone loss of 6 mm to 7 mm and was significant. Boileau and colleagues studied 90 patients and stated that glenoid bone loss greater than 25% was associated with an increased recurrence rate.[8] The amount of bone loss was estimated from traditional computed tomography (CT) cuts, and Hill-Sachs lesions were grossly described as clinically "important."[8] Kim and colleagues reviewed a large series of patients treated with an arthroscopic Bankart and felt that more than 30% loss of the entire glenoid circumference was associated with increased recurrence.[9]

Because bone loss can be somewhat difficult to evaluate, in particular in a preoperative setting, preoperative CT imaging has been suggested as a means of helping the evaluation.[10,11] Sugaya and colleagues evaluated anterior glenoid injuries by CT scan and also separately reported on repairing glenoid rim fractures arthroscopically.[12,13]

Abrams JS. *Management of the Unstable Shoulder: Arthroscopic and Open Repair* (pp. 149-154). © 2011 SLACK Incorporated

Figure 11-1. CT exam of the shoulder with 2 prior failed stabilization attempts, including a Bristow procedure. In the CT reconstruction, one can see that less than 50% of the glenoid is intact and present.

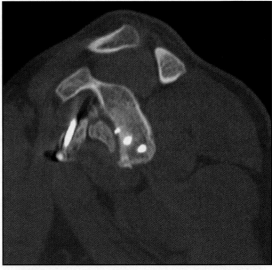

Figure 11-2. This is an arthroscopic view demonstrating an inverted pear and the absence of bone anterior to the bare area of the glenoid. (Reprinted with permission of Stephen Burkhart, MD.)

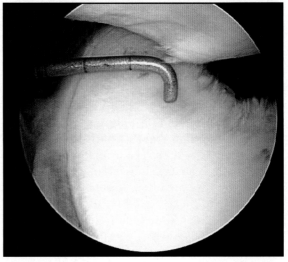

They described methods of measuring bone loss with an "en face" glenoid reconstruction, and further details are provided in other chapters on bone loss. Warner and colleagues also published an approach to measure glenoid bone loss by CT scan where the length of the area of bone loss was greater than the normal radius of the glenoid.[14] All of these methods enable the surgeon to determine, on the glenoid side, if there is significant bone loss in the approximate 25% or more range.

Hill-Sachs lesions have been less extensively measured but also play a role with bone loss. Burkhart and De Beer have described the "engaging" Hill-Sachs lesion and its contribution to increased failure after arthroscopic repair.[6] CT scanning again is a good tool to help evaluate humerus bone loss as well. However, exact quantification of total bone loss of the humeral head that will change treatment has not been determined. For example, a significant Hill-Sachs lesion of the engaging variety with a 10% glenoid bone loss could perhaps be more of a problem than a shoulder with a small Hill-Sachs lesion and 20% of the glenoid absent. In characterizing Hill-Sachs lesions, Boileau and colleagues described them as potentially clinically "important" with no further quantification.[8] So, in summary, it would seem that most authors have felt that having more than about 25% glenoid bone loss would be the level beyond which soft tissue surgery would have a high failure rate and some type of bony replacement would be suggested. The exact amount of humeral bone loss that is critical has been less studied.

So, if more than 25% of glenoid bone loss becomes the area of concern, how often does that really present? Burkhart and De Beer published an article on 194 patients who had arthroscopic anterior shoulder repair and had 21 patients, or 11%, with significant bone loss on the glenoid or humeral side.[6] Multiple other authors have shown that significant bone loss (approximately 25% or more of the glenoid) occurs in approximately 6% to 8% of their patients.[1,13,15,16] Pagnani recently published a study of 119 patients and had only 4% with a glenoid lesion greater than 20%.[17] Obviously, it depends on the surgeon's practice profile, but it would appear from these publications that significant bone loss is not a highly common problem and can range from as little as less than 1% to not much more than 11% of anterior shoulder instabilities that are encountered. So, although a lot has been written on this topic, for practical purposes, the incidence of a significant bone lesion needing to be addressed is low.

The final question in addressing this level of bone loss is whether soft tissue repair can be good enough in some of these cases when bone loss is present. Clearly, patient selection is going to be an issue. In the Burkhart and De Beer article, the bone loss patients had a 67% recurrence rate, but consisted of 88% male patients, and 52% were contact athletes.[6] Ninety-five percent of the contact athletes were South African rugby players, and 89% of the rugby players with bone defect failed. However, this recurrence rate with bone loss might not be as applicable in a less active individual or in an older individual, for example.

So, if significant bone loss is encountered, can soft tissue repair alone be considered? Rowe and colleagues published a study on 158 shoulders with an open soft tissue repair. Seventy-three percent had a damaged glenoid rim, and yet their overall recurrence rate with a soft tissue procedure was only 3.5%.[16] In their patients who they felt had an average glenoid bone loss of 17% to 33%, the patients had 98% good and excellent results with a soft tissue repair and only one recurrence. Bigliani and colleagues evaluated a series of patients with anterior glenoid rim injury.[1] In some of their patients, they were able to repair the bone piece back to the glenoid, but in others, they were only able to do a soft tissue repair back to the glenoid, accepting the amount of bone loss. Only one of their 25 patients with a greater than 25% deficit required a Bristow procedure, thus most of the patients were managed with just a soft tissue repair. Sugaya and colleagues published on placing small fractured glenoid fragments back to the glenoid and have shown that they heal and the recurrence rate with this replacement is very low.[12] In his study, the average bone loss was 25%, and the fragment that was replaced was only 9%. Yet, with replacing the smaller fragment and repairing the soft tissue, they had only a 5% redislocation rate. Mologne and colleagues looked at 21 active-duty military patients who had an inverted pear and so were thought to have at least a 25% bone loss.[15] In half the patients, they were able to re-incorporate a bone fragment as Sugaya had performed and had no failures. In half the patients, they were unable to repair a bone fragment and performed only an arthroscopic soft tissue repair. They had a 15% failure rate with 2 subluxations and one redislocation; however, there was only one reoperation in this group. Again, it would seem that repairing the bone fragment if possible is desirable, but with at least doing a good soft tissue repair, the success rate was far higher than what was shown in the series of Burkhart and De Beer. Finally, Pagnani recently showed very satisfactory results when performing an open pure soft tissue repair even in the presence of

Figure 11-3. AP radiograph of the left shoulder showing multiple aspects of a failed Bristow procedure. There is loose hardware, nonunion, and degenerative change in the shoulder.

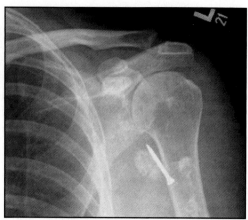

some significant bone loss.[17] He directly questioned the need for bone addition in most cases that present with instability. A final soft tissue adjunct that could be considered to add to a soft tissue repair in lieu of bone grafting is the arthroscopic "Remplissage" introduced by Gene Wolf.[18] This is a way to potentially decrease the negative effects of a Hill-Sachs lesion with significant humeral bone loss. It has yet to be shown how effective this procedure will be when applied to a large patient population, but it is a soft tissue addition that can be considered.

When considering adding bone as part of the procedure, either via a coracoid or iliac graft, there certainly are significant complications, which can include loss of motion, extensive scarring, nonunion, hardware complications, alteration of normal anatomy, increased complexity of revision surgery, and the potential for arthritis with malpositioned bone or screws. Authors such as Young and Rockwood,[19] Allain and colleagues,[20] Zuckerman and Matsen,[21] and Ferlic and DiGlovine[22] have all shown significant hardware problems, nonunions, malunions of bone fragments, and other complications (Figure 11-3). If adding bone might be considered in only 1 in 10 to 20 anterior stabilization procedures, it will be an infrequent technique for most surgeons and therefore can add significant possible morbidity over the more commonly performed soft tissue procedure. There will be cases of major bone loss or bone loss with prior failed surgery where adding bone will be a logical step. However, there will be many more "borderline" cases, and the surgeon has ample published information that soft tissue repair alone can be adequate treatment. This can be done arthroscopically or open depending on the surgeon's experience and preference.

For soft tissue repairs done open or arthroscopically, the repair of bone fragments attached to labrum and capsule are very helpful. When performing open soft tissue repairs, the techniques outlined by Rowe and colleagues[16] and Pagnani[17] have proven track records. For arthroscopic repair, the attention to detail outlined by Mologne and colleagues should be considered.[15] The basic technique of arthroscopic Bankart repair is performed with the inclusion of capsular plication anteriorly and/or posteriorly as needed. This is a case where rotator interval closure may need to be considered as well (see Chapter 11 video). With bone loss, the extra tightening required in the soft tissue will not likely lead to some loss of external rotation. This will not likely cause major restriction, but should be discussed with the patient preoperatively. Otherwise, the techniques are the same as have been shown in many settings and are illustrated in other chapters in this book.

In summary, it would seem that bone loss is a real issue, but the incidence of significant bone loss (more than 25% of the glenoid) requiring attention is fairly low.

Incorporation of glenoid bone fragments in a soft tissue repair gives good results and should be considered preferable to altering local anatomy through bone grafting. Reports of open, or even arthroscopic, soft tissue repairs in the face of bone loss are actually quite reasonable. We might review the literature and feel that recurrent instability is somewhat increased in the setting of bone loss, but the recurrence and reoperation rates are very low when compared with the 67% failure rate of Burkhart and De Beer. Complications of bone replacement procedures are real. This is especially true for an operation that would be infrequently performed by most surgeons. Careful preoperative planning is important in trying to determine if adding bone would be necessary. Clearly, in the failed prior instability case, possibly addressing bone deficiency should be considered much more strongly. However, in the initial treatment, it appears soft tissue procedures in many shoulders still have a good track record.

REFERENCES

1. Bigliani LU, Newton PM, Steinmann SP, Connor PM, McIlveen SJ. Glenoid rim lesions associated with recurrent anterior dislocation of the shoulder. *Am J Sports Med.* 1998;26(1):41-46.
2. Chen AL, Hunt SA, Hawkins RJ, Zuckerman JD. Management of bone loss associated with recurrent anterior glenohumeral instability. *Am J Sports Med.* 2005;33(6):912-925.
3. Itoi H, Lee S, Berglund LJ, Berge LL, An K. The effect of a glenoid defect on anteroinferior stability of the shoulder after Bankart repair: a cadaveric study. *J Bone Joint Surg.* 2000;82A(1):35-46.
4. Millett PJ, Clavert P, Warner JP. Open operative treatment for anterior shoulder instability: when and why? *J Bone Joint Surg.* 2005;87A(2):419-432.
5. Porcellini G, Campi F, Paladini P. Arthroscopic approach to acute bony Bankart lesion. *Arthroscopy.* 2002;18(7):764-769.
6. Burkhart SS, De Beer JF. Traumatic glenohumeral bone defects and their relationship to failure of arthroscopic Bankart repairs: significance of the inverted-pear glenoid and the humeral engaging Hill-Sachs lesion. *Arthroscopy.* 2000;16(7):677-694.
7. Lo IKY, Parten PM, Burkhart SS. The inverted pear glenoid: an indicator of significant glenoid bone loss. *Arthroscopy.* 2004;20(2):169-174.
8. Boileau P, Villalba M, Hery JY, et al. Risk factors for recurrence of shoulder instability after arthroscopic Bankart repair. *J Bone Joint Surg.* 2006;88A(8):1755-1763.
9. Kim S, Ha K, Cho Y, Ryu B, Oh I. Arthroscopic anterior stabilization of the shoulder. *J Bone Joint Surg.* 2003;85A(8):1511-1518.
10. Griffith JF, Antonio GE, Tong CW, Ming CK. Anterior shoulder dislocation: quantification of glenoid bone loss with CT. *AJR.* 2003;180:1423-1430.
11. Provencher MT, Detterline AJ, Ghodadra N, et al. Measurement of glenoid bone loss: a comparison of measurement error between 45° and 0° bone loss models and with different posterior arthroscopy portal locations. *Am J Sports Med.* 2008;36(6):1132-1138.
12. Sugaya H, Moriishi J, Kanisawa I, Tsuchiya A. Arthroscopic osseous Bankart repair for chronic recurrent traumatic anterior glenohumeral instability. *J Bone Joint Surg.* 2006;87A(8):1752-1760.
13. Sugaya H, Moriishi J, Dohi M, Kon Y, Tsuchiya A. Glenoid rim morphology in recurrent anterior glenohumeral instability. *J Bone Joint Surg.* 2003;85A(5):878-884.
14. Warner JP, Gill TJ, O'Hollerhan JD, Pathare N, Millett PJ. Anatomical glenoid reconstruction for recurrent anterior glenohumeral instability with glenoid deficiency using an autogenous tricortical iliac crest bone graft. *Am J Sports Med.* 2006;34(2):205-212.
15. Mologne TS, Provencher MT, Menzel KA. Arthroscopic stabilization in patients with an inverted pear glenoid. Results in patients with bone loss of the anterior glenoid. *Am J Sports Med.* 2007;35(8):1276-1283.
16. Rowe CR, Patel D, Southmayd WW. The Bankart procedure. A long-term end-result study. *J Bone Joint Surg.* 1978;60A(1):1-16.
17. Pagnani MJ. Open capsular repair without bone block for recurrent anterior shoulder instability in patients with and without bony defects of the glenoid and/or humeral head. *Am J Sports Med.* 2008;36(9):1805-1812.
18. Purchase RJ, Wolf EM, Hobgood ER, et al. Technical note: Hill-Sachs "Remplissage": an arthroscopic solution for the engaging Hill-Sachs lesion. *Arthroscopy.* 2008;24(6):723-726.

19. Young DC, Rockwood CA. Complications of a failed Bristow procedure and their management. *J Bone Joint Surg.* 1993;73A(7):969-980.

20. Allain J, Goutallier D, Glorion C. Long-term results of the Latarjet procedure for the treatment of anterior instability of the shoulder. *J Bone Joint Surg.* 1998;80A(6):841-852.

21. Zuckerman JD, Matsen FA. Complications about the glenohumeral joint related to the use of screws and staples. *J Bone Joint Surg.* 1984;66A(2):175-180.

22. Ferlic DC, DiGlovine NM. A long-term retrospective study of the modified Bristow procedure. *Am J Sports Med.* 1988;16(5):469-474.

SUGGESTED READING

Hayashida K, Yoneda M, Nakagawa S, Okamura K, Fukushima S. Arthroscopic Bankart suture repair for traumatic anterior shoulder instability: analysis of the cause of recurrence. *Arthroscopy.* 1998;14(3):295-301.

Ide J, Maeda S, Takagi K. Arthroscopic Bankart repair using suture anchors in athletes. *Am J Sports Med.* 2004;32(8):1899-1905.

Please see video on the accompanying Web site at http://www.slackbooks.com/unstableshouldervideos

12

Arthroscopic Latarjet Graft Technique

Laurent Lafosse, MD and Simon Boyle, MSc, FRCS (Tr and Orth)

Anterior shoulder instability is a common problem for which the operative treatment options have expanded considerably in the past 20 years. Arthroscopy has led to the improved diagnosis of previously unrecognized soft tissue lesions underlying many cases of instability. In combination with radiological investigations, arthroscopy has also improved the awareness of bony lesions of both the glenoid and humeral head and their contribution to shoulder instability.

However, despite the advancement in techniques and instruments and improvements in surgical training, there still remains a significant failure rate when surgical procedures inadequately address the underlying pathology. The open Latarjet procedure has shown excellent and reliable results as published by several authors. The natural evolution of this procedure was to develop an all-arthroscopic technique to confer all the advantages that this type of surgery offers.

PRINCIPLES AND SURGICAL GOALS

Operative Bankart repair, both open and arthroscopic, has demonstrated excellent results when used for isolated soft tissue Bankart lesions. However, in cases of unrecognized soft tissue injury, such as humeral avulsion of glenohumeral ligament (HAGL) lesions, complex labral disruptions, irreparable soft tissue damage, and in cases of bony deficiency, this technique may not be sufficient to stabilize the shoulder. This concern has been raised by a number of authors after several years of follow-up, particularly with regard to young patients (20 years and younger) and those involved in overhead or contact sports.[1]

A study in 2006 by Boileau and colleagues[2] highlighted several reasons for failure of the Bankart procedure for anterior instability. The most important risk factors identified were bone loss on the glenoid or humeral sides and inferior ligament hyperlaxity (as indicated by an asymmetric hyperabduction test). This is often a result of

Abrams JS. *Management of the Unstable Shoulder: Arthroscopic and Open Repair* (pp. 155-170).
© 2011 SLACK Incorporated

stretching from the initial dislocation. A combination of these abnormalities can result in up to a 75% recurrence of instability after soft tissue repair.

It seems clear, therefore, that a simple Bankart repair, which reduces the labrum back onto the glenoid, cannot be expected to return soft tissue stability to the shoulder when the glenohumeral ligaments are torn or attenuated. Further to this, where there is glenoid bone loss or an engaging Hill-Sachs lesion, a soft tissue repair does not lengthen the glenoid articular arc, which is necessary to prevent future engagement and recurrent symptoms. In these situations, another approach must be adopted.

Once it is determined that an isolated soft tissue repair will not be sufficient, then bone block procedures should be considered. In 1954, Latarjet described his technique of transferring the horizontal part of the coracoid to the anteroinferior margin of the glenoid from the 2 o'clock to the 6 o'clock position.[3] The original procedure required the upper part of subscapularis to be detached, but this has since been modified to place the graft through a horizontal split in the subscapularis and to fix this preferably with 2 screws. Patte explained the success of the open Latarjet procedure by virtue of the triple blocking effect. We interpret the triple block effect first by the bony reconstruction of the anterior glenoid, which serves to increase the glenoid articular arc. This prevents an otherwise engaging Hill-Sachs lesion from levering on the potentially deficient anteroinferior glenoid rim. Second, the split subscapularis tendon provides dynamic stability in abduction and external rotation due to the tension created by its intersection with the newly positioned conjoint tendon. Finally, the capsule is attached to the remnant of the coracoacromial (CAL) ligament on the coracoid.

Indications/Patient Selection

After a detailed history, clinical examination, and radiological investigations are performed, the following scenarios may become apparent.

1. *Instability with glenoid bone loss*: This is a common cause for recurrent instability and can be manifested by a bony Bankart lesion or a true fracture of the anterior or inferior glenoid rim. Standard anteroposterior radiographs may show a fracture or a more subtle loss of contour of the anteroinferior glenoid rim. A decrease in the apparent density of the inferior glenoid line often signifies an erosion of the glenoid rim between 3 and 6 o'clock. An axillary view or, better, a Bernageau view may show flattening of this area of the glenoid when bone loss has occurred. CT provides a more detailed imaging modality that is essential to quantify the bone loss[4] preoperatively. These CT reconstructions provide more robust static measurements than those afforded by the arthroscopic view. Arthroscopically, the distance from the glenoid rim as measured from the bare spot can assist the surgeon in identifying an inverted pear glenoid, confirming substantial bone loss[5] and the likely failure of an isolated soft tissue repair.

   Even when the bony fragment is present, replacing it is not always sufficient to restore the bony glenoid articular arc due to the difficulties in healing of this necrotic bone. In these cases, a bone reconstruction as performed by Latarjet procedure should be considered

2. *Instability with humeral bone loss*: The location and size of the Hill-Sachs lesion determines whether the articular arc is reduced and whether this will engage on the glenoid. A dynamic arthroscopy with the shoulder in abduction and external rotation will demonstrate whether the lesion is engaging even within an athletic overhead range of movement. A bone block procedure here will increase the arc of the anterior glenoid, thereby increasing the degree of external rotation that can

be achieved before the lesion approaches the glenoid rim. An alternative to this would be the infraspinatus and posterior capsule Remplissage as described by Purchase and colleagues.[6]

We consider that, by enlarging the glenoid articular arc with a bone graft, there is no increased joint contact pressure during external rotation. A Remplissage, however, can lead to a decrease in external rotation and may give rise to increased contact forces on the articular cartilage during external rotation.

3. *Combinations of glenoid and humeral bone loss*: These 2 lesions usually occur in tandem with varying degrees of severity for each individual lesion. Preoperative radiographs and CT usually detect the lesions, but arthroscopic dynamic evaluation of stability is necessary to determine the likely clinical effects of this combination.

4. *Complex soft tissue injury*: HAGL lesions can be diagnosed on preoperative CT arthrograms or MRI, but often these injuries are discovered on the initial arthroscopic evaluation. There are numerous techniques described for the arthroscopic repair of HAGL lesions; however, most case series are small with only short follow-up periods. Our experience using an all-arthroscopic soft tissue repair technique with anchors has been disappointing due to the postoperative stiffness experienced by some patients.

Furthermore, in patients with multiple dislocations, the intrinsic structure of the glenohumeral ligaments is usually deranged, although this may not be evident macroscopically. Simply repairing this damaged tissue to the glenoid does not restore stability to the shoulder. This has been likened to rehanging a baggy or incompetent hammock.

A final situation is that of the labral tear, often in association with a glenohumeral ligament lesion. In this situation, the ring of the labrum is disrupted, and the strength of a repair will be unable to match that of an intact labral ring.

In these situations, there is a real need for a ligamentoplasty and accompanying bone block.

5. *Revision of Bankart repair*: After an open or arthroscopic Bankart repair, success is often measured by the absence of recurrent dislocations. In some cases, the joint is not sufficiently stabilized, but it does allow function for a more sedentary lifestyle without overt symptoms of instability. This can in part explain the excellent results seen in series with a short follow-up. After 5 to 7 years, we find this particular group of patients can go on to develop instability and/or arthritis. In these cases, the initial operation was considered successful, although the pathological lesion was never truly corrected and the glenoid subsequently becomes increasingly eroded. Again, these patients can be successfully managed with a bone block ligamentoplasty.

6. *Patient activity*: There are some patients who play high-risk sports (climbing, rugby), engage in high-risk occupations (carpentry), or have a high risk of recurrence due to the intensity and action of their activity (throwers). The Latarjet procedure provides a strong stabilization mechanism and fast recovery time for these individuals.

Why a Latarjet Procedure Versus a Free Bone Graft?

It has been previously demonstrated that the sling effect of the conjoint tendon crossing the subscapularis has a significant effect on the shoulder stability.[7] This is best demonstrated by considering that the further the shoulder goes to external rotation, the more the conjoint tendon will stabilize the shoulder through its increased tension and sling effect over the inferior subscapularis muscle. This added important soft tissue stabilizing effect is not seen when free bone block transfers are performed.

Why a Latarjet Versus a Modified Bristow Procedure?

Initially, Bristow's description included only the suturing of the detached tip of the coracoid inside the muscle belly of subscapularis. This was modified to employ a single screw fixation of the coracoid in a standing position. The Latarjet procedure applies the coracoid process in a lying position, allowing the natural shape of the inferior coracoid surface to follow the contour of the anterior glenoid. This is then secured and compressed by a double screw system to encourage bony union and solid fixation. The main advantages of the Latarjet can be seen in the increased surface area of bone-to-bone contact, but also using 2 screws prevents rotation. These differences in technique allow a significantly accelerated rehabilitation postoperatively and favor graft union and stability for the Latarjet procedure.

Why an Arthroscopic Latarjet?

1. Placement of the bone graft is more accurate under arthroscopic control. Several different views can be afforded by the arthroscopic technique that not only improve graft placement but reduce the chances of overhang and impingement.

2. Open surgery does not easily allow the treatment of concomitant pathologies such as SLAP tears and posterior labral lesions. These are much less difficult to deal with using an arthroscopic approach.

3. Double instabilities can be treated during the same surgical procedure using both anterior and posterior bone blocks when employing arthroscopic methods. This is not possible through a single open approach.

4. Even though the strength of the bone block fixation allows early mobilization, the risk of adhesions and shoulder stiffness is higher with an open technique over arthroscopy.

5. If, during an intended Bankart repair, the tissue is determined to not be reconstructible, then an arthroscopic Latarjet offers an alternative solution to traditional open surgery and potentially having to reposition the patient.

6. As in other joints, arthroscopy offers the advantages of less postoperative pain, earlier mobility, quicker rehab, and faster return to sports.

7. Improved cosmetic result for the patients with an all-arthroscopic technique.

SURGICAL TECHNIQUE

We first performed the arthroscopic Latarjet in 2003, and since then it has been the subject of continued modification and refinement. Initially, the procedure took 4 hours, but since the development of specialized instrumentation, it now more frequently takes 45 minutes. At any stage, the procedure can be converted to an open technique using the same instruments or can be changed to perform a modified Bristow procedure instead.

It can be conveniently broken down into 5 steps[8] (see Chapter 12 video):

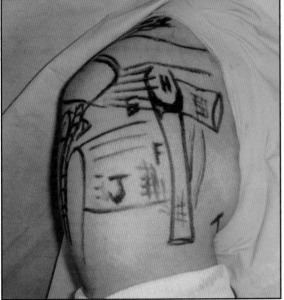

Figure 12-1. Note the I portal at the apex of the anterior axillary fold.

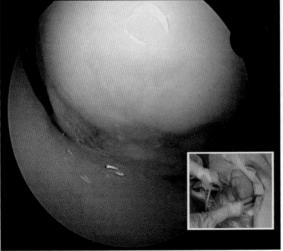

Figure 12-2. An engaging Hill-Sachs lesion as seen from the A portal.

Joint Evaluation/Achieving Exposure

The intra-articular approach commences through the standard posterior A portal, and a probe is introduced through the RI. This probe uses the anterolateral D portal, which is established using an outside-in technique (the anterior portals can be seen in Figure 12-1). A dynamic stability assessment is made (Figure 12-2), and the internal structures are further assessed with the probe (glenoid defects, humeral defects, HAGL, etc).

Open the RI and Expose Both Sides of Subscapularis

The glenohumeral joint is opened at the upper border of subscapularis (Figure 12-3), and the anteroinferior labrum and MGHL are resected between 2 and 5 o'clock to expose the glenoid neck (electrocautery). The intended graft site is marked, and the

Figure 12-3. Rotator interval opened with the coracoid seen in the background.

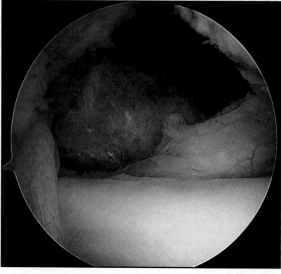

capsule between glenoid neck and subscapularis is split. To provide a healthy base for graft healing, the glenoid neck is abraded with the burr. Both sides of the subscapularis tendon are then exposed, with particular attention to the articular side of subscapularis. These releases are necessary to facilitate the transfer of the coracoid graft.

If there is any other intra-articular pathology, it can be dealt with at this stage (eg, a SLAP repair). If the IGHL or posterior labrum is damaged but reparable, this can be achieved with suture anchors.

The intra-articular preparation is now completed. We now move on to the extra-articular preparation.

Coracoid Soft Tissue Preparation

The coracoacromial ligament (CAL) is located and followed down to the coracoid where it is detached. The anterior aspect of the conjoint tendon is liberated from the fascia on the deep aspect of the deltoid, and the lateral side of conjoint tendon is released, the inferior limit of which is the pectoralis major tendon.

Behind the conjoint tendon exists a medial tissue barrier that separates the plexus from the subcoracoid bursa. This is opened to reveal the nerves to subscapularis, and further gentle inferior dissection exposes the axillary nerve. It is important to see these nerves and appreciate their location when it comes to placing future portals. Any further soft tissue attachments to the coracoid in the bursa are released to free the coracoid for its later transfer.

The scope is moved from the posterior A portal to the lateral D portal.

Subscapularis Split

Establish the I Portal in Apex of Axillary Fold

This portal gives excellent access to the anterior glenoid neck in the correct direction to place the screws for the graft. First, place a needle in the apex of the anterior axillary fold and guide this under direct vision to pass lateral to the conjoint tendon and above subscapularis. Advance the needle to the glenoid neck at the intended graft site, and make a 2-cm incision in the skin for the I portal.

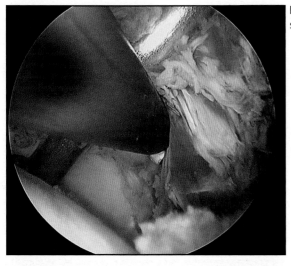

Figure 12-4. Subscapularis split. Note the switching stick elevating the muscle.

Determine the Level of the Subscapularis Split

The switching stick is inserted through the A portal at the level of the glenoid defect. This is then advanced through subscapularis to establish the level of the split. The conjoint tendon and plexus are retracted medially to prevent neurological injury upon the further advancement of the switching stick. The switching stick now holds the plexus and conjoint tendon medially while penetrating subscapularis at the level of the split.

Establish the J Portal

This portal is placed midway on an arc between the I and the D portals using an outside-in technique. It gives a more head-on view of the coracoid, whereas the D portal gives a better lateral view. Two perpendicular views are necessary to ensure optimum coracoid preparation.

Subscapularis Split

Elevate the subscapularis with the switching stick, introducing the electrocautery through the J portal, and commence the split (Figure 12-4.) Move the scope to J portal and the electrocautery to the I portal to complete the split. The split is completed down to the glenoid neck in the line of fibers of subscapularis, extending from the lateral insertion of subscapularis on the lesser tuberosity, passing medially close to the axillary nerve.

At this point, you could place an iliac crest graft if this was revision surgery, as the subscapularis split is done and the glenoid neck exposed.

Harvesting the Coracoid Graft

At this point, the scope is in the J portal and the electrocautery in I portal. Place a trocar in the D portal, and elevate the space above the coracoid (like using a retractor in open surgery).

Define the H Portal

This portal is necessary to allow instrument access to the superior coracoid. Two needles are placed to locate both the tip and the midpoint of the coracoid (Figure 12-5). Next, rotate the arthroscope to give a perpendicular view of the coracoid to

Figure 12-5. Needles placed to define the tip of the coracoid and midpoint of the graft.

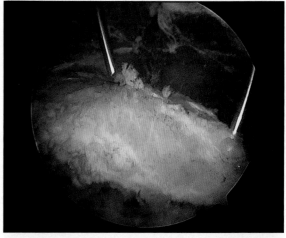

Figure 12-6. Releasing pectoralis minor from the medial coracoid.

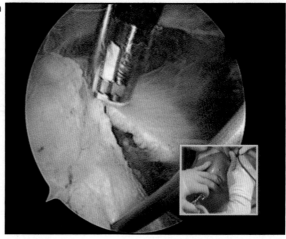

ensure correct needle alignment. This will serve to guide the position of the coracoid drill guide. Once satisfied, make a superior incision for the H portal.

The pectoralis minor tendon on the medial border of the coracoid is now released, taking care to remain on bone at the coracoid level (Figure 12-6). Below this, the conjoint tendon can be released medially with blunt dissection with special care taken to prevent damage to the musculocutaneous nerve and plexus.

With this dissection completed and having an awareness of the position of the nerves, we can proceed with the knowledge that everything lateral to the conjoint tendon is safe.

Drilling the Coracoid

It is important to regularly change the viewing angle of the scope by rotation to ensure mediolateral alignment of the now-inserted coracoid drill guide. Place the guide over the junction of the lateral two-thirds and medial one-third of coracoid, and drill the α hole (inferior and distal) with a K-wire. It is important while doing this to visualize under the coracoid to verify that the direction of the K-wires are perpendicular to the superior surface of the coracoid and to avoid penetrating too deep into subscapularis. Rotationally align the coracoid drill guide, and then drill β (proximal) wire (Figure 12-7).

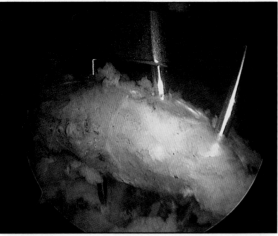

Figure 12-7. Coracoid drill guide with both K-wires in place. Needle remains at the tip of the coracoid.

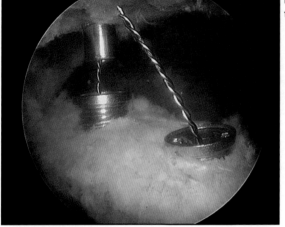

Figure 12-8. Placing the top hat screws over the Chia wire.

Remove the drill guide, and check the wire positions with the scope in both the D and J portals. Overdrill both holes with the coracoid step drill, and remove the drills and K-wires.

Inserting the Top Hats

The drill holes are now tapped to prepare for the top hat and glenoid screws (5.0/3.5 mm). The taps are cannulated and allow the placement of the coracoid-securing Chia wire, which is brought out of the H portal.

The top hats are then inserted over the Chia wire, and a portal plug is placed in the H portal to prevent water escaping (Figure 12-8).

The Sub Scap Channeler is a large trocar now used through the I portal to pass through the subscapularis split and onto the glenoid neck in the intended graft location. This step serves to judge whether the earlier soft tissue split is adequate to allow transfer of the coracoid to the glenoid neck.

Retrieving the Chia Wires Through the I Portal

The coracoid will ultimately be controlled and directed from the I portal, and, as such, the Chia wires must be transferred there. To do this, we pass the crochet hooks through the coracoid positioning cannula in the I portal to retrieve these (Figure 12-9).

Figure 12-9. Retrieving the Chia wires using the crochet hooks.

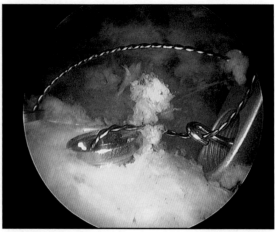

Slotted pegs with specific narrow channels are placed over both Chia wires to prevent water being lost.

Coracoid Osteotomy

Once the coracoid is prepared, we are now ready to make the osteotomy. We use the burr on the inferior and lateral aspects of the coracoid, proximal to the β hole, to create a stress riser. The top of the osteotomy site can be burred by placing it in the H portal. The osteotome is now placed in the H portal, and a controlled osteotomy is made (Figure 12-10).

Coracoid Transfer

To gain control of the graft, it must be reduced onto the coracoid positioning cannula. This is achieved by placing gentle traction on both limbs of the Chia wire (Figure 12-11) and then passing the coracoid 3.5 screw over the Chia wires. The screw advances through top hat and into coracoid where it engages the bone. The coracoid should now be secure on the coracoid positioning cannula.

Graft Trimming

The freshly harvested graft is mobilized, and all remaining adhesions of the pectoralis minor and the medial fascia are removed. Particular attention must be paid to secure the musculocutaneous nerve while this is done. The mobile coracoid usually has a medial spike arising from its base that must be trimmed to permit good bony contact with the glenoid. To do this, the scope is held by the assistant, and using a 2-handed technique, the graft is controlled on the cannula with one hand and trimmed with the burr with the other. Ideally, the burr is held stationary while the coracoid is manipulated around the burr both to allow the accurate debridement of the graft and to minimize any risk to the plexus.

The graft is now ready for transfer and fixation to the glenoid. Manipulate the coracoid on the coracoid positioning cannula (I portal) to the glenoid neck. This is made easier by elevating the subscapularis split with the switching stick.

Coracoid Fixation

Once the graft is sited on the glenoid neck in the desired position, then fixation is undertaken (Figure 12-12). Two long K-wires are passed through the coracoid

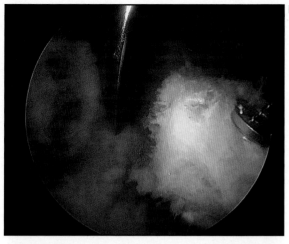

Figure 12-10. Coracoid osteotomy.

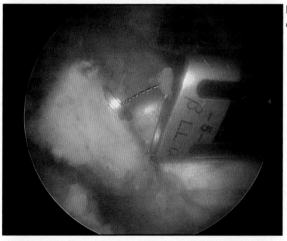

Figure 12-11. Reducing the coracoid onto the coracoid positioning cannula.

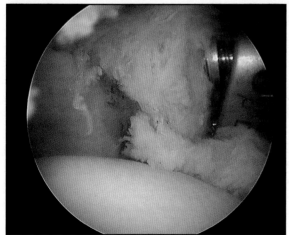

Figure 12-12. Graft positioned on the glenoid neck.

Figure 12-13. Definitive screw being inserted in α hole while coracoid screw remains in β hole.

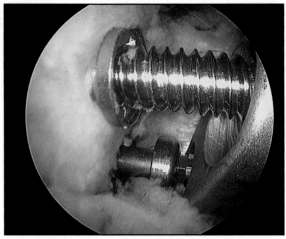

positioning cannula to gain temporary fixation. The scapula must be pulled posteriorly by the assistant using a posterior drawer on the upper arm in order to decrease the relative glenoid anteversion. The handle of the cannula must be pushed medially to obtain a minimum angulation between the K-wires and the glenoid surface. These wires will emerge through the skin of the posterior shoulder, at which stage a clip is placed on them.

The position of the graft is then checked from different portals to ensure the best vertical and horizontal position. We prefer to place the graft from 3 to 5 o'clock and flush with the glenoid.

Drill and Screw the Graft

The α coracoid 3.5 screw (inferior) is removed, and the 3.2 glenoid drill is passed over K-wire. The length of the screw can be read from the depth gauge on the drill. Remove the drill (K-wire remains), and place the screw in the α hole (Figure 12-13). Again, the same action is repeated for the β hole, and the screws are inserted and alternately tightened to reduce the graft in compression onto the glenoid neck. The K-wires can then be removed posteriorly.

Final Checks

The graft and screw position are checked graft through the D and J portals, and any final trimming can be done at this stage with the burr (Figure 12-14).

TIPS AND PEARLS

The all-arthroscopic Latarjet is a reliable but difficult technique with a steep learning curve. Excellent knowledge of the anatomy of this area and of the instrumentation is mandatory. We also feel that saw bone practice is crucial before commencing the first surgeries. To make this technique possible, it is important to start the surgery using an open technique using the instrumentation set used for arthroscopic surgery. Once the surgeon is familiar with these instruments, one should progress to begin the first stage of the surgery arthroscopically. After this first stage is concluded, the rest of the surgery should be performed by reverting to the open technique. The surgeon should not move on to the next stage arthroscopically until he or she feels comfortable and is competent with the present stage. This process should continue until the procedure is being performed all arthroscopically.

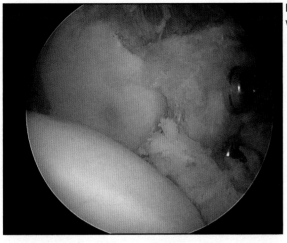

Figure 12-14. Coracoid graft secured and flush with the anterior glenoid.

The ultimate goal of the surgery is a successful coracoid transfer with sound healing and stability restored. There is no shame in opening the shoulder at any stage in case of problems or to aid visualization.

Managing Complications

Despite the complexity of this procedure and its proximity to the neurovascular structures of the upper limb, we have had no neurovascular complications. Problems with graft malposition tend to be minimized due to the excellent view afforded by the arthroscope and its magnification. Where a graft is found to be in a suboptimal position, this is detected intraoperatively after temporary K-wire fixation to the glenoid. At this stage, the position can be modified prior to drilling and definitive fixation. Any prominence of the graft thereafter can be burred flush to the glenoid.

Graft nonunion rarely occurs, and this complication is featured prior to the use of the top hat washer. This can be revised to use the top hat, as this allows greater compression to be applied to the graft. When this has been accomplished, successful union has always occurred within 6 weeks. Graft resorption, however, has been a more common problem, leading to uncovering of the screw heads anteriorly. This has resulted in pain and tendon impingement in some patients, which later resolved with arthroscopic removal of the screws.

Recurrent instability is a difficult problem to manage after a Latarjet procedure and has not occurred in any of the first 100 cases. We have revised cases of previous failed Latarjet procedures by arthroscopic revision bone grafting using a free iliac crest graft. This has resulted in stability being restored in all cases.

Postoperative Management

Postoperatively, the patients require no immobilization and may begin full active range of movements immediately. They can return to work as soon as pain allows and to low-risk sports at 3 weeks. For high-risk (throwing) and collision sports, we recommend that they do not resume these activities before 6 weeks (Figures 12-15 and 12-16).

Figure 12-15. Six weeks postop.

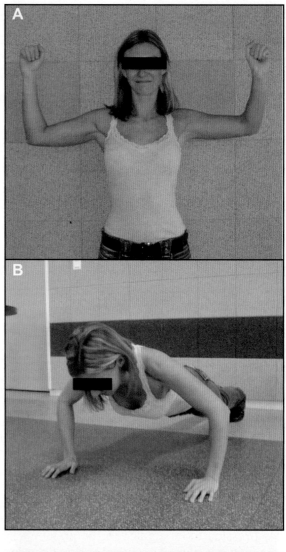

Figure 12-16. Six weeks postop.

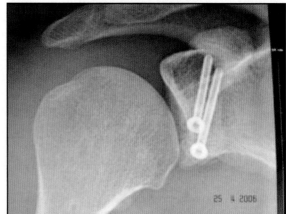

REFERENCES

1. Balg F, Boileau P. The instability severity index score. A simple pre-operative score to select patients for arthroscopic or open shoulder stabilisation. *J Bone Joint Surg Br.* 2007;89-11:1470-1477.
2. Boileau P, Villalba M, Hery JY, Balg F, Ahrens P, Neyton L. Risk factors for recurrence of shoulder instability after arthroscopic Bankart repair. *J Bone Joint Surg Am.* 2006;88-8:1755-1763.
3. Latarjet M. Treatment of recurrent dislocation of the shoulder. *Lyon Chir.* 1954;49-8:994-997.
4. Sugaya H, Moriishi J, Dohi M, Kon Y, Tsuchiya A. Glenoid rim morphology in recurrent anterior glenohumeral instability. *J Bone Joint Surg Am.* 2003;85-A-5:878-884.
5. Burkhart SS, De Beer JF. Traumatic glenohumeral bone defects and their relationship to failure of arthroscopic Bankart repairs: significance of the inverted-pear glenoid and the humeral engaging Hill-Sachs lesion. *Arthroscopy.* 2000;16-7:677-694.
6. Purchase RJ, Wolf EM, Hobgood ER, Pollock ME, Smalley CC. Hill-sachs "Remplissage": an arthroscopic solution for the engaging hill-sachs lesion. *Arthroscopy.* 2008;24-6:723-726.
7. Wellmann M, Petersen W, Zantop T, et al. Open shoulder repair of osseous glenoid defects: biomechanical effectiveness of the Latarjet procedure versus a contoured structural bone graft. *Am J Sports Med.* 2009;37-1:87-94.
8. Lafosse L, Lejeune E, Bouchard A, Kakuda C, Gobezie R, Kochhar T. The arthroscopic Latarjet procedure for the treatment of anterior shoulder instability. *Arthroscopy.* 2007;23-11:1242 e1-5.

**Please see video on the accompanying Web site at
http://www.slackbooks.com/unstableshouldervideos**

13

Treatment of Superior Labral Tears in the Unstable Shoulder

Joseph P. DeAngelis, MD and John E. Kuhn, MD

A comprehensive understanding of the anatomy of the glenoid labrum is essential to effective treatment of pathology of the shoulder. Central to this knowledge is an understanding of the function of the glenoid labrum, not only as the anchor of the long head of the biceps, but also as a fibrocartilaginous extension of the articular cartilage.

The labrum surrounds the glenoid at its periphery and serves as an extension of the articular cartilage, blending with the normal articular surface in a seamless interface in the vast majority of individuals. Below the equator of the glenoid, the labrum is firmly attached to the glenoid. However, above the equator, this fibrous ring is more mobile, and many common variations can affect its appearance. Most often, a meniscus-like variant is seen, in which a thick band of tissue drapes over the superior margin of the glenoid. On careful inspection, the elevation of this tissue will reveal a normal articular margin on the superior glenoid, which transitions to fibrocartilage directly. The absence of frayed tissue or exposed cortical bone at the interface confirms this configuration as a normal variant, rather than a traumatic presentation.

Understanding the normal labral anatomy is challenging because there are so many subtle variations. When 191 consecutive patients were evaluated prospectively using arthroscopy to quantify the dimensions of the labrum, some 49 (26%) were identified with articular cartilage that extended to the supraglenoid tubercle beneath a mobile labrum, in the absence of fibrous tearing or injury (Figure 13-1).[1]

To compound the problem, there is also substantial variation in the biceps anchor (Figure 13-2). In most people, the fibers for the long head of the biceps invest in the labrum posterior to the 12 o'clock position and are designated posterior-dominant. This anatomic difference is important to identify because it contributes to the pathogenesis of labral tears and is essential for subsequent repair of these lesions. As the labrum extends anterior, different anatomic presentations may be encountered where the middle glenohumeral ligament attaches to the labrum. Originally described by Williams and colleagues, a Buford complex consists of a bare anterosuperior glenoid (no anterior labrum) with a cord-like middle glenohumeral ligament that attaches to

Abrams JS. *Management of the Unstable Shoulder: Arthroscopic and Open Repair* (pp. 171-180). © 2011 SLACK Incorporated

Figure 13-1. Meniscoid variant of the superior labrum.

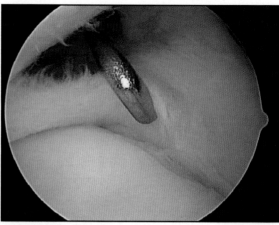

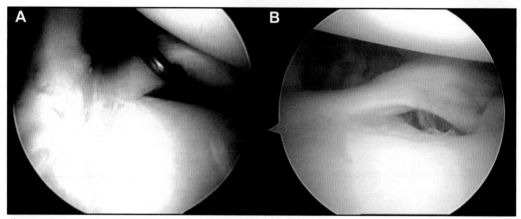

Figure 13-2. Variations in normal labral anatomy. (A) Sub-labral foramen. (B) Buford complex.

the base of the biceps tendon.[2] This variation has an anteroinferior labrum that is normal in appearance and occurs 2% to 6% of the time. In contrast, a sub-labral foramen presents with a detached anterosuperior labrum to which a cord-like middle glenohumeral ligament attaches. The incidence of this pattern is estimated to be 8% to 15%.

Superior labral tears in throwing athletes were first described by Andrews and colleagues in a consecutive series of 73 throwing athletes.[3] Snyder and colleagues offered a 4-part classification system of superior labral tears based on a larger series of patients (700 arthroscopies, 27 injuries; Figure 13-3).[4] This system was then expanded to include other common variants, including superior labral tears associated with classic lesions of instability.[5]

BIOMECHANICS

The superior labrum has many functions. It serves as an attachment site for glenohumeral ligaments, a restraint to superior translation of the humeral head, and is the anchor for the long head of the biceps. The long head of the biceps is an important restraint to external rotation of the abducted arm.[6] In throwing athletes, torque on the biceps anchor is generated with abduction and external rotation as the arm is placed in a cocked position. This resulting traction is transmitted to the posterior labrum,

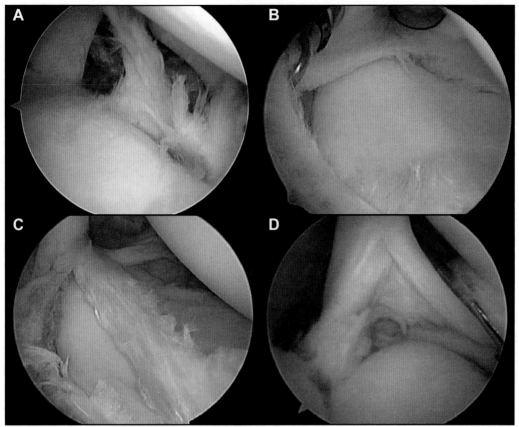

Figure 13-3. Snyder classification of superior labral tears.

peeling the labrum away from the posterior glenoid.[7] In a cadaveric study attempting to model the throwing motion, an external rotation moment (cocking) was found to produce a type II SLAP lesion more often than an early deceleration position.[6]

ASSOCIATED PATHOLOGY

With SLAP tears, periglenoid cysts may form as joint fluid flows through defects in the labral tissue. Additionally, rotator cuff disease may be seen in up to 41% of patients.[4] In athletes with shoulder instability, SLAP tears can coincide with labral pathology (anterior labral tears and bony Bankart lesions) and has been reported in 20% to 32% of patients with instability.[8,9]

Because these lesions occur in overhead athletes, it is important to evaluate the patient for scapular dysfunction, posterior capsular tightness, core strength, and single-leg stability as these elements form the foundation of the kinetic chain in throwers.[10]

MECHANISMS OF INJURY

Many different mechanisms can result in an injury to the superior labrum. Trauma from lifting a heavy object, a motor vehicle accident, a shoulder dislocation, or a fall can result in a SLAP tear. Similarly, repetitive motion induces microtrauma to the relatively avascular area when throwing, serving, or lifting for repetitions. In throwing athletes, anterior capsular laxity often develops. The resulting anterior shoulder instability may place additional strain on the superior labrum, resulting in a SLAP tear.[11] Alternatively, SLAP tears may occur following a shoulder dislocation, with an incidence of 5% to 27%.[8,12,13]

PRESENTATION

Patients with SLAP tears often complain of shoulder pain associated with overhead activity. The pain may be accompanied by weakness, a sense of instability, or mechanical symptoms. Symptoms of instability may result from the increased translation of the humeral head that accompanies the loss of normal restraint provided by the superior labral complex.[14]

On physical examination, a formal evaluation of strength and range of motion can guide the evaluation, paying particular attention to core stability, scapular function, and the presence of an internal rotation deficit. In addition to a thorough examination including tenderness to palpation and neurovascular status, there are different provocative tests designed to test the integrity of the superior labrum. Unfortunately, no single provocative physical exam test has been shown to accurately diagnosis a SLAP tear. In a level III, systematic review, both O'Briens and the crank test were found to have inconsistent positive and negative predictive values.[15]

Different imaging modalities have been employed to aid in the diagnosis of SLAP tears. Lee and colleagues reported on the use of Grashey-view arthrography in 28 patients with arthroscopically confirmed lesions.[16] In this investigation, the sensitivity, specificity, and accuracy were 50%, 86%, and 79%, respectively. Other studies have examined the role of magnetic resonance imaging (MRI), computed tomography (CT), and MR arthrography, which seems to be the best imaging modality to identify SLAP lesions (Figure 13-4).[17-20]

In light of the limitations of physical examination and radiographic studies in the diagnosis of SLAP tears, a surgeon must be ready for the unexpected SLAP lesion identified during arthroscopy.

PATIENT SELECTION

Unlike isolated shoulder instability, one the most challenging elements in dealing with superior labral pathology in the setting of instability is determining who will benefit from a surgical repair. Multiple studies have demonstrated a wide range of labral abnormalities in asymptomatic patients, with the incidence of pathology ranging from 7.5% to 100%.[21-25] To further confound the issue, a recent level III study of the *nonoperative* treatment of SLAP tears found 18 of 18 patients were able to return to sport with less pain at 3.1 years of follow-up. The rehabilitation protocol emphasized pain control with anti-inflammatory medication and eliminating posterior capsular tightness.

Interestingly, in a level I, randomized controlled trial of operative repair versus biceps tenotomy in patients older than 50 years of age, patients undergoing a rotator cuff repair with tenotomy only had significantly better outcomes than those patients who had a rotator cuff repair with a SLAP repair.[26]

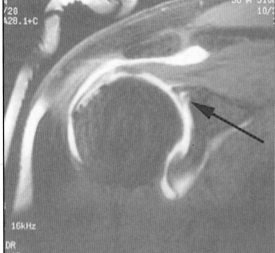

Figure 13-4. MRI arthrography of SLAP lesion.

It would seem that a formal SLAP repair is best indicated in younger, athletic patients who present following acute injury to the biceps anchor. Older patients with pain, who fail conservative management, may benefit from a biceps tenotomy alone, particularly if their nondominant arm is affected or if their body habitus masks the potential for deformity. Chronic SLAP tears that demonstrate intra-articular changes in the biceps tendon or signs of wear on the humeral head are also well-served by an arthroscopic tenotomy, especially if they demonstrate no pain in the bicipital groove. On the other hand, individuals who work vigorously with their upper extremities (manual laborers) or who are sensitive to the cosmesis of the upper arm will benefit from a formal biceps tenodesis. This is also the case for chronic SLAP tears with biceps changes that have pain in the bicipital groove. Clearly, the best approach to the patient with superior labral and/or biceps tendon pathology is continuing to evolve.

In patients with shoulder instability, the effect of a SLAP tear warrants careful consideration, and its treatment may be part of the larger (global) plan of care. In these challenging cases, the superior labral pathology should be considered in the context of instability, and the SLAP repair should be performed after addressing the Bankart lesion in accordance with the clinical presentation.

TREATMENT OPTIONS

In the treatment of SLAP tears, arthroscopy is the gold standard. (In fact, an open technique has never been reported.) After the induction of anesthesia, an examination under anesthesia should be conducted to identify deficiencies in the range of motion or signs of instability not elucidated preoperatively (see Chapter 13 video). In throwing athletes in particular, the posterior capsule should be evaluated by internally rotating the arm with the humerus abducted to 90 degrees. Posterior tightness that accompanies scapular dysfunction and weakness of the abdominal core musculature can contribute to poor mechanics and the development of SLAP lesions. At the same time, throwing athletes may demonstrate anterior capsular laxity that contributes to their instability. Rare patients may present with some element of both posterior capsular contracture and anterior laxity, with a concomitant superior labral lesion.

Like arthroscopic stabilization procedures, SLAP lesion repairs can be performed in the beach chair or lateral decubitus position. Once appropriately prepared for surgery, a thorough diagnostic arthroscopy of the glenohumeral joint should be completed. A careful exam will probe the labrum for variant anatomy and identify perilabral cysts, signs of instability, tearing of the rotator cuff, or biceps pathology. Additional helpful maneuvers include switching the arthroscope from the posterior portal to the anterior portal for a different perspective. Finally, a dynamic examination is performed by abducting and externally rotating the humerus and observing the superior labrum from posterior. The "Peel Back Sign" exists when this maneuver causes the labrum to peel back from its anatomic attachment (see Chapter 13 video). Returning the arm to a neutral, or internally rotated, position relieves the tension, and the labrum reapproximates the glenoid margin.

Portal Placement

The close proximity of the superior labrum to the rotator cuff limits the effective arthroscopic working space, and precise positioning of anchors and instruments can be challenging. For these reasons, careful portal placement is critical to the success of a superior labral repair. A surgeon needs enough room for examination and manipulation of the tissues, without injuring the overlying rotator cuff or biceps tendon.

The standard posterior portal is usually for introduction of the arthroscope and for viewing and is typically made parallel to the glenohumeral joint surface. If the surgeon knows that the patient has a superior and/or posterior labral tear that needs to be addressed, the first posterior portal can be created more laterally than normal. In doing so, this portal could also be used as a working portal to place anchors at an ideal angle (see Chapter 13 video).

In most cases, a working portal should be placed high in the rotator interval at the leading edge of the supraspinatus tendon, creating a high anterosuperior rotator interval portal (see Chapter 13 video). From this position, it is possible to manipulate the superior labrum, probe the biceps tendon, and place suture anchors in the superior glenoid. This portal also helps in docking and tying sutures because it is easily manipulated to gain access to the sublabral surface of the glenoid.

A trans-tendonous approach will produce a portal that helps with access to the region just posterior to the biceps tendon. To avoid injuring the supraspinatus, this portal is made using a guide needle and is dilated using a cannulated switching stick. This portal is used for the anchor insertion cannula for anchor placement—not for large-bore cannulas typically used for suture management. This portal is also placed medial to the rotator crescent to avoid damaging the supraspinatus tendon (see Chapter 13 video).

Labral Repair

The approach to the labrum is determined by the type of labral tear that is encountered. If the labral tissue is degenerated and will not tolerate a formal repair (Snyder Type I, Type II), gentle débridement is helpful in eliminating loose tissue that can cause mechanical symptoms. However, if the fibrocartilage is in good condition, as is usually the case in younger, throwing athletes, an arthroscopic shaver can be used to prepare the tissue edges for repair and to remove soft tissue from the superior glenoid (see

Chapter 13 video). If a bone-cutting shaver is available, the same instrument can decorticate the point of labral attachment on the glenoid. Otherwise, a small burr should be used to decorticate the glenoid until small areas of punctate bleeding are easily seen. At this point, the suture anchors can be introduced.

ANCHOR PLACEMENT

Restoration of the normal superior glenoid labral anatomy is essential to the success of the surgical repair. In this way, it is important to reapproximate the fibrocartilage to the articular margin without significant advancement or excessive tethering of the biceps tendon and to establish an environment for the tissue to heal. Having prepared the labral tissue and glenoid, suture anchors should be placed at the articular margin with the appropriate angle to gain good purchase in the bone.

In shoulder instability, when superior labral pathology is addressed at the same time as a Bankart lesion, a careful assessment of the native anatomy is imperative, as anatomic variants are common. Repairing a normal sublabral foramen or securing a Buford lesion to the glenoid may result in an unintended restriction in external rotation.

Depending on the type of anchor used, the sequence of steps for insertion will vary according to the manufacturer's specification, but their position will be approximately the same. In throwing athletes, it is imperative that the repair does not overly constrain biceps anchor. For this reason, when the lesion extends anterior to the biceps tendon, suture anchors should not be placed any farther anterior than the anterior edge of the tendon itself.

Access to the superior glenoid can be obtained using a percutaneous, cannulated technique to minimize trauma to the rotator cuff or from a working portal in the rotator interval. With one anchor at the leading edge of the biceps, a second is placed at the posterior edge of the biceps (see Chapter 13 video). When necessary, a third or fourth suture anchor can be employed on the posterior edge of the glenoid through the posterior portal (see Chapter 13 video).

FIXATION OF THE LABRUM

Different instruments are available to aid in passing suture through the detached labrum, and they range in cost and specialization. The simplest tool is a spinal needle with or without a looped passing wire. Similarly, a set of curved meniscal repair needles (meniscus mender) can pass through the rotator cuff tendon with minimal injury. Longer cannulated instruments can be used through portals or percutaneously to accurately place a suture through the labrum.

With preloaded anchors, careful suture management is essential to complete the repair efficiently, particularly if multiple single-loaded anchors or double-loaded anchors are used. A process of passing and tying individual sutures sequentially can be used to minimize the risk of tangling the sutures within the joint. While somewhat tedious, the stepwise introduction of an anchor, passing of its suture, and securing the tissue does limit the opportunity for suture entrapment. Alternatively, a second working portal can be positioned low in the rotator interval at the leading edge of the subscapularis tendon. In this portal, sutures can be docked until they are transferred to the superior portal for tying. While many anchors required knot tying, knotless anchors are also available and have been found to be useful in repairing SLAP lesions.

When knotless anchors are used with a mattress suture configuration, they are thought to better reproduce the native labrum-glenoid anatomy.

Regardless of the number of portals or type of anchors used, it is important to have a systematic method for gaining access and securing the tissue in order to best address the labral tear. Once repaired, the biceps anchor should be firmly held in place, as evidenced by attempted manipulation, and the "peel back" should be resolved (see Chapter 13 video).

Outcomes

In general, the outcomes following repair of SLAP lesions have been good. Many of the patients reported in the literature have had concurrent pathology addressed, introducing performance bias and making it unclear as to the effect of repairing the SLAP lesion. Brockmeier and colleagues reported 87% good to excellent results in repairing isolated SLAP lesions with suture anchor techniques.[27] Patients with a discrete traumatic event did better than patients with a more insidious onset of pain. Interestingly, patients with workers' compensation claims do not fare as well, with only 43% returning to their previous work level. Similarly, of 42 major league baseball players, only 29 returned to play for one or more seasons, suggesting that high-demand performers may not fare as well.

In considering the results of SLAP repairs in the setting of shoulder instability, the outcomes data are limited to case series. Lo and Burkhart reported 86% patient satisfaction in their series of "Triple Labral" lesion, while Takase found a significant decrease in postoperative external rotation.[28,29]

Complications

Following arthroscopic repair of a SLAP tear, the surgical complications are most often related to a few common areas: anchor-related, failure to heal, stiffness, and entrapment of a pathologic biceps. A prominent suture anchor or suture knot may produce an audible squeak in a reproducible range of motion. A more pronounced mechanical presentation usually accompanies gross failure (pull-out) of the anchor and will require removal of the loose fragment, as significant chondral damage may occur.

A recurrent SLAP tear is often seen when the anatomic lesion is repaired, but the contributing deficits in a thrower's mechanics are unaffected by rehabilitation. Persistent scapular motion abnormalities, posterior capsular tightness, abdominal core weakness, and poor single-leg stability all compromise a thrower's ability to generate power. The former 2 elements limit the efficient transfer of energy to the ball, while the latter 2 deficits impede the development of torque between the shoulders and hips. As a result, the individual tends to compensate for the resulting shortfall by throwing harder, straining the repaired labrum, and recreating the original pathology. For this reason, it is very important for the postoperative rehabilitation protocol to address these deficiencies and improve the thrower's mechanics prior to his or her return to play.

Though rare in young adults, postoperative stiffness can hamper the recovery following a SLAP repair, particularly in the treatment of an unstable shoulder. Failure to regain full and symmetric range of motion after surgery will limit the recovery of strength and prevent the humerus from rotating normally in the glenoid. However, early range of motion may affect the results of arthroscopic stabilization. As with most presentations of arthrofibrosis, infection needs to be excluded as a cause of the disability, and recovery efforts must focus on adequate pain control and the re-establishment of normal shoulder kinematics. When truly recalcitrant, a repeat arthroscopy may be required to address capsular adhesions and to improve the range of motion. However, this intervention should only be undertaken when conservative efforts have been exhausted.

An additional source of disability following repair of a SLAP tear is unrecognized pathology in the biceps tendon. This frequent source of discomfort can be aggravated if the intra-articular segment of the tendon is overly constrained in the bicipital groove as it passes through the rotator interval. Once reattached at the superior glenoid, an incarcerated biceps tendon is subject to considerable tension between the repaired labrum and the point of entrapment in the groove. If the tendon is unable to slide, there will be little or no retraction if the biceps anchor is incised for tenotomy. If a formal, open biceps tenodesis is undertaken, an hourglass deformity may be seen in the cut tendon before fixing it to the humerus. Both examples help illustrate how undiagnosed biceps pathology can limit a patient's recovery from a SLAP repair.

CONCLUSION

Lesions of the superior labrum are a disease of the arthroscopic era. While difficult to diagnose clinically, they represent an important source of shoulder pain and dysfunction and may be more problematic in the unstable shoulder. The approach to the patient is evolving, but many patients will benefit from an arthroscopic repair of the torn labrum. In patients with instability and SLAP lesions, repair of the labrum at both sites is warranted. Technical aspects of the repair include minimizing damage to the supraspinatus, preparing a bed for healing, and repairing the labrum anatomically without overconstraining the biceps tendon. While the results of repair are generally good, the indications for surgery and the surgical approach continue to evolve.

REFERENCES

1. Davidson PA, Rivenburgh DW. Mobile superior glenoid labrum: a normal variant or pathologic condition? *Am J Sports Med.* 2004;32(4):962-966.
2. Williams MM, Snyder SJ, Buford D Jr. The Buford complex—the "cord-like" middle glenohumeral ligament and absent anterosuperior labrum complex: a normal anatomic capsulolabral variant. *Arthroscopy.* 1994;10(3):241-247.
3. Andrews JR, Carson WG Jr, McLeod WD. Glenoid labrum tears related to the long head of the biceps. *Am J Sports Med.* 1985;13(5):337-341.
4. Snyder SJ, Karzel RP, Del Pizzo W, Ferkel RD, Friedman MJ. SLAP lesions of the shoulder. *Arthroscopy.* 1990;6(4): 274-279.
5. Maffet MW, Gartsman GM, Moseley B. Superior labrum-biceps tendon complex lesions of the shoulder. *Am J Sports Med.* 1995;23(1):93-98.
6. Kuhn JE, Lindholm SR, Huston LJ, Soslowsky LJ, Blasier RB. Failure of the biceps superior labral complex: a cadaveric biomechanical investigation comparing the late cocking and early deceleration positions of throwing. *Arthroscopy.* 2003;19(4):373-379.
7. Burkhart SS, Morgan CD. The peel-back mechanism: its role in producing and extending posterior type II SLAP lesions and its effect on SLAP repair rehabilitation. *Arthroscopy.* 1998;14(6):637-640.
8. Yiannakopoulos CK, Mataragas E, Antonogiannakis E. A comparison of the spectrum of intra-articular lesions in acute and chronic anterior shoulder instability. *Arthroscopy.* 2007;23(9):985-990.

9. Kim DS, Yoon YS, Kwon SM. The spectrum of lesions and clinical results of arthroscopic stabilization of acute anterior shoulder instability. *Yonsei Med J.* 2010;51(3):421-426.

10. Ben Kibler W, Sciascia A. Kinetic chain contributions to elbow function and dysfunction in sports. *Clin Sports Med.* 2004;23(4):545-552, viii.

11. Mihata T, McGarry MH, Tibone JE, Fitzpatrick MJ, Kinoshita M, Lee TQ. Biomechanical assessment of Type II superior labral anterior-posterior (SLAP) lesions associated with anterior shoulder capsular laxity as seen in throwers: a cadaveric study. *Am J Sports Med.* 2008;36(8):1604-1610.

12. Hintermann B, Gachter A. Theo van Rens Prize. Arthroscopic assessment of the unstable shoulder. *Knee Surg Sports Traumatol Arthrosc.* 1994;2(2):64-69.

13. Antonio GE, Griffith JF, Yu AB, Yung PS, Chan KM, Ahuja AT. First-time shoulder dislocation: high prevalence of labral injury and age-related differences revealed by MR arthrography. *J Magn Reson Imaging.* 2007;26(4):983-991.

14. Morgan CD, Burkhart SS, Palmieri M, Gillespie M. Type II SLAP lesions: three subtypes and their relationships to superior instability and rotator cuff tears. *Arthroscopy.* 1998;14(6):553-565.

15. Jones GL, Galluch DB. Clinical assessment of superior glenoid labral lesions: a systematic review. *Clin Orthop Relat Res.* 2007;455:45-51.

16. Lee JH, Van Raalte V, Malian V. Diagnosis of SLAP lesions with Grashey-view arthrography. *Skeletal Radiol.* 2003;32(7):388-395.

17. Gusmer PB, Potter HG, Schatz JA, et al. Labral injuries: accuracy of detection with unenhanced MR imaging of the shoulder. *Radiology.* 1996;200(2):519-524.

18. Tuite MJ, Cirillo RL, De Smet AA, Orwin JF. Superior labrum anterior-posterior (SLAP) tears: evaluation of three MR signs on T2-weighted images. *Radiology.* 2000;215(3):841-845.

19. Applegate GR, Hewitt M, Snyder SJ, Watson E, Kwak S, Resnick D. Chronic labral tears: value of magnetic resonance arthrography in evaluating the glenoid labrum and labral-bicipital complex. *Arthroscopy.* 2004;20(9):959-963.

20. Waldt S, Metz S, Burkart A, et al. Variants of the superior labrum and labro-bicipital complex: a comparative study of shoulder specimens using MR arthrography, multi-slice CT arthrography and anatomical dissection. *Eur Radiol.* 2006;16(2):451-458.

21. Chandnani V, Ho C, Gerharter J, et al. MR findings in asymptomatic shoulders: a blind analysis using symptomatic shoulders as controls. *Clin Imaging.* 1992;16(1):25-30.

22. Liou JT, Wilson AJ, Totty WG, Brown JJ. The normal shoulder: common variations that simulate pathologic conditions at MR imaging. *Radiology.* 1993;186(2):435-441.

23. Miniaci A, Mascia AT, Salonen DC, Becker EJ. Magnetic resonance imaging of the shoulder in asymptomatic professional baseball pitchers. *Am J Sports Med.* 2002;30(1):66-73.

24. Connor PM, Banks DM, Tyson AB, Coumas JS, D'Alessandro DF. Magnetic resonance imaging of the asymptomatic shoulder of overhead athletes: a 5-year follow-up study. *Am J Sports Med.* 2003;31(5):724-727.

25. Jost B, Zumstein M, Pfirrmann CW, Zanetti M, Gerber C. MRI findings in throwing shoulders: abnormalities in professional handball players. *Clin Orthop Relat Res.* 2005;434:130-137.

26. Franceschi F, Longo UG, Ruzzini L, Rizzello G, Maffulli N, Denaro V. No advantages in repairing a type II superior labrum anterior and posterior (SLAP) lesion when associated with rotator cuff repair in patients over age 50: a randomized controlled trial. *Am J Sports Med.* 2008;36(2):247-253.

27. Brockmeier SF, Voos JE, Williams RJ III, et al. Outcomes after arthroscopic repair of type-II SLAP lesions. *J Bone Joint Surg Am.* 2009;91(7):1595-1603.

28. Lo IK, Burkart SS. Triple labral lesions: pathology and surgical repair technique-report of seven cases. *Arthroscopy.* 2005;21(2):186-193.

29. Takase K. Risk of motion loss with combined Bankart and SLAP repairs. *Orthopedics.* 2009;**32**(8).

Please see video on the accompanying Web site at http://www.slackbooks.com/unstableshouldervideos

14

Arthroscopic Revision Surgery and Treatment of Complications in Shoulder Stabilization

Jeffrey S. Abrams, MD

There has been a great deal of enthusiasm for using arthroscopic techniques to repair the unstable shoulder. Results with early techniques provided surgeons with experience in recognizing multiple articular lesions, but outcomes were inferior to open procedures in reducing the chance of recurrence. Modern suture anchor techniques with additional capsular tensioning have reduced the risk of recurrence and are comparable to stabilization rates found with open repairs.[1-4] Complications of shoulder stiffness, return to overhand throwing sports, absence of subscapularis dehiscence or dysfunction, and reduced risk of infection have made arthroscopic stabilization the most common stabilization technique performed today.[5,6] With a greater percentage of athletes returning to sport, there continues to be a risk of recurrence, and surgeons need to be able to treat patients who underwent prior surgery.[7-11]

Recurrence of instability following surgical stabilization can create a complex situation. There is often a recreation of the Bankart lesions in addition to capsular changes. In addition, there is additional trauma to the glenohumeral joint, raising concern due to degenerative arthritis, rim fractures, and advancing glenoid and humeral deficiency.[12,13] Revision surgeons have blamed anchors placed medially as the cause of failure referring to the index surgery. This may not have actually occurred, but following addition of glenoid loss, anchors *appear* to be medial to the glenoid rim (Figure 14-1).

Successful management includes 1) proper patient selection for nonoperative, arthroscopic, and open procedures; 2) techniques used to address multiple articular lesions; and 3) time for healing and postoperative rehabilitation. The results of revision surgery have not been as favorable as initial surgery, suggesting difficulty in correcting articular defects, limiting excessive translation, and preventing the development of degenerative arthritis.[9,14-16]

This chapter will address arthroscopic approaches to patients with failure due to recurrence of instability, failure due to pain with a stable shoulder, and management of complications. Certain arthroscopic techniques have been abandoned, including prolonged thermal shrinkage and articular pain pumps using potential chondrolytic agents due to reports of chondrolysis and premature degenerative arthritis. As with many forms of "new technology," problem recognition and early management are essential.[16]

Abrams JS. *Management of the Unstable Shoulder: Arthroscopic and Open Repair* (pp. 181-196).
© 2011 SLACK Incorporated

Figure 14-1. Suture anchors appear too close to the glenoid rim due to additional bone loss after instability recurrence.

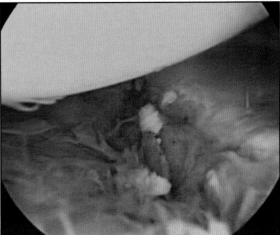

PATIENT SELECTION

Patient selection is an important aspect when managing individuals with continued or recurring problems after previous surgery. We should not assume that the same procedure should be repeated because additional pathologic changes may be present and patients' expectations and activities may have changed. A careful history, physical examination, radiographic evaluation, and additional imaging studies may be helpful in guiding your patients. The treatment options include nonoperative treatment; arthroscopic management; open reconstruction; and possible grafting deficiencies of the glenoid, humerus, or capsular ligaments.

NONOPERATIVE

Nonoperative treatment is rarely described when suggesting treatment to a young patient with recurrent instability, due to high risk of failure.[17,18] This may not be the same situation in a patient who fails following surgical repair. Patients who have had a long interval between surgery and recurrence may have success with nonoperative management. There may be a number of reasons, including cicatrix in the anterior capsule, older patients approaching the end of an athletic career, changing expectations from student athlete to employed weekend warrior, and early degenerative changes.

Nonoperative treatment consists of rest in a sling until minimal discomfort, followed by protective range of motion. Strengthening of rotators and scapular stabilization with closed kinetic chain exercises are started to limit proprioceptive changes in the shoulder. Avoiding the provocative position that recreates instability is important, but may be started 10 to 12 weeks after history of trauma. Slight stiffness may be protective in this situation.

Patients with an acute glenoid rim fracture create a situation that may require a surgical approach. This presents an opportunity to anatomically repair the glenoid inferior rim. Because bone loss is a risk factor for arthroscopic failure, intervention should be considered if an arthroscopic approach is being considered. Late treatment with bone loss often uses open surgery and possibly bone grafting. The opportunity for arthroscopy has the greatest chance of success in patients who can maintain maximal glenoid width.

Sport-specific exercises begin when range of motion approaches normal and strength of the cuff and scapular stabilizers are approaching the uninjured shoulder. Use of braces or harnesses may be considered in sports that normally wear shoulder pads or do not require maximal elevation and external rotation. Results of this treatment are difficult to quantitate because some of these athletes may choose an operation at the end of their playing season, even if instability events have not recurred.[19]

ARTHROSCOPY

There are patients who have had prior arthroscopic and open surgery who are disabled by recurrent instability. Arthroscopy allows for careful inspection of the articulation and appreciation of the orientation and degree of bone changes that have resulted from prior surgery and subsequent trauma. The ideal patient to consider an arthroscopic approach is a patient who has had success with previous surgery, had a recurrence following a traumatic onset, plays sports that require maximum abduction and external rotation, and has had minimal bone loss.

Important features from the history include the disability and treatment that led to the index surgery. An operative report and possibly photos, if available, are helpful in appreciating the degree of instability that led to the decision for surgery. Operative findings and treatment are important to understand whether the original surgery was likely to succeed or not. Open surgery details should include how the subscapularis was mobilized and whether a tenotomy or a horizontal split was performed. This may raise suspicion of subscapularis detachment and whether there was limited inferior capsular mobilization.

The history reveals the level of satisfaction prior to recurrence and what additional factor created the failure. Was failure due to a significant trauma or was there a minor injury or positional factor that caused the redislocation? When recurrent instability follows a minor event, it is often preferable to not repeat the same surgical approach for revisions. For example, if a patient who had arthroscopic repair redislocated rolling over in bed or lifting his or her arm, additional fixation is important and may be best achieved with an open approach. It is also helpful to understand what was done to reduce the shoulder and whether assistance was needed.

The physical exam begins with observation of range of movement and whether the patient is apprehensive to position in the provocative posture. Internal rotation strength is an important factor, particularly if prior open surgery was performed on the subscapularis.[20] Strength can be measured with a lift-off test behind the back or belly press sign pressing on the upper abdomen and seeing whether the elbow can maintain the distance from the trunk. Apprehension occurs when the patient either verbalizes, looks concerned, or uses muscle reaction to avoid positioning the shoulder in a position that may allow subluxation. The load-and-shift test is helpful in understanding degree of translation, directions of increased translation, and static stabilizer integrity. Repeat the test with the arm 45 degrees externally rotated and 45 degrees abducted to partially tension the inferior glenohumeral ligament. A reduction maneuver may relieve apprehension and permit further external rotation.

Radiographs should include at least 2 views—anteroposterior to the glenoid or scapular and axillary view. Additional views, such as an anteroposterior view with humeral internal rotation to visualize head defects or a West Point view of the glenoid to identify glenoid rim pathology, are helpful. Many shoulders will benefit from further imaging with CT scan or MRI. Reconstruction views of the face of the glenoid allow for an estimate of bone loss or recognition of rim fracture.[21,22] It may be helpful to arthroscopically evaluate the degree of bone loss and decide on whether repair should be performed arthroscopically or with open techniques.[23]

As bone loss exceeds 20% of the width of the glenoid, the anatomic arthroscopic repair has increased risk of failure, particularly if the athlete is playing a contact or collision sport. An arthroscopic option is still available for defects up to 30%, but additional tensioning is required and loss of external rotation is a likely consequence. Because preservation of external rotation is a significant benefit of an arthroscopic approach, over-tensioning may make this a less effective approach.

Soft tissue deficiency is not easy to appreciate with preoperative studies. The recurrence of a Bankart lesion is common. The lateral and mid-capsular injuries can be missed, even with contrast studies. Patients with prior thermal treatment are at risk for capsular necrosis, and open reconstruction and grafting may be indicated when capsular closure cannot be achieved. Select capsular tears and detachments can be repaired arthroscopically if a safe interval can be established from adjacent neurologic structures (Figure 14-2).

OPEN BANKART REPAIR

The indications for an open soft tissue repair include moderate bone loss, failure of an arthroscopic repair with minor trauma, subscapularis dehiscence, and lateral capsule injury. Capsular injury in the anteroinferior quadrant is close to the axillary nerve. Anchor placement in the humeral head to repair capsular avulsion may place the nerves in the pathway.[24] There are techniques to address this arthroscopically, and they are safer when this occurs in the posterior quadrant.[25] Certain sports (ie, wrestling) have increased middle and lateral capsular injuries and may have greater success with open repairs that allow medial suture anchor repair combined with lateral criss-crossing capsular flaps.

Bone loss of 25% or less has been successfully treated with an open Bankart repair.[26] There may be many factors that will impact whether there is a need for additional grafting. Glenoid rim fractures requiring screw internal fixation may be approached by an open or arthroscopic approach, depending on the preference of the surgeon.

The most common reason for choosing an open repair is that patient who has had a recurrence following a well-done arthroscopic procedure with minimal trauma. If there is a biological reason why there was incomplete healing after the first surgery, repeating the process may not be successful. Interestingly, an open approach (ie, Bristow) that fails may be approached arthroscopically with less risk of injury to the musculocutaneous nerve.

BONE GRAFTING

Glenoid rim loss and humeral head impression defects are often combined. Experts do not agree on an actual glenoid loss that necessitates a bone augmentation procedure, but the range is between 20% and 30%.[27,28] The engaging Hill-Sachs lesion becomes more critical when the shoulder can lock out of the joint in positions of 0 to 45 degrees of abduction. This will affect activities of daily living as well as physical activities.

Bone grafting is most commonly performed along the anteroinferior glenoid when combined lesions are present. The Latarjet procedure indications are described in this

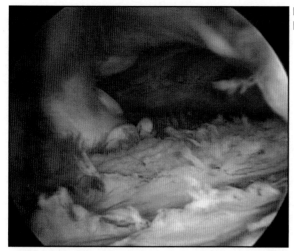

Figure 14-2. Large inferior capsular tear following recurrent dislocation.

text and will not be repeated. Patients with prolonged dislocation following seizures may have excessive humeral head impression with a relatively small glenoid rim injury. Open grafting or prosthetic augmentation of the humeral head may be helpful. The arthroscopic Latarjet is a technique to graft the glenoid and has had early success.[29,30] Direction of drilling and screw placement is a challenge, especially for patients in the lateral decubitus position. Currently, the open approach is being done more frequently due to proximity of neurovascular structures. For more information on indications and techniques, see Chapters 17 and 18.

TECHNIQUE

Diagnostic Arthroscopy

Examination under anesthesia is performed in neutral position, as well as with various degrees of abduction and rotation, to place important ligaments in position to see if they effectively limit translation. The degree of compromised static stabilizers is compared to the unaffected shoulder.

Arthroscopic stabilization can be performed in the lateral decubitus or beach chair position. Surgeons need to be able to adjust patients if they feel that an open approach is beneficial. A diagnostic arthroscopy is helpful, even if the plan is to perform an open repair.

Most surgeons prefer to create 3 portals, although additional portals may be needed in selected cases. The posterior portal is 2 cm inferior to the angle of the acromion and scapular spine and directed at the mid-glenoid. An outside-to-inside technique with a spinal needle allows palpation for potential portal development. The anterosuperior portal is inferior to the acromioclavicular joint, and the anteroinferior portal is lateral to the coracoid and enters above the superior border of the subscapularis. If you are too far lateral, injury to the humeral head can occur when trying to place an anchor along the anterior glenoid rim. An assistant distracts and posteriorly translates the humerus, reducing the dislocation and maximizing access to the glenoid. If the working inferior portal is too medial, inferior anchors are difficult to place without injuring the glenoid articular surface.

Figure 14-3. Metallic suture anchors are exposed following recurrence and glenoid rim fracture.

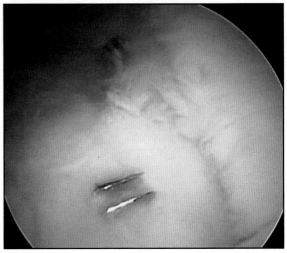

The diagnostic steps begin at the biceps and use the light cord rotation when using a 30-degree arthroscope to view superiorly and inferiorly. Inspection includes the superior labrum, rotator cuff, anterior labrum, subscapularis insertion, and pouch. An anterior view may be necessary to visualize the inferior aspect of the glenoid rim. If the plan is to open, portals are closed with nylon interrupted sutures, and the patient is positioned for the arthrotomy.

Suture Anchor Repair

Following examination under anesthesia and a diagnostic arthroscopy, débridement of capsule, labral mobilization, and preparation of the glenoid neck should follow (see Chapter 14 video). Fractured and displaced hardware may be adjacent to the repair and should be removed (Figure 14-3).

The liberator is used to separate the labrum from the bone. Carefully preserve the quality of the labrum, which may be challenging superiorly, near the interval. Concentrate on the inferior ligament, including the pouch and the thickened capsular bands superiorly (Figure 14-4). Next, use a shaver and suction punch to divide attachment to the subscapularis. Expose the subscapularis to its inferior border (Figure 14-5). This will begin with the viewing portal posteriorly and be completed with the anterosuperior viewing portal. A shaver is placed in the anteroinferior portal, and devitalized tissue is removed.

A special situation may present when there is a rim fracture with attached labrum. If this can be mobilized as a unit, then perform the repair by securing the labrum and fragment in its original location. However, if the bone has healed to the glenoid neck, use a liberator, and separate the labrum and periosteum from the fractured rim, allowing for mobilization. The bone fragment is decorticated, and soft tissue is transferred, covering the surface.

Define the inferior and superior extent of the injury while viewing from both posteriorly and anteriorly. Place the scope in the anterior portal, and visualize inferiorly to the posterior extent of the lesion. Pass a shaver in the posterior portal, and abrade the capsule and pouch. Use a curved hook, grasp the posteroinferior capsule, and pass suture under the intact labrum. If the labrum is deficient, place a posterior anchor through a puncture hole 3 cm lateral to the posterior portal. Sutures can be placed that retension the posterior band of the IGHL (Figure 14-6).

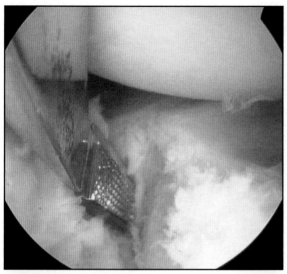

Figure 14-4. A liberator is used to dissect labrum and capsule from the glenoid neck.

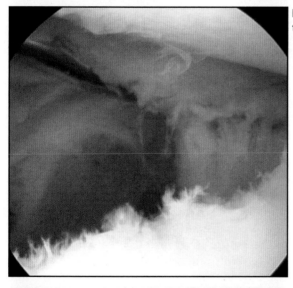

Figure 14-5. Divide capsular attachments to the subscapularis.

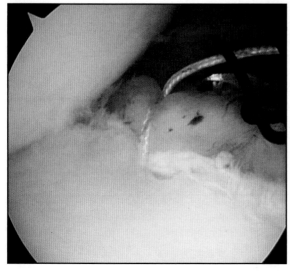

Figure 14-6. A posterior suture anchor is percutaneously placed, reinforcing the posterior band of the IGHL.

Figure 14-7. An anterior anchor (right shoulder) is approached through a posterior portal to retrieve the suture.

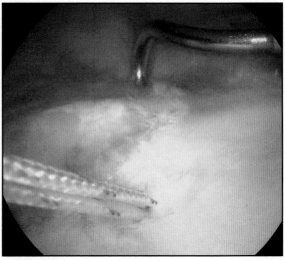

The most anteroinferior anchor is placed through the portal lateral to the coracoid. The anchor hole should be as inferior as possible and should be placed on the articular surface. There should be less than 1 cm between the posterior sutures and this anchor. Rather than using the anterior portal that will create a modest capsule shift, place a suture hook through the posterior portal. Grasp the capsule, and rotate the hook under the labrum. Advance a shuttle or monofilament suture, and retrieve out through the anterior portal. Shuttle a braided suture under the labrum and out through the posterior cannula. Securing this suture will reduce the inferior pouch and labrum (Figure 14-7).

The next anchor is placed 1 cm above the previous. Exchange curved suture hooks to the opposite direction of curvature, and place in the anterior inferior cannula. A right hook will be used on a right shoulder. Puncture the capsule inferior and lateral to the anchor. It should be adjacent to the previous suture to provide additional tension to the capsule. After retrieving the suture, a second hook is placed superior and parallel to the anchor; a second arm of the suture is retrieved, creating a mattress suture. This combines an inferior-to-superior shift and tensions the capsule as well. The mattress suture is secured, transferring the labrum on top of the glenoid and reapproximating the capsule against the abraded glenoid (Figure 14-8).

A third anterior anchor is placed more superiorly. This anchor is generally at 2 o'clock for a right shoulder and 10 o'clock for a left shoulder. A simple suture is passed through the middle ligament, which is adjacent to the superior aspect of the defect, completing the labral repair (Figure 14-9). Do not attempt suture anchor closure of a large fovea or Buford complex. In cases where there is a congenital alteration of the superior capsule, plan an inferior-to-superior capsular plication superior to the suture anchor repair.

In patients with a combined SLAP lesion, you should consider repair rather than resect to maximize stability. If you are planning to perform a suture anchor repair, it is preferable to do this at this time to avoid loss of visualization as swelling and tensioning progresses.

There are instances where the Hill-Sachs lesion appears adjacent to the articular surface, raising concern that the head remains in an anteriorly translated position and engagement may occur. A surgical option is a Remplissage or arthroscopic Connolly procedure, securing the infraspinatus into the defect.[31] This can be performed by

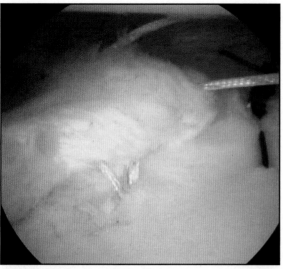

Figure 14-8. A mattress suture can be created with a suture anchor to reinforce the capsule.

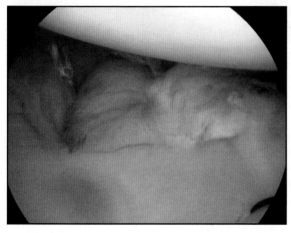

Figure 14-9. A completed labral repair includes a combination of mattress and simple sutures.

initially débriding the bursal tissue overlying the infraspinatus. Return the scope to the anterior portal or a posterosuperior portal. Rotator cuff suture anchors are placed percutaneously into the defect approximately 3 mm from the articular edge. Retrieve the cannula so that it no longer enters the capsule and the infraspinatus. Now use a piercing instrument to retrieve sutures in a spread fashion. The scope can be placed in the subacromial space, and sutures are secured. During tying, place a posterior force on the humeral head to optimize soft tissue approximation (Figure 14-10).

Rotator interval closure has been controversial, and results are mixed in contributing to shoulder stability.[32] In revision surgery, the addition of closure of the superior and middle glenohumeral ligaments can improve reduction of anterior translation.[5] This will also incorporate the coracohumeral ligament into the repair.

Remove one of the anterior cannulas. Through the second cannula, place a suture hook, and grasp the full thickness of the middle glenohumeral ligament. Do not include the subscapularis. Back out the cannula, and use a piercing instrument to pass through the superior ligament and retrieve the free end of the suture. Sutures can be tied as they are placed. Generally, 2 or 3 sutures are used and can be nonabrasive permanent sutures or monofilament sutures.

Figure 14-10. Posterior infraspinatus insertion into the enlarged Hill-Sachs defect. (Reprinted with permission from Abrams JS. Revision instability surgery. In: Angelo RL, Esch JC, Ryu RKN. *AANA Advanced Arthroscopy: The Shoulder.* Philadelphia, PA: Saunders; 2010:147-156. Copyright Elsevier 2010.)

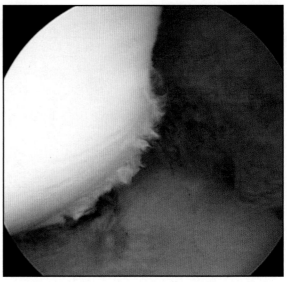

PAINFUL SHOULDER FOLLOWING STABILIZATION

Revision surgery may be used to manage shoulders that have pain, in spite of restoring stability. The major concern here is the viability of the articular cartilage. This viability can be compromised due to suture impingement, anchor abrasion, or chondrolysis.

Suture impingement is important to distinguish from anchor impingement. The "squeaky" shoulder may improve with temporary reduction of activities. The concern raised with exposed anchors is very real and can cause irreversible changes to the glenoid or humeral head.[33] Confirmation of anchor location with radiographs (metal anchors) or MRI (absorbable or plastic anchors) is important to allow for early intervention (Figure 14-11). Removal of sutures can be performed if surgery has adequate time to heal and may be replaced with new anchors if the healing process is early. It is often preferable to delay suture removal until after 4 to 6 months, allowing healing and avoiding additional need for hardware (Figure 14-12). Prominent anchor removal should not be delayed if causing injury to the humeral head.

Stiffness is an uncommon problem with arthroscopic repairs. Anatomic reasons for significant loss of motion include closing fovea or middle capsule defects to the glenoid. Allow the patient to heal for 3 to 6 months, and consider arthroscopic release. Manipulation may cause damage to the articular structures and will likely recreate labral separation from the glenoid. Arthroscopic removal of superior sutures, interval release, and a limited capsulotomy should re-establish the desired range of motion (Figure 14-13). Early appropriate rehabilitation is an important component of release of adhesions. Stiffness may be an early finding in patients with chondrolysis. Removal of foreign bodies (ie, sutures) and capsulotomy may limit the compressive forces if performed early. More advanced degenerative changes and delays in treatment may require prosthesis or resurfacing procedures.

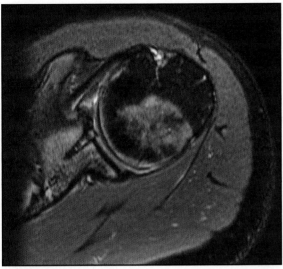

Figure 14-11. MRI of a patient with pain following stabilization demonstrating a proud absorbable suture anchor.

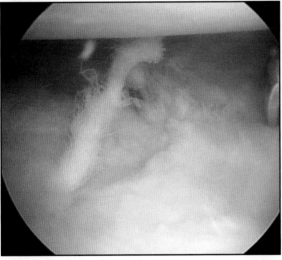

Figure 14-12. Suture is damaging articular cartilage on the glenoid and should be removed.

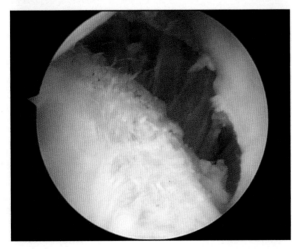

Figure 14-13. The stiff shoulder can undergo selective arthroscopic release without disrupting the Bankart repair. (Reprinted with permission from Abrams JS. Revision instability surgery. In: Angelo RL, Esch JC, Ryu RKN. *AANA Advanced Arthroscopy: The Shoulder*. Philadelphia, PA: Saunders; 2010:147-156. Copyright Elsevier 2010.)

MANAGING COMPLICATIONS

Complications can occur with revision surgery as well. Patients may present with pain, stiffness, and continued loss of function. A systematic approach to evaluation includes a detailed history, physical examination, radiographs, and advanced imaging.

The most common complication is recurrence of instability. The success of revision stabilization is approximately 70% to 80%.[7-11,16] Additional concern with volition or habitual subluxators, seizures, greater degrees of bone loss, and returning to athletics prematurely can contribute to poor outcomes. Structural problems will require a different approach, with the possible addition of bone augmentation. If a patient is continuing to have seizures, then medical management needs to achieve success before shoulder surgery is considered. Behavioral problems and scheduled return to sport need additional discussion and treatment to optimize the chance of success.[14]

Degenerative arthritis can be detected on imaging studies and diagnosis arthroscopy (Figure 14-14). It may be difficult to decide if additional surgery will permit physical activity and possibly accelerate degenerative arthritis. From a joint mechanical perspective, you need to decide which is worse: compression forces or shearing forces due to additional subluxation. From a personal standpoint, if the range of motion allows an athlete to return to sport, then stabilization seems to be a reasonable option. Allowing instability events to continue will make reconstructive surgery less reliable as well.

Painful shoulders with a stable joint are often seen with chondral injury. This can be due to isolated glenoid or humeral head lesion or be diffuse as in chondrolysis. Early intervention with repeat arthroscopy, release of adhesions, possible removal of sutures or foreign bodies, and select capsulotomy may limit the progression of this potential disaster. Foreign bodies may include prominent suture anchors and suture material (see Figures 14-11 and 14-12). As normal articular cartilage rubs against these materials, deterioration of the surrounding cartilage becomes evident. This may stay localized or extend to a larger region. Removal of symptomatic foreign bodies is important to limiting permanent damage.

Pain pumps placed within the articulation have been associated with chondrolysis. This uncommon, but devastating, complication occurs when catheters have been in place for 2 days and bupivacaine of various concentrations has been used.[34] A chondrolytic effect of analgesics have been shown, but certain individual shoulders are more sensitive to this effect than others. It is best to avoid the prolonged pain pump with marcaine until better options are available or science is able to identify significant risk factors.

Stiffness is not uncommon after multiple surgeries to the shoulder. Surgery and instability events can traumatize the capsular ligaments. Repairing a torn, contracted ligament may leave a patient with a reduction of external rotation. As we choose to "retension" the ligaments, we are reducing rotation while attempting to alter humeral translation. We often rely on physical therapy and exercise to correct stiffness. This is not always possible, and the combination of articular changes is a concern. Arthroscopic evaluation and potential selective release is occasionally necessary (see Figure 14-13). Surgeons may choose a labral repair without significant capsular transfer in patients at risk for stiffness.

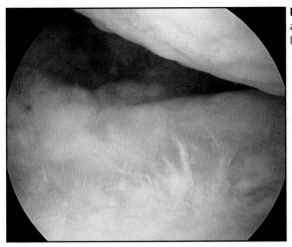

Figure 14-14. Degenerative articular changes are detected in shoulders with recurrent subluxation.

POSTOPERATIVE TREATMENT

Revision surgery may heal more slowly than the initial surgery. This is due to soft tissue vascularity compromise, use of bone grafts, older patients, or compromise of fixation. In spite of risk factors, success can be achieved arthroscopically in approximately 3 out of 4 patients.[8-11] Patients are placed in a sling for 4 to 6 weeks. The brace is used to limit activities and ideally places the shoulder in neutral, avoiding significant internal or external rotation. Daily exercises to improve posture and core strength will limit the potential contribution from the scapula and chest wall.

Shoulder exercises postoperatively include pendulum exercises beginning with small circles and gradually increasing the radius, performed without the use of weights. Shoulder shrugs can help avoid contracted pectoralis muscles that may promote forward positioning of the humeral head on the glenoid. Additional exercise to the elbow and hand can begin early, but should not position the shoulder in a position that stresses the repair.

At 4 to 5 weeks, the sling can be weaned, and external rotation can begin. This should be limited to 30 degrees to avoid maximum stress. More advanced external rotation is not started until 6 to 8 weeks. During the initial period, forward elevation is allowed passively and actively. At 4 weeks, patients can touch the top of their head and progress to near-normal elevation by 8 to 12 weeks. Cross-chest motion can begin at 4 weeks, but behind the back should not begin until 6 weeks following arthroscopy, possibly longer if an open procedure was performed.

Strengthening and resistive exercises may begin at 8 weeks. This may begin as isometrics and progress to rotators and scapular stabilizers. A series of closed-chain exercises will coordinate core strength with arm strength and improve the proprioceptive awareness of the articulation. Exercises for the cuff include internal and external rotation with thick bands of rubber or light weights. Scapular strength includes seated-rows, shrugs, latissimus pulls to the chest, and neutral grip push-ups.

More advanced training should be sport-specific, and return to athletics can be considered after 5 to 6 months following arthroscopic revision surgery. If bone grafting procedures are performed, radiographic evidence of healing should occur prior to returning to sports. Shoulder bracing may be helpful in high-risk sports, particularly those that require shoulder pads. The additional security has been helpful to some athletes who do not depend on the abducted posture for performance. Throwing and catching athletes do not always like this additional restraint and choose a longer duration of healing prior to return to sports.

TIPS AND PEARLS

- Additional trauma creating recurrence may produce glenoid rim fractures and degenerative joint changes.

- Failed arthroscopic surgery with minor trauma may have better chance of success with open revision surgery. Failed open surgery with minor trauma may be better treated with arthroscopy.

- Imaging studies are less reliable after prior surgical procedures. Intraoperative evaluation may change surgical approach.

- Capsular mobilization is essential to reposition the labrum and capsule. Capsular attachments to the subscapularis may create medial traction on the capsule during external rotation and should be released.

- Glenoid preparation is light burring and débridement. Healed bone fragment on anterior glenoid can be repositioned or "freshened" to transfer capsule and labrum on top.

- Posterior and posterior inferior portals allow improved access to the inferior pouch.

- Sutures and suture anchors should include the entire IGHL, including the posterior band.

- Using additional anchors is common in revision procedures.

- Painful shoulders raise concern with prominent anchors and sutures that may impinge inside the joint. This may require early intervention to minimize joint damage.

- Rotator interval closure between superior and middle glenohumeral ligaments is routinely done with revision surgery. You may consider avoiding in overhead throwers.

REFERENCES

1. Carreira DS, Mazzocca AD, Oryhon J, Brown FM, Hayden JK, Romeo AA. A prospective outcome evaluation of arthroscopic Bankart repairs minimum 2-year follow-up. *Am J Sports Med.* 2006;34(5):771-777.
2. Bottoni CR, Smith EL, Berkowitz MJ, et al. Arthroscopic versus open stabilization for recurrent instability: a prospective randomized clinical trial. *Am J Sports Med.* 2006;34:1730-1737.
3. Fabbricianni C, Milano G, Demontis A, et al. Arthroscopic versus open treatment of Bankart lesion of the shoulder, a prospective randomized study. *Arthroscopy.* 2004;20:456-462.
4. Larrain MV, Montenegro HJ, Mauas DM, et al. Arthroscopic management of traumatic anterior shoulder instability in collision athletes: analysis of 204 cases with a 4- to 9-year follow-up and results with the suture anchor technique. *Arthroscopy.* 2006;12(12):1283-1289.
5. Abrams JS. Role of arthroscopy in treating anterior instability of the athlete's shoulder. *Sports Med Arthrosc Rev.* 2007;15:230-238.
6. Kropf EJ, Tjoumakaris FP, Sekiya JK. Arthroscopic shoulder stabilization: is there ever a need to open? *Arthroscopy.* 2007;23(7):779-784.
7. Zabinski SJ, Callaway GH, Cohen S, Warren RF. Revision shoulder stabilization: 2- to 10-year results. *J Shoulder Elbow Surg.* 1999;8(1):58-65.
8. Pelet S, Jolles BM, Farron A. Bankart repair for recurrent anterior glenohumeral instability: results of twenty-nine years' follow up. *J Shoulder Elbow Surg.* 2006;15(2):203-207.

9. Kim SH, Kwon-Ick HA, Kim YM. Arthroscopic revision Bankart repair: a prospective outcome study. *Arthroscopy.* 2002;18(5):469-482.

10. Creighton RA, Romeo AA, Brown FM, et al. Revision arthroscopic shoulder instability repair. *Arthroscopy.* 2007;23(7):703-709.

11. Franceschi F, Longo UG, Ruzzini L, et al. Arthroscopic salvage of failed arthroscopic Bankart repair: a prospective study with a minimum follow-up of 4 years. *Am J Sports Med.* 2008;36(7):1330-1336.

12. Meehan RE, Petersen SA. Results and factors affecting outcome of revision surgery for shoulder instability. *J Shoulder Elbow Surg.* 2005;14(1):31-37.

13. Sugaya H, Moriishi J, Dohi M, et al. Glenoid rim morphology in recurrent anterior glenohumeral instability. *J Bone Joint Surg.* 2003;85A:878-884.

14. Levine WN, Arroyo JS, Pollock RA, et al. Open revision stabilization surgery for recurrent anterior glenohumeral instability. *Am J Sports Med.* 2000;28(2):156-160.

15. Neri BR, Tuckman DV, Bravman JT, et al. Arthroscopic revision of Bankart repair. *J Shoulder Elbow Surg.* 2007;16(4):419-424.

16. Abrams JS, Bradley JP, Angelo RL, Burks R. Arthroscopic management of shoulder instabilities: anterior, posterior, and multidirectional. *Instr Course Lect.* 2010;59:141-155.

17. Robinson CM, Howes J, Murdoch H, et al. Functional outcome and risk of recurrent instability after primary anterior shoulder dislocation in young patients. *J Bone Joint Surg.* 2006;88:2326-2336.

18. Arciero RA, Wheeler JH, Ryan JB, et al. Arthroscopic Bankart repair versus nonoperative treatment for acute initial anterior dislocation of the shoulder. *Am J Sports Med.* 1994;22:589-594.

19. Buss DD, Lynch GP, Meyer CP, Huber SM, Freehill MQ. Nonoperative management for in-season athletes with anterior shoulder instability. *Am J Sports Med.* 2004;32(6):1430-1433.

20. Greis PE, Dean M, Hawkins RJ. Subscapularis tendon disruption after Bankart reconstruction for anterior instability. *J Shoulder Elbow Surg.* 1996;5:219-222.

21. Itoi E, Lee SB, Amrami KK, et al. Quantitative assessment of classic anteroinferior bony Bankart lesions by radiography and computed tomography. *Am J Sports Med.* 2003;31(1):112-118.

22. Sugaya H, Moriishi J, Kanisawa I, Tsuchiya A. Arthroscopic osseous Bankart repairs for chronic recurrent traumatic anterior glenohumeral instability. *J Bone Joint Surg.* 2005;87:1752-1760.

23. Burkhart SS, De Beer JF, Tehrany AM, Parten PM. Quantifying glenoid bone loss arthroscopically in shoulder instability. *Arthroscopy.* 2002;18(5):488-491.

24. Arciero RA, Mazzocca AD. Mini-open repair technique of HAGL (humeral avulsion of the glenohumeral ligament) lesion. *Arthroscopy.* 2005;21(9):1152.e1-1152.e4.

25. Abrams JS. Arthroscopic repair of posterior instability and reverse humeral glenohumeral ligament avulsion lesions. *Orthop Clin North Am.* 2003;34(4):475-483.

26. Pagnani MJ, Dome DC. Surgical treatment of traumatic anterior shoulder instability in American football players. *J Bone Joint Surg.* 2002;84A:711-715.

27. Burkhart SS, De Beer JF. Traumatic glenohumeral bone defects and their relationship to failure of arthroscopic Bankart repairs: significance of the inverted-pear glenoid and the humeral head engaging Hill-Sachs lesion. *Arthroscopy.* 2000;16(7):677-694.

28. Chen AL, Hunt SA, Hawkins RJ, Zuckerman D. Management of bone loss associated with recurrent anterior glenohumeral instability. *Am J Sports Med.* 2005;33(6):912-925.

29. Lafosse L, Lejeune E, Bouchard A, Kakuda C, Gobezie R. The arthroscopic Latarjet procedure for the treatment of anterior shoulder instability. *Arthroscopy.* 2007;11:1242-1245.

30. Boileau P, Bicknell RT, El Fegoun AB, Chuinard C. Arthroscopic Bristow procedure for anterior instability in shoulders with a stretched or deficient capsule: the "belt-and-suspenders" operative technique and preliminary results. *Arthroscopy.* 2007;23(6):593-601.

31. Purchase RJ, Wolf EM, Hobgood ER, Pollock ME, Smalley CC. Hills-Sachs "Remplissage": an arthroscopic solution for the engaging Hill-Sachs lesion. *Arthroscopy.* 2008;24(6):723-726.

32. Mologne TS, Zhao K, Hongo M, et al. The addition of rotator interval closure after arthroscopic repair of either anterior or posterior shoulder instability: effect on glenohumeral translation and range of motion. *Am J Sports Med.* 2008;36(8):1123-1131.

33. Rhee YG, Lee DH, Chun IH, Bae SC. Glenohumeral arthropathy after arthroscopic anterior shoulder stabilization. *Arthroscopy.* 2004;20(4):402-406.

34. Gomoll AH, Kang RW, Williams MJ, et al. Chondrolysis after continuous infra-articular bupivacaine infusion: an experimental model investigating chondrotoxity in the rabbit shoulder. *Arthroscopy.* 2006;22:813-819.

Please see video on the accompanying Web site at
http://www.slackbooks.com/unstableshouldervideos

Arthrotomy and Repair of the Unstable Shoulder

15

Bankart Repair
and Capsule Shift

J. Douglas Haltom, MD and Gary W. Misamore, MD

Glenohumeral instability is a common problem that affects predominantly young, active individuals. The direction of dislocation and subsequent instability is anterior in 95% of these patients.[1,2] Bankart was one of the first to describe the essential anterior glenoid rim lesion and a surgical technique to repair such. In his 1939 article, he stated, "the only rational treatment is to reattach the glenoid ligament to the bone from which it has been torn."[3] The avulsion of the anterior/inferior capsulolabral complex, the Bankart lesion, is shown in the magnetic resonance image (MRI) in Figure 15-1. A bony Bankart lesion, in which a portion of the glenoid is fractured with the capsulolabral complex, is shown in the image in Figure 15-2.

Anatomic and nonanatomic repairs for anterior instability have been described. Capsulolabral reconstructions, or anatomic repairs, are largely synonymous with the Bankart repair. Significant variation exists, however, in the technique in which the subscapularis muscle and capsule are taken down and repaired. Surgical techniques are also tailored intraoperatively to treat the identified pathology. The ultimate goal of surgery is to reduce and secure the labrum to the glenoid face with the appropriate amount of capsular tension so that these structures may heal in an anatomic manner.

INDICATIONS

Indications for an open Bankart repair are largely dependent on the patient's symptoms and do not differ significantly from an arthroscopic repair. Patients who participate in high-demand sports or activities or have high-demand vocations may require a repair after an initial dislocation. Other possible indications may include recurrent episodes of instability despite adequate nonoperative therapy or pain and disability associated with subluxation episodes. Midseason athletes may choose to brace the shoulder, continue to play if possible, and consider a repair after the season depending on their instability symptoms.

Abrams JS. *Management of the Unstable Shoulder: Arthroscopic and Open Repair* (pp. 199-208).
© 2011 SLACK Incorporated

Figure 15-1. The red arrow indicates the Bankart lesion.

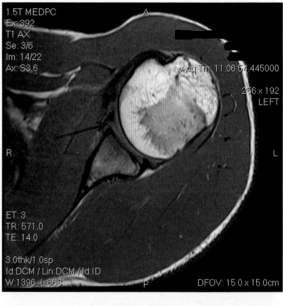

Figure 15-2. The red arrow indicates the bony Bankart lesion.

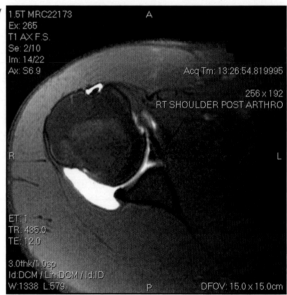

Open and arthroscopic repair techniques are discussed with the patient. MRI is not always necessary, but an identified Bankart lesion on MRI supplies more information that allows a treatment plan to be formulated. In most situations, both techniques are acceptable, and the benefits of each are explained to the patient. Both are outpatient procedures with similar postoperative rehab programs. The cosmetic difference is discussed along with the implications of a subscapularis incision that has to be performed in the open repair. Outcomes are also discussed. In our experience, the patient has a 95% success rate with the open repair compared to 90% with the arthroscopic repair. This difference can more than likely be explained in the capsular tensioning portion of the open procedure, which will be explained later in the chapter. Finally, if significant glenoid bony deficiency is present, then an open procedure would be favored.

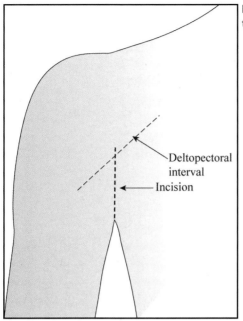

Figure 15-3. This more cosmetic incision is in line with the axillary fold.

Deltopectoral interval

Incision

SURGICAL SET-UP/APPROACH

The patient is positioned supine on the operating room table. A thorough examination under anesthesia is undertaken, including the uninvolved shoulder for comparison. Particular attention is paid to the amount of external rotation that is present in both adduction and abduction. These measurements can be used as a reference for the capsular closure portion of the procedure. After the examination under anesthesia, the patient is placed in a semi-beach chair position, and a shoulder arthroscopy can be performed if desired.

A standard deltopectoral approach is performed. A more cosmetic incision in line with the anterior axillary line can be used (Figure 15-3). If this is chosen, it is important to sufficiently undermine the subcutaneous tissue in the superomedial and inferolateral portion of the incision to gain access to the deltopectoral interval. The cephalic vein is usually retracted laterally with the deltoid because of its large feeding vessels into that muscle. Blunt dissection is used to develop the interval, and large retractors are used to gain exposure of the conjoined tendon. Once the fascia is divided lateral to the muscular portion of the coracobrachialis, a large retractor can be placed beneath the conjoined tendon, and it is retracted medially. The subdeltoid fascia must also be incised so a retractor can be placed beneath the deltoid to retract it laterally. With external rotation of the arm, the subscapularis and its tendon are identified. The arm is kept in a position of adduction to protect the axillary nerve.

SUBSCAPULARIS AND CAPSULAR INCISIONS

The subscapularis tendon and capsule are incised and taken down separately in this procedure. The rotator interval is identified, and approximately 1-cm medial to the medial aspect of the lesser tuberosity, a vertical tenotomy is made in the subscapularis

Figure 15-4. As shown in this diagram, the tenotomy (dotted line) ends just superior to the anterior humeral circumflex vessels.

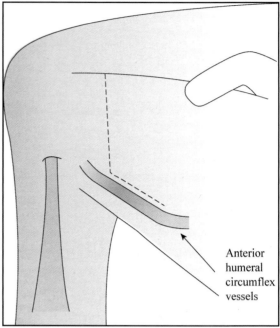

Anterior
humeral
circumflex
vessels

tendon. The incision begins superiorly at the rotator interval and continues inferiorly to the anterior circumflex humeral vessels, which lie on the inferior portion of the tendon. This inferior-most portion of the tendon is left undisturbed, protecting the anterior humeral circumflex vessels and the axillary nerve. Care is taken not to disturb the underlying capsule. This tenotomy is very similar to one described by Matson and colleagues[4] and is depicted in Figure 15-4.

Several other options exist for dividing the subscapularis tendon. Rowe and colleagues[5] describe a technique in which the entire tendon is excised in a vertical fashion 2-cm medial to the lesser tuberosity, ligating the vessels inferiorly (Figure 15-5). The advantage includes better visualization of the glenohumeral joint. The subscapularis muscle and its tendon can also be incised transversely in line with its fibers (Figure 15-6). This provides less external rotation restrictions in the early post-operative period and avoids the risk of postoperative rupture. Glenoid visualization, however, is more difficult.[6]

After the tendon has been incised, the underlying capsule has to be exposed. An elevator is used to carefully develop this plane, usually in an inferior-to-superior direction. It is often helpful to use the medial muscular portion of the subscapularis to develop this plane between the subscapularis and capsule. Once this is accomplished, a tag stitch is placed in the subscapularis tendon, and the muscle is carefully freed from the underlying glenoid and scapular neck. A scapular neck retractor is then placed, exposing the underlying shoulder capsule. Placing the retractor medially on the scapular neck allows the capsule to be mobilized for later repairs and/or shifts.

A transverse capsular incision is then made. The capsular interval can often be used, which is just superior to the middle glenohumeral ligament (Figure 15-7). The transverse capsulotomy is continued medially to the glenoid. The capsule is then incised horizontally, usually from a superior-to-inferior direction, approximately 1-cm medial to the humerus (Figure 15-8). The inferior limit of the dissection is determined by the glenoid pathology. When the most inferior portion of the glenoid can be visualized,

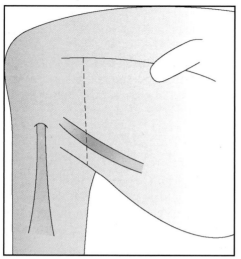

Figure 15-5. This tenotomy involves the entire subscapularis tendon, and the vessels are sacrificed.

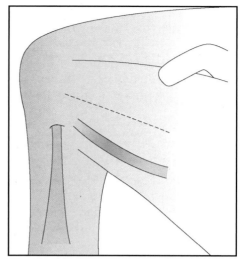

Figure 15-6. A transverse incision is made in the tendon and muscle belly, leaving the insertion intact.

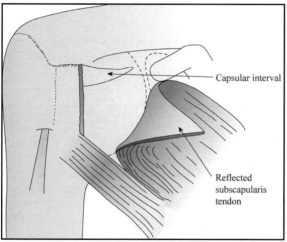

Figure 15-7. After the subscapularis tenotomy, the tendon is reflected and the capsular interval is identified.

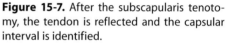

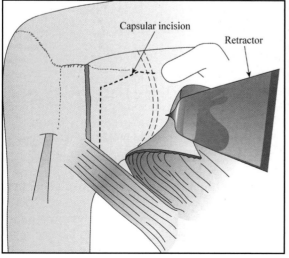

Figure 15-8. A glenoid retractor has been placed, which helps retract the subscapularis. The capsulotomy is continued transversely from the capsular interval to a point approximately 1 cm medial the humerus, and then is continued horizontally (dotted line). Tag sutures are placed in medial lateral corners at the apex of the capsulotomy.

the capsular incision is stopped. Tag stitches are placed in the both the medial and lateral corners of the capsule at the apex of the capsular incision, and the capsule is reflected medially. The glenoid and labrum are now exposed.

There are options for incising the capsule as well. Vertical,[7] transverse,[8] or T-shaped[9] capsulotomies have been described. The vertical portion of the T-shaped incision can be based medially toward the glenoid or laterally toward the humerus.

BANKART REPAIR

The anterior and inferior aspect of the glenoid and labrum are inspected. The area in which the labrum and capsule have been avulsed from the glenoid is identified. If there has been significant scarring, a soft tissue elevator may be used to elevate the labrum so that it can be reduced to the glenoid rim. A burr may also be used to prepare the glenoid bony bed. Two or 3 double-loaded suture anchors, depending on the size of the lesion, are then placed in the glenoid. The anchors are placed at the edge of the glenoid cartilage and angled approximately 45 degrees. Bone tunnels with a similar suture configuration can be used as an alternative to the suture anchors.

The avulsed capsule is addressed first. Two sister limbs from the most inferior suture anchor are taken out medially through the capsule in a horizontal mattress fashion. It is important that these sutures are appropriately placed so that the capsule is not tethered medially. Lateral retraction on the capsule while placing the sutures is helpful in preventing this medial tethering. This is continued superiorly with the remaining anchors. Attention is then turned to the labrum. One limb from the remaining suture of each anchor is taken and placed around the labrum in a simple suture fashion. This is also more easily done in an inferior-to-superior direction. The horizontal mattress capsular sutures are then tied, followed by the simple labral sutures. This is done in an inferior-to-superior direction as well. The repair and suture configuration is depicted in Figure 15-9.

Bony Bankart lesions can also be addressed with this technique. If the bone is of sufficient size, screw fixation can be used. Once the glenoid is reduced and secured, the repair can proceed as above. If the bone is too small and screw fixation cannot be achieved, then the suture anchors can be placed in the fracture bed. The bony glenoid fragment is then captured with the sutures to reduce and secure it.

CAPSULAR REPAIR/CAPSULAR SHIFT AND SUBSCAPULARIS REPAIR

The glenohumeral joint is copiously irrigated prior to capsular closure. A heavy non-absorbable suture is used to close the capsule. Closure is started at the inferior-most aspect of the capsular incision and is continued superiorly. The previously placed tag stitches at the superior apices of the capsule are used for reference. If there is no significant capsular redundancy, then no shift is performed, and a standard capsular closure is undertaken. If there is significant redundancy or laxity in the capsule, then a shift can be instituted by superior and/or lateral elevation of the medial capsular leaflet, referencing the tag stitches. Once the vertical portion of the capsule is closed, stability and external rotation are tested in both adduction and abduction. If either is unacceptable, then the sutures can be removed and the capsule retensioned accordingly.

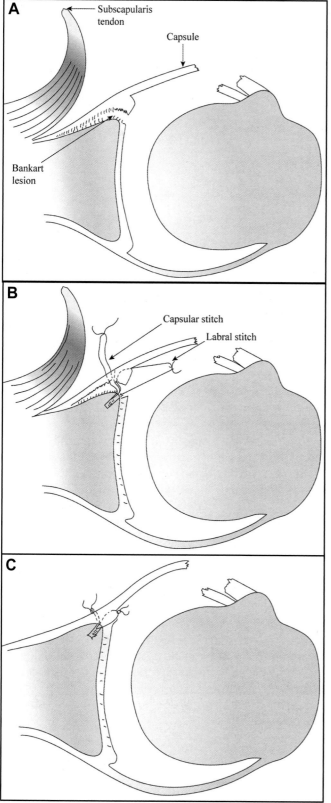

Figure 15-9. (A) In this axial schematic, the Bankart lesion is shown on the anterior glenoid face. The double-loaded suture anchor has been placed. (B) The horizontal mattress suture is shown through the capsule and the simple suture configuration around the labrum. (C) Completed repair.

Figure 15-10. Depiction of the caplusar repair and capsulotomy closure.

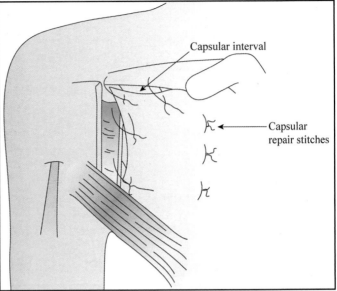

Capsular interval

Capsular repair stitches

Following this, the capsular interval is closed with nonabsorbable sutures as well. Capsular closure, as well as the medial capsular repair stitches, is depicted in Figure 15-10.

Again, in our experience, the open procedure has a 95% success rate compared to the 90% success rate in the arthroscopic procedure. This portion of the open procedure, in which stability and range of motion can be checked and the capsule retensioned if needed, is the likely explanation for this difference.

The subscapularis tendon is closed using the stump that was left laterally on the humerus. Figure-of-eight nonabsorbable sutures are again used. Particular attention is paid to the amount of external rotation present after subscapularis closure. This is compared to preoperative range of motion values so as to not over-tighten the shoulder. Finally, the rotator interval can be closed if needed. The wound is then irrigated, hemostasis is ensured, and standard wound closure is undertaken.

For a complete surgical demonstration, please see Chapter 15 video.

COMPLICATIONS

Although rare, a wide array of complications exists. These include superficial wound infections, deep infections, nerve injury (particularly the axillary nerve), stiffness, and ultimately surgical failure with recurrent instability. Recurrent instability is managed case specifically and is dependent on the cause of the failure. If a traumatic dislocation occurs, then a repeat Bankart repair with or without a capsular shift may be in order. If glenoid deficiency is the cause, then a bone grafting procedure (ie, coracoid transfer, iliac crest autograft, allograft) may be needed.

REHABILITATION

The operative arm is placed in a protective sling. The exact postoperative regimen is dependent on the patient as well as the nature of the repair. However, in general, the arm is left in the sling for 3 to 4 weeks with "thigh to face" activities (eg, eating, writing, bathing, keyboarding) allowed. Physical therapy is usually started at the time of suture removal. The sling is discontinued at 4 weeks, and cautious use of the involved extremity for normal activities of daily living is encouraged. Active and passive range of motion exercises are advanced at that time, as well as some very light strengthening. Regaining shoulder range of motion is the primary goal for this period, and this should be conveyed to the patient. At the 2- to 3-month period, as long as shoulder range of motion has been restored, progressive resistance exercises are increased. Generally speaking, 4 to 6 months is required for return to full activity. A throwing progression for dominant arm athletes will not begin prior to 6 months postoperatively. Bracing is usually recommended for athletes returning to contact or collision sports up to 12 months postoperatively.

REFERENCES

1. Burkhead WZ Jr, Rockwood CA Jr. Treatment of instability of the shoulder with an exercise program. *J Bone Joint Surg.* 1992;74A:890-896.
2. Goss TP. Anterior glenohumeral instability. *Orthopedics.* 1988;11:87-95.
3. Bankart ASB. The pathology and treatment of recurrent dislocation of shoulder joint. *Br J Surg.* 1939;26:23-39.
4. Matsen FA, Thomas SC, Rockwood CA, et al. Glenohumeral instability. In: Rockwood CA, Matsen FA, eds. *The Shoulder.* New York, NY: Churchill Livingstone; 1998:717.
5. Rowe CR, Patel D, Southmayd WW. The Bankart procedure. A long-term end-result study. *J Bone Joint Surg.* 1978;60A:1-16.
6. Zarins B, Rowe CR. Modifications of the Bankart procedure. In: Post M, Morrey BF, Hawkins RJ, eds. *Surgery of the Shoulder.* St. Louis, MO: Mosby-Year Book; 1990:170-177.
7. Andrews JR, Satterwhite YE. Anatomic capsular shift. *J Orthop Tech.* 1993;1:151-160.
8. Zarins B, Faulks CR, Satterwhite YE. Open operative procedures for shoulder instability in the baseball player. In: Andrews JR, Zarins B, Wilk KE, eds. *Injuries in Baseball.* Philadelphia, PA: Lippincott-Raven Publishers; 1998:175-188.
9. Altchek DW, Warren RF, Skyhar MJ, et al. T-plasty modification of the Bankart procedure for multidirectional instability of the anterior and inferior types. *J Bone Joint Surg.* 1991;73A:105-112.

Please see video on the accompanying Web site at
http://www.slackbooks.com/unstableshouldervideos

16

Subscapularis Tears and Capsular Deficiency in Shoulder Instability

Bojan Zoric, MD and Peter J. Millett, MD, MSc

SUBSCAPULARIS TEARS

Making a clinical diagnosis of a tear of the subscapularis tendon can often be difficult, which can frequently result in a delayed repair attempt.[1] A diagnostic delay often means that surgical repair is no longer possible. The subscapularis muscle is important for normal shoulder function and stability.[2] It is a strong internal rotator of the glenohumeral joint, particularly with the shoulder in an adducted and extended position.[3,4] Loss of subscapularis function can result in pain, weakness, instability, and impairment of shoulder function, which may require surgical treatment.[1,5] Isolated subscapularis tears are relatively uncommon. Warner and colleagues found involvement of the subscapularis tendon in 4.7% of a series of 407 rotator cuff tears.[6] The majority of these subscapularis injuries were associated with tears of the superior rotator cuff.[6-8] Isolated subscapularis tears are less common and are frequently associated with trauma.[1,9] Traumatic subscapularis tendon tears have also been associated with recurrent anterior glenohumeral dislocation.[10-13] Gerber and Krushell[14] reported on a group of 16 patients who sustained isolated complete subscapularis tears as the result of forced external rotation with the arm at the side. However, the greatest force can be applied to the subscapularis tendon when an external rotation and abduction force is applied with the arm maximally rotated and abducted 60 degrees.[15] Subscapularis deficiency is also a well-documented complication of open anterior instability surgery and prosthetic humeral head replacement.[10] Anterior instability after shoulder arthroplasty is multifactorial and can be due to a deficiency of the subscapularis.[16] Over-stuffing the shoulder with placement of a large glenoid component or oversized humeral component will lateralize the lesser tuberosity and will place the subscapularis tendon under increased tension, which increases the risk for rupture. When diagnosed early, it may be amenable to surgical repair (an Achilles tendon allograft may be considered for augmentation). Failure to restore proper deltoid tension, proper retroversion (normally 20 to 30 degrees) of the humeral component may lead to subscapularis failure and anterior dislocation. Moeckel and colleagues[16] looked at shoulder arthroplasties

Abrams JS. *Management of the Unstable Shoulder: Arthroscopic and Open Repair* (pp. 209-222).
© 2011 SLACK Incorporated

performed in 236 shoulders from 1984 through 1989. They described the findings and results of reoperation in 7 patients complicated by anterior instability following a total shoulder arthroplasty. At the time of reoperation, all 7 were found to have a disruption of the repaired subscapularis tendon, which was subsequently repaired. Anterior instability recurred in 3 shoulders, all of which were treated with an additional procedure in which an Achilles allograft was used as a static constraint.

The literature does not clearly establish the true incidence of failed tendon repairs after open shoulder stabilization or shoulder replacement surgery. In a retrospective study, Greis and colleagues[17] reported on 88 patients who underwent an open Bankart procedure using a complete subscapularis tenotomy approach. Of these patients, 4 (4.5%) required reoperation for subscapularis tendon repair failure. However, other series do not report any revisions due to postoperative subscapularis tendon disruption. Maynou and colleagues[18] found 3 cases (3.9%) of failed repairs in a group of 77 patients who underwent a Latarjet procedure using an inverted L-shaped tenotomy. Two patients had marked fatty infiltration on arthrogram computerized tomography (CT; stages 3 and 4 according to Goutallier); however, reoperation was not required.

Unlike an isolated rupture of the supraspinatus tendon, a rupture of the subscapularis tendon can be associated with marked retraction of the tendon. This is primarily thought to occur due to lack of intact tendon tissue alongside of the rupture site to checkrein the retraction. After delay of several months, this retraction makes repair very difficult.[6,9] Gerber and colleagues[1] reported improved outcomes in patients who underwent surgery after a short delay between the ensuing traumatic event and the repair compared to those who had a considerable delay prior to having an operation.

The delay caused by difficulties in diagnosis results in a situation where mobilization of the retracted tendon is no longer possible or repair is not indicated because of the degree of atrophy in the muscle.[11,19] On the other hand, patients with persistent pain, shoulder dysfunction, or continued anterior instability call for some form of intervention. Muscle transfers have become useful salvage options for patients with irreparable tears of the subscapularis. Several different options exist, including transfer of the pectoralis major, pectoralis minor, trapezius, latissimus dorsi, teres major, as well as allograft reconstruction.[7,16,20-22] The pectoralis major tendon transfer has produced the most reliable clinical results when compared to other reconstructive options, although this is not always successful.[23]

Evaluation

The clinical presentation of patients with subscapularis tears is variable. The majority of subscapularis tears do not occur as isolated tears but instead are often seen in combination with tears of the superior and posterior cuff. Isolated injuries of the subscapularis often result from isolated trauma to the shoulder with a forced external rotation moment. Anterior shoulder dislocation in middle-aged patients can also result in subscapularis disruption and recurrent instability. The majority of the patients with subscapularis tears will complain of pain, usually localized to the anterior shoulder. Most patients will also notice increased weakness and pain with overhead activities. Activities requiring forced or resisted internal rotation are difficult, and sensations of glenohumeral anterior instability are common. The physical examination of patients with subscapularis tears can be significantly influenced by the integrity of the remaining cuff. The majority of patients with isolated tears of the subscapularis can still elevate the arm to the overhead position. Subscapularis tears will often result in increased passive external rotation compared to the opposite shoulder. The belly-press and lift-off test are excellent clinical examination tools that are highly accurate for detecting subscapularis disruption. Apprehension in abduction may be seen in those patients with instability. Tears of the subscapularis are also often associated with instability of the long head of the biceps tendon.

Radiographic Evaluation

Preoperative evaluation should include radiological imaging in 3 planes (anteroposterior [AP], axillary, Y-view) and magnetic resonance imaging (MRI) or MR arthrogram to assess soft tissue anomalies and to evaluate for retraction of subscapularis tendon and amount of fatty degeneration and atrophy.

Radiographs of the shoulder in patients with isolated subscapularis tears are typically normal. Occasionally, subtle anterior translation can be appreciated on an axillary view with the patients who have a subscapularis deficiency. If the patient has an associated posterior rotator tear, superior migration of the humeral head can be noted on an AP radiograph. Ultrasound and MRI can be used to accurately identify tears of the subscapularis and associated rotator cuff. Associated MRI findings are frequently encountered, including subluxation or dislocation of the biceps tendon, fluid collections local to the subscapular recess, and tears of the supraspinatus or posterior rotator cuff.

Subscapularis Arthroscopic Repair

Surgery is performed with regional plus general anesthesia, with the patient in a beach-chair position with assistance of a pneumatic arm holder (authors' preference). The surgery can also be performed in the lateral decubitus position. Glenohumeral arthroscopy is performed through a standard posterior arthroscopy portal with a pump pressure maintained at 60 mm Hg. Visualization of the subscapularis tendon and its footprint on the lesser tuberosity is performed through the posterior viewing portal. Often, improved visualization of the subscapularis insertional footprint can be achieved by placing the arm in 45 degrees of abduction and 30 degrees of internal rotation. Sometimes, a 70-degree arthroscope may be needed to help look over the proximal humerus and lend an aerial view of the subscapularis footprint and its attachment onto the lesser tuberosity. Using these maneuvers, subtle and partial-thickness articular side tears can now be identified at the lesser tuberosity.

In chronic complete tears of the subscapularis tendon, the tendon is often retracted medially to the glenoid and can be found scarred into the deltoid fascia. This makes identification of the tendon edge extremely difficult. Burkhart and Lo have described cases such as this and identification of the comma sign, which is essential in identifying a retracted edge of the subscapularis tendon. The comma sign represents a combination of the superior glenohumeral ligament and coracohumeral ligament complex that has torn off the humerus at the upper part of the subscapularis footprint. This ligament complex remains attached to the superolateral portion of the subscapularis and forms a comma-shaped arc with a torn edge of the subscapularis tendon. Often, by pulling with a tendon grasper on the tissue that is lateral and forms a comma sign, the superior portion of the subscapularis will come into view and will be visualized.

When identifying subscapularis tears, the relationship with the biceps tendon pulley has to be explored. The biceps tendon can be evaluated by internally and externally rotating the arm and noting its relationship to the subscapularis tendon. Normally, the biceps tendon is anterior to the plane of the subscapularis. If it is noted to be posterior, subluxation of the biceps tendon is present. Attempts to repair or stabilize the biceps sling are most often unsuccessful, and redislocation of the biceps tendon can disrupt the repair that is performed in the subscapularis. If there is any biceps subluxation, we prefer to perform a biceps tenodesis.

To perform an arthroscopic subscapularis tendon repair, we use 3 portals. A posterior viewing portal and an anterior portal for suture anchor placement are used, and an anterolateral portal, which is made just anterior to the biceps tendon, is used for bone bed preparation and suture passage. Any time there is evidence of a subscapularis tear, evaluation for subcoracoid stenosis should be performed. The coracoid can be found just anterior to the subscapularis tendon, and by removing and excising a portion of the rotator interval capsule, the coracoid can be visualized directly. Using an instrument of known size, the coracohumeral space can be measured. If the coracohumeral space is less than approximately 6 mm, we perform a coracoplasty. Using a radiofrequency ablation device, the soft tissues are removed from the undersurface of the coracoid, and the rotator interval space is cleared. A 4-mm burr or shaver (depending on bone quality) is introduced through the anterolateral portal, and the posterolateral aspect of the coracoid is resected parallel to the subscapularis tendon. Once there is more than 8 to 10 mm of space between the reconfigured coracoid and the subscapularis tendon, there should be no further subcoracoid impingement. Dynamic intraoperative evaluation with cross-arm testing is helpful to evaluate this.

In retracted tears, mobilization of the retracted subscapularis tendon has to be performed first. For large retracted tears, an extra-articular viewing portal parallel to and in line with the anterior border of the acromion can help. The scope is placed just posterior to the coracoacromial ligament and can follow this down to the coracoid and the subscapularis fossa. When the subscapularis is retracted, a traction suture can be used to provide tension on the subscapularis, and an arthroscopic elevator through the anterolateral portal and the anterior, posterior, and superior portions of the subscapularis tendons can be used to mobilize the tendon. Dissection along the inferior border of the subscapularis should be avoided to minimize any risk for neurologic or vascular injury. Furthermore, releasing the coracohumeral ligament from the coracoid base can significantly increase the lateral excursion of the subscapularis tendon. The lesser tuberosity bone bed is prepared through the anterolateral portal using an arthroscopic shaver and burr. It should be roughened up until there is bleeding bone but not decorticated. If there is a retracted immobile tear, the insertional footprint bed can be medialized up to between 3 to 5 mm in order to decrease tension on the subscapularis repair. Suture anchors loaded with #2 super strong sutures (Fiberwire, Arthrex, Naples, FL) with metal or bioabsorbable anchors are placed through the anterior portal for complete tears of the subscapularis tendon. Two anchors are used for tears involving the upper half, while partial tears are repaired often with just one double-loaded suture anchor. For large tears, the authors prefer a double row technique to completely restore the surface area of the insertion. Once anchors are placed, we use a spinal needle to penetrate the subscapularis tendon at the desired position. We often use a nontraumatic grasper to retract the subscapularis toward the lesser tuberosity and then penetrate the subscapularis with the spinal needle. A #1 monofilament suture is brought through the spinal needle, grabbed intra-articularly and taken out through the anterolateral portal. The suture from the anchor is subsequently tied to the #1 monofilament suture, and using the #1 monofilament suture, it is shuttled through the subscapularis tendon. A second suture is subsequently shuttled in the similar position with the spinal needle, creating a mattress suture over the subscapularis tendon at the footprint. Using the second suture in a double-loaded anchor, this process can be repeated to create a mattress suture repair. Various other types of suture passing instruments may also be used depending on surgeon preference. The tissue of the subscapularis may be grasped and pulled toward the bone bed prior to suture delivery to ensure that proposed suture location is satisfactory. We subsequently tie a sliding knot followed by 3 to 4 alternating half-hitches to anchor the tendinous insertion. Subsequently, the subscapularis tendon is palpated and evaluated for its integrity. After the repair, the shoulder is taken through a range of motion to evaluate how much tension is applied at various degrees of external rotation, and a safe zone for rehab is determined.

Postoperative Care

The shoulder is protected in a sling with an abduction pillow for 6 weeks, and pendulum and passive range of motion exercises are initiated starting on day 1. Cryotherapy is used from day 0 to minimize postoperative pain and reduce swelling. External rotation is limited to protect the repair to neutral or 10 degrees with the arm at the side depending on the assessment performed intraoperatively, at the time when the subscapularis was repaired. Early motion helps to prevent scarring of the tendon, and passive elevation as tolerated is allowed with the shoulder in a slight internal rotation. At 6 weeks, progressive active and passive range of motion is allowed with no limits to external rotation. Isometric exercises on the shoulder and strengthening exercises are started at 6 weeks, excluding any internal rotation, and internal rotation exercises can be started approximately 8 to 10 weeks postoperatively.

Irreparable Subscapularis Tears

Indications for pectoralis transfer include patients with pain, instability, and associated impaired function in whom a primary subscapularis repair is unlikely to be successful or has been attempted and has been unsuccessful. The indication for pectoralis major tendon transfer is related to the likelihood of success for primary subscapularis repair. We prefer to treat all acute subscapularis tears with a primary repair when possible. Attempted subscapularis repair in the presence of advanced muscle shortening, atrophy, and fatty infiltration is unlikely to be successful. If preoperative MRI findings demonstrate retraction of the tendon to the edge of the glenoid or medial to it, or if there is extensive fatty infiltration of the subscapularis muscle, we recommend a pectoralis major transfer over a primary repair.[19]

Contraindications to performing a pectoralis tendon transfer include the presence of a repairable subscapularis tendon tear or inadequate pectoralis major tissue. The repair is also contraindicated in patients who are medically unstable or are unable to comply with a vigorous postoperative rehabilitation protocol. Other relative contraindications include an associated massive tear of the anterosuperior and posterior cuff with pseudoparalysis of the shoulder. In these cases, normal shoulder elevation is unlikely to be restored after just a pectoralis tendon transfer.

Split Pectoralis Major Transfer Surgical Technique

All surgeries are performed under general anesthesia with a regional block to supplement postoperative pain control. The patient is seated in a beach-chair position with an assistance of a pneumatic arm holder. In cases of clinical or radiographic evidence for additional intra-articular pathologies such as suspicion of an engaging Hill-Sachs defect, diagnostic glenohumeral arthroscopy prior to the open surgery can be helpful. Subsequently, an extended delta pectoral approach is performed to expose the glenohumeral joint. The skin incision extends from the coracoid process down to approximately 12 to 15 cm inferolaterally. Full-thickness subcutaneous flaps are elevated, and the medial flap is developed such that the inferior border of the pectoralis muscle is fully exposed. The cephalic vein is taken laterally as the deltopectoral interval is developed. Blunt dissection proceeds to the level of a clavipectoral fascia. Any fascial adhesions are swept off the lateral aspect of the pectoralis major muscle with a dry sponge exposing the insertion of the pectoralis tendon into the humerus. The clavipectoral fascia is split inferior to the coracoacromial ligament, and this interval is developed with blunt dissection lateral to the conjoint tendon with the arm externally rotated to expose any remaining subscapularis tendon. At this point, the anterior humeral circumflex vessels should be well visualized. The torn subscapularis tendon is usually found retracted medially under the conjoint tendon. The anterior humerus circumflex vessels are identified and ligated with suture and bovie. The remaining subscapularis tendon is marked with a stay suture. Often, inferior fibers of the subscapularis will be found attached to the most inferior portion of the lesser tuberosity, and these fibers should be left intact. Following the inferior border of the subscapularis, the axillary nerve is identified. A thin blunt retractor can be placed between the axillary nerve and subscapularis while the tendon is mobilized.

The subscapularis muscle is subsequently freed from the anterior glenoid and subscapularis fossa with the inferior border of the muscle mobilized from surrounding adhesions while protecting the axillary nerve and anterior neurovascular structures. At this point, mobility and integrity of the muscle of the subscapularis muscle and tendon are evaluated. If it is of poor quality or too retracted, this is when the decision is made to proceed with a pectoralis major tendon transfer.

It is important to understand the anatomical makeup of the pectoralis major muscle and tendinous insertion. The pectoralis major is composed of 2 heads: the sternal and clavicular head. The sternal head of the pectoralis major lies inferior and deep to the clavicular head. The interval between the muscles and orientation of the tendon can often be identified at the inferior edge of the muscle developed bluntly through superficial fascia. The sternal portion of the tendon rotates deep to the clavicular tendon and forms the posterior aspect of the pectoralis major insertion. This deep sternal head of the pectoralis major tendon is more tendinous and has a more appropriate vector of pull for a subscapularis repair. The inferior and superior aspects of the sternal portion of the pectoralis tendon are tagged with suture, and the sternal head is then released sharply off the humerus.

Anatomic studies have demonstrated that the muscle can safely be split for a distance of approximately 8.5 cm from the lateral edge of the tendon before risking damage to the medial pectoral nerve. The lateral pectoral nerve is located medial to the pectoralis minor muscle and innervates the upper portion of the pectoralis major muscle. If you avoid dissection medial to the pectoralis minor, both the lateral and medial pectoral nerves will be protected. The pectoralis major tendon is then secured with a whip-stitched suture (Fiberwire) down toward the musculotendinous junction and back up the opposite side. The insertion of the pectoralis minor tendon is identified at the tip of the coracoid, and the pectoralis minor is partially released for improved exposure. The interval at the medial aspect of the conjoined tendon is identified and developed by sweeping a finger bluntly and inferiorly. The musculocutaneous nerve can be identified as it enters on the undersurface of the coracobrachialis and should be visualized prior to tendon transfer. The average distance from the coracoid tip to the point where the nerve penetrates the coracobrachialis is approximately 5 to 6 cm. The released sternal head tendon is then passed deep to the clavicular head and under the conjoint tendon while remaining superficial to the musculocutaneous nerve. Excursion of the transferred pectoralis major tendon is assessed by pulling on the stay sutures. Often, the pectoralis tendon can be tensioned so it inserts 2 to 3 cm lateral to the bicipital groove with the arm in neutral position. This allows for fixation of the pectoralis major to the anterolateral aspect of a greater tuberosity. The surface of the area of the greater tuberosity where the tendon will be attached is roughened to a healthy bleeding surface, and the tendon is repaired using transosseous sutures with a wide bone bridge or bone anchors. Bone anchors can also be used more medially to augment the repair at the level of the lateral aspect of lesser tuberosity. This furthermore increases the area of tendon-to-bone healing by enlarging the footprint of the repair. The muscle transfer should be tensioned so that 30 degrees of external rotation is achieved with the arm at the side. The shoulder can then be placed through range of motion, and its stability can be tested intraoperatively. The wound is irrigated copiously and closed in a standard fashion. A compressive sterile dressing is placed over the shoulder and over the incision to minimize any hematoma formation. Postoperatively, the patient is placed in an abduction sling for 6 weeks.

Pearls and Pitfalls

Excessive tension on the neurovascular structures must be assessed by direct palpation after tendon transfer. Placing the tendon under the musculocutaneous nerve risks neurapraxic injury from tension created by the bulky pectoralis major tendon.

Rehabilitation

The rehabilitation for pectoralis tendon transfer is similar to rotator cuff repair. The shoulder is protected in a sling for 6 weeks, and pendulum and passive range of motion exercises are initiated starting on day 1. External rotation is limited to protect the repair to 10 to 20 degrees with the arm at the side depending on the assessment performed intraoperatively at the time when the pectoralis major was tensioned. Early motion helps to prevent scarring of the tendon, and passive elevation to as tolerated as is allowed with the shoulder in a slight internal rotation. At 6 weeks, progressive active and passive range of motion is allowed with no limits to external rotation. Isometric exercises on the shoulder and strengthening exercises are started at 6 weeks, excluding any internal rotation, and internal rotation exercises can be started approximately 8 to 10 weeks postoperatively.

Elhassan and colleagues[23] looked at 30 patients and divided them into 3 groups. Group I comprised 11 patients with a failed procedure for instability of the shoulder, group II included 8 with a failed shoulder replacement, and group III included 11 with a massive tear of the rotator cuff. All underwent transfer of the sternal head of pectoralis major to restore the function of subscapularis. Improvement in pain was shown in 7 of the 11 patients in groups I and III, but in only 1 of 8 in group II. Failure of the tendon transfer was highest in the arthroplasty group and was associated with preoperative anterior subluxation of the humeral head. They concluded that, in patients with irreparable rupture of subscapularis after shoulder replacement, there is a high risk of failure of transfer of pectoralis major, particularly if there is preoperative anterior subluxation of the humeral head. Jost and colleagues[19] reported on 28 patients who underwent a total of 30 consecutive pectoralis major transfers. There were 12 isolated subscapularis tears and 18 subscapularis tears associated with a tear of the supraspinatus or the supraspinatus and infraspinatus. The mean relative constant score increased from 47% preoperatively to 70% at an average of 32 months postoperatively ($P<0.0001$). Thirteen patients (14 shoulders) were very satisfied, 10 patients (11 shoulders) were satisfied, 2 patients (2 shoulders) were disappointed, and 3 patients (3 shoulders) were dissatisfied with the result. The average subjective shoulder value increased from 23% preoperatively to 55% postoperatively ($P=0.0009$). In patients with a massive tear, the outcome was less favorable when the torn supraspinatus tendon was irreparable, as determined preoperatively or intraoperatively, than when it was reparable (average relative constant scores, 49% and 79%, respectively; *P*=0.002). They concluded that pectoralis major transfer results in improvement for patients with an irreparable subscapularis tear with or without an associated reparable supraspinatus tear. If an irreparable subscapularis tear is associated with an irreparable supraspinatus tear, they found the results less favorable, and pectoralis major transfer may not be warranted.

CAPSULAR DEFICIENCY AND INSUFFICIENCY IN SHOULDER INSTABILITY

Background

Patients with an attenuated or absent glenohumeral capsule pose one of the toughest challenges in the surgical management of glenohumeral instability.[24,25] These patients fall into 2 broad categories: patients failing multiple prior stabilization procedures and patients with connective tissue disorders such as Ehlers-Danlos syndrome. Moreover, the recurrence of instability is related to the number of prior surgeries. Deficiency of the subscapularis, the capsule, and the important enforcing structures (the middle glenohumeral ligament [MGHL] and the anterior band of the inferior glenohumeral ligament [IGHL]) is often noted after multiple open surgical attempts to stabilize the joint. It can also occur as a complication of electrothermal capsulorrhaphy.

Glenohumeral capsule augmentation and reconstruction have been described with autogenous hamstring or long head of the biceps tendon, autogenous iliotibial band, and reconstruction using Achilles, tibialis anterior, and hamstring allografts.[16,26-28] The technique described here focuses on the treatment of recurrent anterior glenohumeral instability secondary to soft tissue insufficiency. This is especially pertinent to patients who have undergone multiple unsuccessful surgeries in the past and to those who have soft tissue/collagen disorders. The main structures that are reconstructed by the tibialis anterior allograft in this technique are the anterior labrum, the MGHL, and the anterior band of the IGHL. Because of the complexity of the reconstruction, the technique is performed as an open surgery, which allows precise placement and tensioning of the allograft tendon.

Evaluation

Evaluation begins with ascertaining history of instability, including the initial instability episode; whether it was traumatic or atraumatic, voluntary or involuntary; the activity level of the patient; any family history of connective tissue disorders; the number and nature of instability occurrences; and the specifics of prior surgical treatment.

Physical examination should focus on the direction of apprehension and glenohumeral instability. Preoperative evaluation should include assessment of the coracohumeral ligament, rotator interval, an assessment of generalized ligamentous laxity, and the level of deltoid and rotator cuff functioning. In cases of prior thermal treatment, MRI with intra-articular contrast may help the treating surgeon quantify the amount of remaining capsule and the tissue quality.

Indications

Indications for allograft capsular reconstruction include cases of failed treatment for multidirectional instability, failures after anterior instability reconstruction with insufficient capsule for standard capsulolabral reconstruction, and cases of attenuated capsule after undergoing thermal capsulorrhaphy. The technique presented here is regarded as a salvage procedure for patients with recurrent shoulder instability and dislocations after multiple surgical attempts at stabilization. Indications are recurrent shoulder instability in the setting of capsulolabral deficiency without associated bone loss. We sometimes refer to this as "end-stage" instability. This may result from either traumatic or atraumatic etiology. The technique addresses the soft tissues and is therefore useful in soft tissue disorders, such as Ehlers-Danlos syndrome, electrothermal capsular necrosis, the multiply operated shoulder, and labral deficiency.

Absolute contraindications to allograft capsular reconstruction include active glenohumeral joint infections, patients with recurrent voluntary subluxations, and cases of instability coupled with brachioplexopathy. Although capsular augmentation may be appropriate for selected patients with connective tissue disorders and pathologic ligamentous laxity, patients with sufficient capsular tissue should undergo a standard inferior capsular shift and labral repair when possible, even if additional allograft capsular augmentation is required.

Radiographic Evaluation

Preoperative evaluation should include radiological imaging in 3 planes (anteroposterior, axillary, Y-view) and MR arthrogram or CT to assess soft tissue anomalies and to evaluate for any bone deficiency or bony pathologies, such as pathologic glenoid anteversion or retroversion.

Patients with deficiencies of the capsulolabral structures frequently present in MRI with wide joint capsules, hypotrophic anterior labrum, and either stretched or very thin superior, middle, and/or IGHL. MRI also helps in estimating the status after previous surgical interventions. Attention should be turned to the status of the anterior labrum and the width of the capsule.

Surgical Technique

Surgery is performed with regional plus general anesthesia, with the patient in a beach-chair position with assistance of a pneumatic arm holder. In cases of clinical or radiographic evidence of any additional intra-articular pathology, such as an engaging Hill-Sachs defect, diagnostic glenohumeral arthroscopy prior to the open surgery can be advantageous.

A standard deltopectoral approach is performed to expose the glenohumeral joint (Figure 16-1). In many cases, there is extensive scarring and altered soft tissue planes due to prior surgeries. The bicipital groove is identified and opened, and a tenodesis of the long head of the biceps is performed. The subscapularis tendon can then be taken down from the insertion at the lesser tuberosity with the capsule in one layer. This simplifies the exposure. In many cases, the capsule is scarred to the subscapularis. The tendon is secured with stay sutures for later repair. The rotator interval is opened, and thus full exposure of the glenohumeral joint is achieved. This enables accurate inspection of the glenohumeral joint.

Figure 16-1. A standard deltopectoral approach is performed to expose the glenohumeral joint.

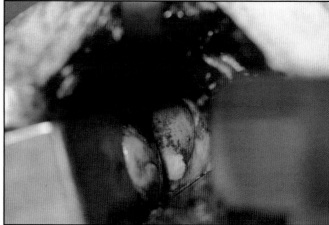

Labral Reconstruction

Once good exposure of the glenoid is obtained, the anterior glenoid neck is roughened up with a burr to expose healthy raw bone. Any residual labrum is removed. Three or preferably 4 suture anchors are placed at the glenoid rim. They are used as points of fixation of the labral reconstruction at the anterior glenoid rim. The anchors are placed at approximately 2 o'clock, 3 o'clock, 4 o'clock, and 5:30 in a right shoulder and 10 o'clock, 9 o'clock, 8 o'clock, and 6:30 in a left shoulder (Figure 16-2). A 6- or 7-mm thick tibialis anterior allograft is prepared on the side table by whip-stitching at either end with #2 Fiberwire. This allograft is placed so that it is centered along the anterior glenoid rim to reconstruct the labrum. The allograft is then secured using the suture ends from the anterior glenoid rim anchors starting at the middle and working superiorly and inferiorly (Figure 16-3). In this way, the tibialis anterior allograft is used to recreate the anterior labrum. The remaining native capsule and labrum are then sewn into the allograft with #2 suture (Fiberwire) to reinforce the neolabrum and also to bring in vascularity to help with healing and graft incorporation.

Capsular Reconstruction

The 2 free limbs of the tibialis anterior allograft are then used to reconstruct the MGHL and the anterior band of the IGHL. The graft will be secured by bioabsorbable interference screws both inferiorly and superiorly in bone tunnels drilled in the humerus. The tunnels should be placed just lateral to the articular margin of the humerus where the native capsule attaches. The drill's diameter for the tunnel is chosen according to the thickness of the graft, typically 6 mm, such that the interference screw provides good compression of the tendon in the bone tunnel. One tunnel is created for each limb of the allograft.

The 2 free superior and inferior limbs of the graft are appropriately sized in length and finally fixed to the humerus with 2 bioabsorbable interference screws (BioTenodesis screw, Arthrex) in bone tunnels in the technique similar to that used for biceps tenodesis (Figure 16-4).

Instead of 2 blind-ended tunnels, alternatively, 2 complete tunnels (one superior and one inferior) can be created so that they span the bicipital groove. The graft ends can then be passed through each tunnel, respectively, tensioned, and tied to themselves lateral to the bicipital groove. Tensioning of the graft should occur with the shoulder in 30 degrees of external rotation and 30 degrees of elevation.

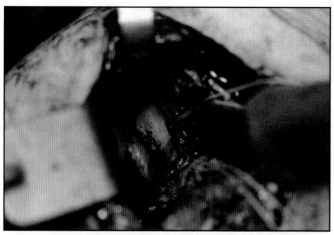

Figure 16-2. The anchors are placed at approximately 2:00, 3:00, 4:00, and 5:30 in a right shoulder and 10:00, 9:00, 8:00, and 6:30 in a left shoulder.

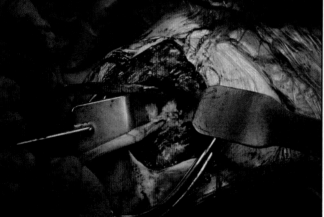

Figure 16-3. The allograft is then secured using the suture ends from the anterior glenoid rim anchors starting at the middle and working superiorly and inferiorly.

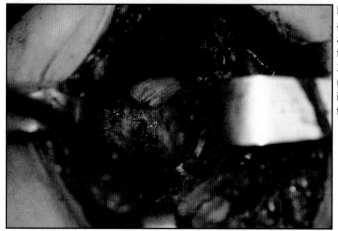

Figure 16-4. The 2 free superior and inferior limbs of the graft are appropriately sized in length and finally fixed to the humerus with 2 bioabsorbable interference screws (BioTenodesis screw) in bone tunnels in the technique similar to that used for biceps tenodesis.

This technique allows the surgeon to reconstruct both the MGHL and the anterior band of the IGHL. For additional security, if there is residual native capsular tissue, it can be sewn to the neocapsular ligaments with #2 sutures. Then, the shoulder can be placed through a range of motion, and stability can be tested intraoperatively.

The subscapularis and the adherent underlying capsule are then meticulously repaired to the lesser tuberosity through bone tunnels or directly to the allograft (Figure 16-5). The rotator interval is closed in a pants-over-vest fashion to provide additional resistance against inferior translation. The remainder of the wound is closed in standard fashion. A compressive sterile dressing is placed over the shoulder and over the incision to minimize any hematoma formation (see Chapter 16 video).

Postoperative Care

Postoperatively, the patient's arm is placed in a sling for 6 weeks. Pendulum exercise with limited passive range of motion is started at approximately 4 weeks. Patients may have a persistent loss of external rotation and forward flexion, but the goal is to obtain at least 45 degrees of external rotation and 140 degrees of forward flexion. Active range of motion is started around 8 to 10 weeks postoperatively. Patients should achieve maximal functional return by 4 to 6 months postoperatively.

Results and Prognosis

Chronic shoulder instability and recurrent dislocations because of soft tissue deficiency are difficult problems to address. The presented technique of capsulolabral reconstruction with an allograft tendon is a salvage procedure to restore stability and therefore can avoid glenohumeral fusion as a last and much more invasive option. Although there are many other techniques described to restore stability with open or arthroscopic soft tissue reconstruction, there are some advantages of the presented procedure: the reconstruction of the anterior labrum is anatomical and increases the depth of the cavity. Moreover, the most important ligaments for anteroinferior stability, the MGHL and IGHL, are reconstructed, and tensioning and fixation of the structures can be obtained in a biomechanical, reliable, and secure fashion. A precise diagnosis based on a complete physical examination and sufficient radiological imaging helps in selecting patients with soft tissue insufficiency and disorders and without relevant bony defects or malformations. As patient selection fits the indication, the clinical results in this difficult patient population have been favorable. So far, 13 patients with severe recurrent dislocations after multiple surgeries have been treated with the above-described technique. Nine of these procedures were successful. These patients were highly satisfied with the outcome; did not have clinical evidence for instability; and did not report recurrent instability, subluxations, or dislocations after the procedure. Nevertheless, there were 4 patients who had to be revised. One was revised because of infection and another because of avulsion of the tendon graft from the humeral head. The other 2 had recurrent instability even after the index surgery, and subsequently one had to be converted to a Latarjet procedure and one to a glenohumeral fusion.

Thus, the presented technique of open anterior capsular reconstruction of the shoulder for chronic instability using a tibialis anterior allograft is a feasible salvage procedure that can help avoid much more invasive and lifestyle-limiting procedures, such as fusion of the glenohumeral joint.

Complications

As noted above, recurrent glenohumeral instability is still possible. Stiffness could be a complication after having had the shoulder immobilized for 6 weeks, but in cases of patients with chronic instability and recurrent dislocation, some stiffness is desirable. We have not had a patient with significant limitation in range of motion after 4 to 6 months. Interference screw pull out or fixation failure is another possible cause of

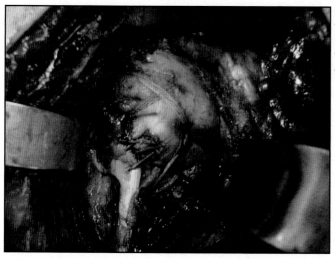

Figure 16-5. The subscapularis and the adherent underlying capsule are meticulously repaired to the lesser tuberosity through bone tunnels or directly to the allograft.

failure. Kilicoglu and colleagues[29] showed that the strength of a biceps tenodesis with bioabsorbable interference screw is achieved after 6 weeks.

Pitfalls and Complications

Alternatives to allograft capsular reconstruction include performing an inferior capsular shift when adequate capsule remains. Massoud and colleagues[30] have shown that even after thermal capsular necrosis, inferior capsule shift may be successful without further capsular reconstruction. However, in cases of prior failed stabilization, intrinsic connective tissue disorders, and after failed thermal capsulorrhaphy, autograft or allograft augmentation of the capsular shift is advised. Alternatives to tibialis anterior allograft reconstruction include other allograft sources, including hamstring and Achilles as well as autograft hamstrings, iliotibial band, or long head of the biceps tendon. Anterior tibialis allograft is reliable for this procedure as it has superior tensile string compared to hamstring tendons, is readily available as a graft source, and has adequate length to use a single graft with no associated donor morbidity.

Complications with this procedure can arise with under-tensioning of the reconstruction. If the patients undergoing this procedure have a history of multidirectional instability, connective tissue disease, or failed prior stabilization, they will tend to stretch the reconstructed capsulolabral complex. The allograft reconstruction should be viewed as an adjunct to a properly tensioned inferior capsular shift to ensure biologic healing and sustainable results after reconstruction. Failure to properly diagnose the pattern of instability preoperatively with an examination under anesthesia may also lead to inferior results.

REFERENCES

1. Gerber C, Hersche O, Farron A. Isolated rupture of the subscapularis tendon. *J Bone Joint Surg Am.* 1996;78:1015-1023.
2. Keating JF, Waterworth P, Shaw-Dunn J, et al. The relative strengths of the rotator cuff muscles: a cadaver study. *J Bone Joint Surg Br.* 1992;75:137-140.
3. Tokish JM, Decker MJ, Ellis HB, et al. The belly-press test for the physical examination of the subscapularis muscle: electromyographic validation and comparison to the lift-off. *J Shoulder Elbow Surg.* 2003;12:427-430.

4. Greis PE, Kuhn JE, Schultheis J, et al. Validation of the lift-off test and analysis of subscapularis activity during maximal internal rotation. *Am J Sports Med.* 1996;24:589-593.

5. Deutsch A, Altchek DW, Veltri DM, et al. Traumatic tears of the subscapularis tendon: clinical diagnosis, magnetic resonance imaging findings, and operative treatment. *Am J Sports Med.* 1997;25:13-22.

6. Warner JJ, Higgins L, Parsons IM, et al. Diagnosis and treatment of anterosuperior rotator cuff tears. *J Shoulder Elbow Surg.* 2001;10:37-46.

7. Warner JJ. Management of massive irreparable rotator cuff tears: the role of tendon transfer. *Instr Course Lect.* 2001;50:63-71.

8. Warner JJ, Gerber C. Treatment of massive rotator cuff tears: posterior-superior and anterior-superior. In: Iannotti JP, ed. *The Rotator Cuff: Current Concepts and Complex Problems.* Rosemont, IL: American Academy of Orthopaedic Surgeons; 1998:59-94

9. Mansat P, Frankle MA, Cofield RH. Tears in the subscapularis tendon: descriptive analysis and results of surgical repair. *Joint Bone Spine.* 2003;70:342-347.

10. Miller BS, Joseph TA, Noonan TJ, Horan MP, Hawkins RJ. Rupture of the subscapularis tendon after shoulder arthroplasty: diagnosis, treatment, and outcome. *J Shoulder Elbow Surg.* 2005;14(5):492-496.

11. Wirth MA, Rockwood CA Jr. Operative treatment of irreparable rupture of the subscapularis. *J Bone Joint Surg Am.* 1997;79:722-731.

12. Neviaser RJ, Neviaser TJ, Neviaser JS. Concurrent rupture of the rotator cuff and anterior dislocation of the shoulder in the older patient. *J Bone Joint Surg Am.* 1998;70:1308-1311.

13. Neviaser RJ, Neviaser TJ, Neviaser JS. Anterior dislocation of the shoulder and rotator cuff rupture. *Clin Orthop.* 1993;291:103-106.

14. Gerber C, Krushell RJ. Isolated rupture of the tendon of the subscapularis muscle: clinical features in 16 cases. *J Bone Joint Surg Br.* 1991;73:389-394.

15. Haas SL. Fracture of the lesser tuberosity of the humerus. *Am J Surg.* 1944;63:253-256.

16. Moeckel BH, Altchek DW, Warren FR, Wickiewicz TL, Dines DM. Instability of the shoulder after arthroplasty. *J Bone Joint Surg Am.* 1993;75:492-497.

17. Greis PE, Dean M, Hawkins RJ. Subscapularis tendon disruption after Bankart reconstruction for anterior instability. *J Shoulder Elbow Surg.* 1996;5(3):219-222.

18. Maynou C, Cassagnaud X, Mestdagh H. Function of subscapularis after surgical treatment for recurrent instability of the shoulder using a bone-block procedure. *J Bone Joint Surg Br.* 2005;87(8):1096-1101.

19. Jost B, Puskas GJ, Lustenberger A, et al. Outcome of pectoralis major transfer for the treatment of irreparable subscapularis tears. *J Bone Joint Surg Am.* 2003;85A:1944-1951.

20. Gerber C, Hersche O. Tendon transfers for the treatment of irreparable rotator cuff defects. *Orthop Clin North Am.* 1997;28:195-203.

21. Resch H, Povacz P, Ritter E, et al. Transfer of the pectoralis major muscle for the treatment of irreparable rupture of the subscapularis tendon. *J Bone Joint Surg Am.* 2000;82:372-382.

22. Gerber A, Clavert P, Millet PJ, et al. Split pectoralis major and teres major tendon transfers for reconstruction of irreparable tears of the subscapularis. *Tech Shoulder Elbow Surg.* 2004;5:5-12.

23. Elhassan B, Ozbaydar M, Massimini D, Diller D, Higgins L, Warner JJ. Transfer of pectoralis major for the treatment of irreparable tears of subscapularis: does it work? *J Bone Joint Surg Br.* 2008;90(8):1059-1065.

24. Flatow EL, Miniaci A, Evans PJ, Simonian PT, Warren RF. Instability of the shoulder: complex problems and failed repairs: part II. Failed repairs. *Instr Course Lect.* 1998;47:113-125.

25. Flatow EL, Warner JI. Instability of the shoulder: complex problems and failed repairs: part I. Relevant biomechanics, multidirectional instability, and severe glenoid loss. *Instr Course Lect.* 1998;47:97-112.

26. Lazarus MD, Harryman DT 2nd. Open repair for anterior instability. In: Warner JJP, Iannotti JP, Gerber C, eds. *Complex and Revision Problems in Shoulder Surgery.* Philadelphia, PA: Lippincott-Raven; 1997:47-64.

27. Warner JPJ, Venegas AA, Lehtinen JT, Macy JJ. Management of capsular deficiency of the shoulder. A report of three cases. *J Bone Joint Surg Am.* 2002;84:1668-1671.

28. Iannotti JP, Antoniou J, Williams GR, Ramsey ML. Iliotibial band reconstruction for treatment of glenohumeral instability associated with irreparable capsular deficiency. *J Shoulder Elbow Surg.* 2002;11(6):618-623.

29. Kilicoglu O, Koyuncu O, Demirhan M. Time-dependent changes in failure loads of 3 biceps tenodesis techniques: in vivo study in a sheep model. *Am J Sports Med.* 2005;33(10):1536-1544.

30. Massoud SN, Levy O, Copeland SA. Inferior capsular shift for multidirectional instability following failed laser-assisted capsular shrinkage. *J Shoulder Elbow Surg.* 2002;11(4):305-308.

Please see video on the accompanying Web site at http://www.slackbooks.com/unstableshouldervideos

---

17

Techniques to Bone Graft the Deficient Anterior Glenoid Rim

Michael J. DeFranco, MD; Monica Morman, MD; Travis G. O'Brien, BA; Laurence D. Higgins, MD; and Jon J. P. Warner, MD

Several surgical procedures have been described to address anterior glenohumeral instability. The technique of using a bone graft to reconstruct the anteroinferior glenoid has been used since the early 19th century. Since that time, many surgeons have reported variations of this technique.[1-5]

The technique described here (Latarjet-Patte procedure) uses the coracoid process as the source for a bone graft, which creates glenohumeral stability in 3 ways. First, primary stability is provided by transferring part of the coracoid process to the antero-inferior aspect of the glenoid in a position that is flush with its articular surface. As the bone graft from the coracoid process is secured in this position, it provides a bone block, preventing anterior dislocation of the humeral head. Second, preservation and inferior shift of the inferior half to one-third of the subscapularis musculotendinous fibers also help prevent anterior dislocation of the humeral head by acting as an inferior sling. Finally, part of the coracoacromial ligament remains attached to the bone graft obtained from the coracoid process. During the final steps of the procedure, this part of the coracoacromial ligament is repaired to the lateral glenohumeral joint capsule in order to provide an additional soft tissue restraint. The combination of these stabilization effects is referred to as the "triple blocking effect."[3]

Alternatives to the coracoid process as a source of a bone graft include autologous iliac crest (Eden-Hybinette procedure) or allogeneic bone.[6] These alternative grafts are used in the same manner as the coracoid process to harvest a bone graft, which restores the concavity of the glenoid and prevents recurrent anterior instability. Alternative grafts are used most commonly in primary cases where the osseous defect is larger than the autologous coracoid process or in revision cases where the coracoid process was used in a previous surgery.

Abrams JS. *Management of the Unstable Shoulder: Arthroscopic and Open Repair* (pp. 223-234).
© 2011 SLACK Incorporated

Figure 17-1. Intraoperative patient position (beach chair).

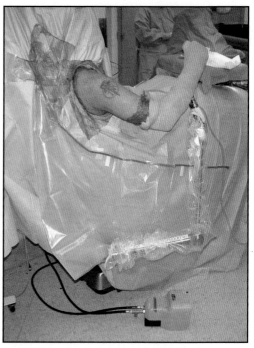

PATIENT SELECTION

Patients who present with recurrent anterior glenohumeral instability and fail to regain stability through nonoperative treatment become candidates for surgical intervention. Factors that must be considered when choosing an open stabilization procedure that requires the use of a bone graft include the etiology of the instability and the resulting pathology. These factors are discussed in more detail in previous chapters. In general, the critical factors to assess are the type of lesion causing the instability, the amount of anterior glenoid bone loss, and a history of failed arthroscopic stabilization procedures.

SURGICAL TECHNIQUE

Anesthesia and Patient Positioning

The procedure is performed under general anesthesia. An interscalene block is used for additional pain control. The patient is positioned in a beach-chair position (Figure 17-1). In cases where the iliac crest bone graft is harvested, the position of the bed should be at approximately 30 degrees to allow for easier access to the iliac crest. A small drape may be used behind the scapula to position the glenoid surface perpendicular to the operating table to assist in screw placement at 90 degrees to the glenoid. The upper extremity is prepped and draped in usual sterile fashion. The affected arm is completely free to move during the procedure. A hydraulic arm holder is used to assist in intraoperative arm positioning.

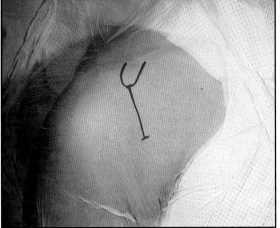

Figure 17-2. Surgical incision (10 to 15 cm starting at tip of coracoid process).

Surgical Approach

A 10- to 20-cm skin incision is made, starting at the tip of the coracoid process (Figures 17-2 and 17-3). The deltopectoral interval is developed, retracting the cephalic vein laterally (see Chapter 17 video). A self-retainer is placed in the deltopectoral interval. A Homan retractor is placed over the top of the coracoid process. Identification of the coracoacromial ligament, coracoid process, conjoint tendon, and pectoralis minor is essential before proceeding with the procedure. The anterior circumflex vessels are kept intact. The clavipectoral fascia is incised to expose the conjoint tendon. Dissection should not extend distal to the tip of the coracoid process in order to preserve the blood supply to the bone graft. The musculocutaneous and axillary nerves are identified and protected throughout the procedure.

Procuring the Bone Block

The first step in harvesting the bone graft from the coracoid process is to release the coracoacromial and coracohumeral ligament (Figures 17-4). The coracoacromial ligament is sectioned as close as possible to its attachment on the acromion. This is the part of the coracoacromial ligament that will be sutured to the lateral glenohumeral joint capsule at the end of the procedure. The coracohumeral ligament is transected as it lies inferior to the coracoacromial ligament. The second step is to release the insertion of the pectoralis minor from the medial aspect of the coracoid process (Figure 17-5). Next, a periosteal elevator is used to expose the base of the coracoid process, which is the location for the osteotomy. (Figure 17-6) The insertion of the coracoclavicular ligaments is identified, and the osteotomy is made just anterior to them. Finally, the osteotomy is performed with a 90-degree saw from medial to lateral at the junction of the horizontal and vertical parts of the coracoid.

In cases where a tricortical bone graft is harvested from the iliac crest, a 3- to 5-cm incision is made starting approximately 5 cm posterior to the anterior superior iliac spine to avoid injury to the lateral femoral cutaneous nerve. The dimensions of the harvested graft are based on the glenoid defect. An oscillating saw is used to make 2 vertical cuts in the iliac crest. A curved osteotome is then used to make a transverse cut in order to release the bone graft from the iliac crest. Bone wax or thrombin-soaked gel foam may be used to control any residual bleeding from the donor site. The soft tissues are closed in layers with absorbable sutures.

Figure 17-3. Key surgical landmarks: coracoid process, coracoacromial ligament, conjoint tendon, pectoralis minor.

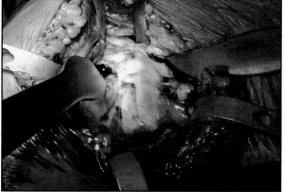

Figure 17-4. Release of the coracoacromial ligament.

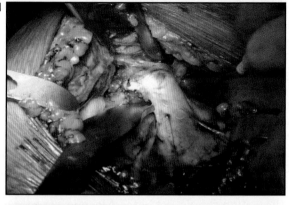

Figure 17-5. Release of pectoralis minor from its insertion on the coracoid process.

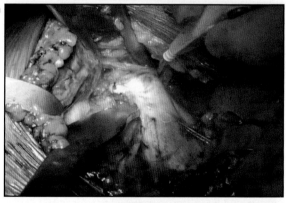

Figure 17-6. Coracoid osteotomy at the junction of the horizontal and vertical parts of the coracoid process.

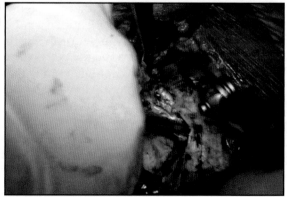

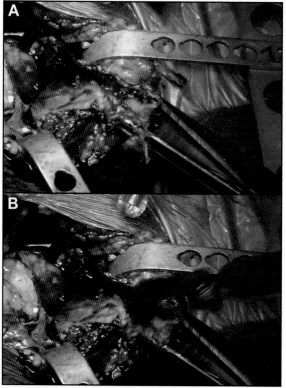

Figure 17-7. (A) Soft tissue removed from bone graft (deep surface). (B) Decortication of the bone graft (deep surface).

Preparation of the Bone Graft

The bone graft is released from any remaining soft tissue attachments (Figure 17-7). Care is taken to preserve the musculocutaneous nerve, which is located 3 to 5 cm distal to the tip of the coracoid process on the deep side of the conjoint tendon. Once the bone graft is released, its deep surface is decorticated using a saw or a burr. The length of the graft should be approximately 3 cm. A 3.2-mm drill is then used to drill 2 holes at 90 degrees to the surface of the bone graft and parallel to each other. The holes should be placed approximately 5 mm from the proximal and distal ends of the graft. There should be approximately 10 mm between the 2 holes (Figures 17-8). The holes will be used for screw placement to secure the bone graft to the glenoid. After drilling the holes in the bone graft, it is placed under the pectoralis major, and attention is directed toward exposure of the anterior glenoid.

Autologous iliac crest bone graft or allogeneic bone is contoured to the dimensions of the defect and to accommodate 2 screws used for fixation. For the iliac crest, the concave inner table is positioned such that it is facing laterally. Regardless of the type of bone graft (autograft or allograft), its position with respect to the glenoid articular surface is critical to the success of the procedure.

Exposure of the Anterior Glenoid

The superior and inferior borders of the subscapularis are identified. The axillary nerve is identified and protected with a blunt retractor placed underneath it and over the subscapularis inferiorly (Figure 17-9). A horizontal split in line with its fibers is made between the junction of the superior two-thirds and inferior one-third of the

Figure 17-8. Placement of drill holes.

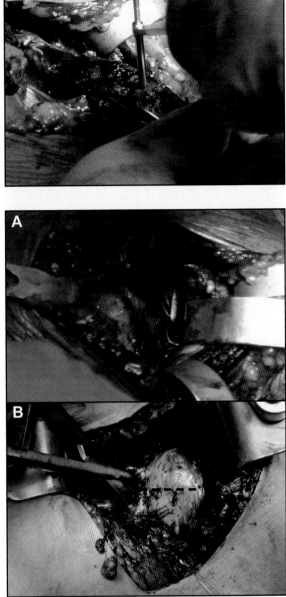

Figure 17-9. (A) Subscapularis and axillary nerve exposure. (B) Subscapularis exposed (line indicates location of subscapularis split).

musculotendinous unit (Figure 17-10). The division is continued to, but not through, the glenohumeral joint capsule. Traction sutures may be placed in the subscapularis superior and inferior to the split to assist in retraction of the subscapularis and visualization of the glenohumeral joint. A Homan retractor is placed in the subscapularis fossa. A vertical incision is made in the glenohumeral joint capsule at the level of the anteroinferior glenoid. A humeral head retractor is placed into the joint to retract it laterally. At this point, the anteroinferior glenoid should be visible. The damaged labrum, bone, and capsule are removed from this area. The bone is then decorticated with an osteotome or burr in preparation for placement of the bone block (Figure 17-11).

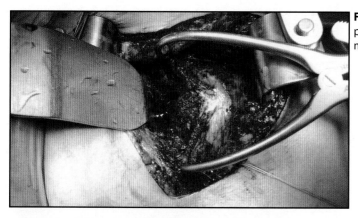

Figure 17-10. A Gelpi retractor is placed in the split subscapularis muscle and tendon.

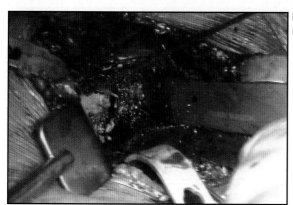

Figure 17-11. Decortication of injured antero-inferior glenoid.

Fixation of the Bone Block to the Glenoid

A 3.2-mm drill is used to drill a bicortical hole through the neck of the glenoid parallel to the articular surface and about 5 to 10 mm from the articular margin. On the right shoulder, the position of this hole should be at the 5 o'clock position and on the left shoulder at the 7 o'clock position. The inferior hole of the bone graft is aligned with the inferior hole of the glenoid, and a depth gauge is used to measure the length of the screw. A 4.5-mm malleolar screw is inserted into the inferior hole. A 3.2-mm cortical screw may be used if a 2.7-mm drill is used for the holes. The bone graft should be flush or just medial (1 to 2 mm) to the articular surface of the glenoid (Figure 17-12). There should be no lateral overhang of the bone graft. These same steps are repeated for placement of the superior screw through the bone graft and glenoid. The superior hole should also be parallel to the articular surface of the glenoid. Screws should be gently tightened. Over-tightened screws can cause the bone graft to fracture.

Various techniques (screw sizes, screw types) may be used to secure the bone graft to the glenoid (Figure 17-13). An alternative to the one described here is to secure the bone graft to the glenoid with 2 terminally threaded K-wires placed medial and parallel to the articular surface and parallel to each other. Direct visualization confirms correct placement of the graft. The 2.7-mm cannulated drill bit is used to drill over one of the K-wires. The K-wires are then removed, and the hole is enlarged with a 3.2-mm drill bit. A 4.5-mm malleolar screw is then inserted. Prior to tightening the screw, a #2 nonabsorbable braided suture is placed around the screw head and is later used to

Figure 17-12. Positioning of bone graft to the anteroinferior glenoid.

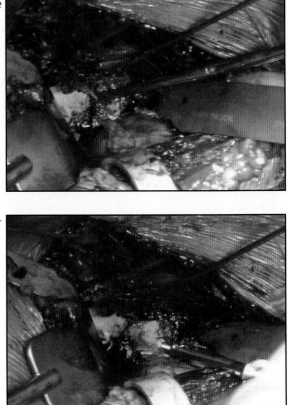

Figure 17-13. Fixation of bone graft to anteroinferior glenoid.

reattach the capsule to the graft. Care must be taken to prevent rotation of the graft while the screw is inserted. The second screw is placed in a similar fashion parallel to the first screw. Both screws are tightened, and the graft is inspected. If necessary, a small burr may be used to make any final adjustments to ensure correct graft fit. When smaller screws are needed, 4.0-mm partially threaded cannulated cancellous screws can be used for fixation of the graft.

Soft Tissue Fixation

After the bone graft is secured to the anteroinferior glenoid, the remnant of the coracoacromial ligament on the coracoid is sutured to the lateral glenohumeral capsule using two absorbable sutures (Figure 17-14). The sutures should be placed with the arm in external rotation. The stability and range of motion of the glenohumeral joint is then assessed.

Wound Closure

The operative area is inspected to achieve hemostasis before the wound closure. The subscapularis is not closed with suture. A drain is not used in the wound. The subcutaneous tissue is closed with an absorbable suture. The subcuticular layer is also closed with an absorbable suture.

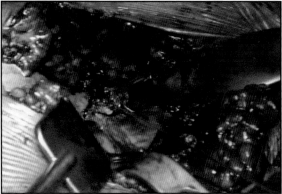

Figure 17-14. Suturing coracoacromial ligament to lateral glenohumeral joint capsule.

TIPS AND PEARLS

- *Correct indications for open anterior glenoid reconstruction:* Successful reconstruction of the anteroinferior glenoid to prevent recurrent instability requires appropriate patient selection. A thorough history, physical examination, and imaging studies are required to decide if a patient is a candidate for this procedure. A CT scan (axial and sagittal images) is essential to assess the degree of osseous injury to the anteroinferior glenoid and to determine which graft type should be used for reconstruction.

- *Patient positioning:* Patients are placed in a beach-chair position. Mobilizing the entire upper extremity is essential during the procedure. A sheet or towel under the operative scapula positions the glenoid in a more favorable position for screw placement.

- *Exposure:* When the bone graft is harvested from the coracoid process, exposure of the key structures is critical. The exposure should allow for clear visualization of the coracoid process, coracoacromial ligament, insertion of the pectoralis minor, conjoint tendon, and subscapularis. The musculocutaneous and axillary nerves should be identified and protected to prevent nerve injury.

- *Drill holes:* Drill holes in the bone graft should be placed appropriately to allow for placement of 2 screws. Malpositioned drill holes can result in poor bone graft fixation and fracture.

- *Placement of bone graft flush or medial to the articular surface of the glenoid:* In order to create a stable glenohumeral joint and to avoid unnecessary impingement of the humeral head, the bone block should be flush with or 1- to 2-mm medial to the articular surface of the glenoid. Placement of the bone block lateral to the articular surface is unacceptable. Impingement between the bone block and the humeral head will lead to degeneration of the articular cartilage and failure of the procedure. Placement of the bone block more than 1- to 2-mm from the articular surface of the glenoid can result in recurrent instability.

- *Screw fixation:* For optimal fixation, screws securing the bone block should be bicortical through the glenoid. Screws should be tightened gently as the bone graft is secured to the glenoid. Over-tightening of the screws can lead to fracture of the bone graft.

MANAGING COMPLICATIONS

- *Nerve injury:* Intraoperative nerve injuries should be addressed immediately. An intraoperative consult with a hand surgeon should be obtained, and transected nerves should be repaired. Identification and protection of the musculocutaneous nerves during the procedure is essential. In order to avoid nerve injury, the nerves should be located and checked during the steps of the procedure.

- *Subscapularis injury:* Damage to the subscapularis or release of it from the lesser tuberosity may occur during the procedure. The continuity of the subscapularis musculotendinous unit should be restored before the completion of the procedure. Normal function of the subscapularis is essential to achieving a successful clinical outcome.

- *Size of the bone graft:* If the harvested bone graft from the coracoid process is too small to accommodate 2 fixation screws or is inadequate to fill an osseous glenoid defect, then the iliac crest should be used as an alternative graft source. The patient should be consented for this procedure at the preoperative visit. Screw sizes may be adjusted to provide fixation for smaller grafts.

- *Intraoperative fracture of bone graft:* The bone graft may fracture as it is harvested, drilled, or fixed to the glenoid. An assessment needs to be made if the bone graft can be salvaged and provide adequate stability. If it becomes too small or cannot hold the appropriate fixation, then an alternative graft must be used to complete the procedure.

POSTOPERATIVE MANAGEMENT

Initially, patients are placed in a shoulder immobilizer for 4 weeks. Pendulum exercise may begin immediately. Passive range of motion starts at 2 weeks following surgery. Limitations for passive range of motion include 120 degrees of flexion, 30 degrees of external rotation, and 80 degrees of abduction in the plane of the scapula. There are no limitations on internal rotation. The shoulder immobilizer is removed after 4 weeks. At 4 weeks after surgery, full range of motion is allowed without limitations. Strengthening begins at 2 months after surgery. Return to full activity is allowed at 3 months after surgery.

ACKNOWLEDGMENT

The authors acknowledge Gilles Walch, MD, for his development and teaching of the Latarjet-Patte surgical procedure.

REFERENCES

1. Helfet A. Coracoid transplantation for recurring dislocation of the shoulder. *J Bone Joint Surg.* 1958;40B:198-202.
2. May VR Jr. A modified Bristow operation for anterior recurrent shoulder dislocation. *J Bone Joint Surg.* 1970;52(5):1010-1016.

3. Walch G, Boileau P. Latarjet-Bristow procedure for recurrent anterior instability. *Tech Shoulder Elbow Surg.* 2000:256-261.
4. Hovelius L, Korner L, Lundberg B, et al. The coracoid transfer for recurrent dislocation of the shoulder: technical aspects of the Bristow-Latarjet procedure. *J Bone Joint Surg.* 1983;65A:926-934.
5. Boileau P, Bicknell R, El Fegoun AB, Chuinard C. Arthroscopic Bristow procedure for anterior instability in shoulders with a stretched or deficient capsule: the "belt and suspenders" operative technique and preliminary results. *Arthroscopy.* 2007;23:593-601.
6. Provencher M, Ghodadra N, LeClere L, et al. Anatomic osteochondral glenoid reconstruction for recurrent glenohumeral instability with glenoid deficiency using distal tibia allograft. *Arthroscopy.* 2009;25:446-452.

Please see video on the accompanying Web site at
http://www.slackbooks.com/unstableshouldervideos

18

Hill-Sachs Injuries of the Shoulder
When Are These Important and How Should I Manage Them?

CDR Matthew T. Provencher, MD, MC, USN;
LT Matthew Rose, MD, MC, USN; and William Peace, MD

Glenohumeral stability is dependent upon the close bony relationship of the humeral head with the glenoid and inherent congruency of these structures. Deficiencies in the native osseous topography of the glenoid or humerus are important to recognize, as they may contribute to early failure of instability repair. Bony loss or injury to the humerus, known as a Hill-Sachs lesion, is an example of the importance of the bony structure of the glenohumeral joint. Although many Hill-Sachs lesions can largely be ignored, there are several characteristics of the Hill-Sachs injury that need to be carefully evaluated in order to optimize glenohumeral instability treatment. The focus of this chapter is to identify when a Hill-Sachs injury becomes important to the management of instability, to present current surgical techniques that address the Hill-Sachs lesion, and to identify the advantages and disadvantages unique to each approach.

HOW DOES A HILL-SACHS INJURY OCCUR?

The Hill-Sachs lesion occurs when a dislocating force displaces the humeral head outside the concavity of the glenoid. Once the humeral head is dislocated from the glenoid, the ligamentous structures are tensioned, building potential energy that is released, thus sending the soft spongiform bone of the posterior humeral head back against the much harder cortical bone of the anterior glenoid rim. The frequency of these episodes in addition to the force generated upon dislocation determine the severity of the ultimate Hill-Sachs fracture.[1] In addition, the position of the humerus at the time of injury is also important with regard to location, depth, and orientation of the Hill-Sachs injury.[2,3] A Hill-Sachs lesion is felt to become important if it symptomatically engages the anterior rim at a position of function (abduction at 90 degrees and 0 to 135 degrees of external rotation) either by patient history during activities or examination findings. This is also supported by radiographic findings of the size and orientation of the Hill-Sachs deficiency.[2] A Hill-Sachs injury pattern that is generally unstable will

Abrams JS. *Management of the Unstable Shoulder:*
Arthroscopic and Open Repair (pp. 235-252).
© 2011 SLACK Incorporated

Figure 18-1. Arthroscopic image of a Hill-Sachs injury to the humeral head demonstrating some chondral damage and impaction of the relatively soft bony humeral surface.

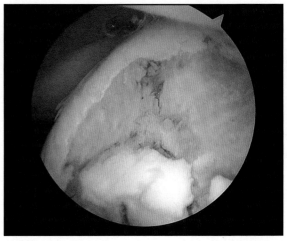

be orthogonal to the long axis of the humerus and align itself longitudinally with the anterior glenoid rim when the humerus is in a position of function (Figure 18-1).[3,4]

The prevalence of a Hill-Sachs lesion occurring in a population with a history of anterior shoulder instability ranges from 40% to 90%.[1,5-13] For the patient presenting with an initial anterior dislocation, the incidence is 25%.[11] The presence and size of a Hill-Sachs injury also increases with recurrent instability episodes as well as total time of symptomatic instability.[11,14] It should be kept in mind that the majority of Hill-Sachs injuries are not clinically significant[4]; however, if a Hill-Sachs is moderately large and is associated with a combined glenoid bone defect, the Hill-Sachs defect becomes clinically more important.[4,15]

SPECIFIC EXAMINATION FINDINGS IN A PATIENT WITH A CLINICALLY IMPORTANT HILL-SACHS INJURY

On physical examination, in addition to positive apprehension test findings, crepitus and catching may be felt with ranging the shoulder through various positions of abduction and external rotation. The patient will likely find these motions uncomfortable and may resist the examiner during the physical exam. Palpable and audible crepitus may be present. The suspicion for an engaging defect is supported by findings of an audible or palpable clunk in abduction/external rotation or the patient's sensation of instability through mid-ranges of motion.

CLASSIFICATION AND BIOMECHANICS OF A HILL-SACHS DEFECT

There are numerous proposed classification systems for the delineation of Hill-Sachs injuries to the shoulder. One of the classification systems used for Hill-Sachs lesions proposed by Rowe is graded as the following: mild is a defect that is 2.0-cm wide and 0.3-cm deep, a moderate defect is 4-cm wide and 0.5-cm deep, and a severe defect is 4-cm wide and 1-cm deep.[16] Franceschi and colleagues proposed 3 classifications based upon surface involvement. Grade I is strictly cartilaginous, grade II has superficial bony scuffing, and grade III lesions are described as a "hatchet fracture."[17] Calandra and colleagues graded lesions arthroscopically on the 32 shoulders in their study, which was also based on the surface involvement. Grade I (8/32) lesions had articular surface involvement that did not include subchondral bone. Grade II (5/32) included the subchondral bone, and grade III (2/32) had large subchondral bone defects.[5] Flatow and Warner felt that the significance of the lesion is related to the percentage of the articular cartilage involved.[18] They described the following: clinically insignificant involved less than 20% of the articular surface, variably significant had 20% to 40%, and clinically significant were lesions with more than 40% articular involvement. Although these classification systems have been proposed, the relative infrequency of the symptomatic Hill-Sachs deficiency makes it difficult to make definitive treatment decisions regarding the use of the classification systems above. However, it has been advocated that the larger defects and those at the largest of size in each respective classification system may be more important to recognize and treat.

It is pretty well accepted that those patients with a long history of instability episodes or those who have had numerous dislocations have more extensive injuries to the glenoid, the labrum, and development of a Hill-Sachs. In a study that compared frequency of instability, one episode of instability versus 2 or more, the cohort with 2 or more instability episodes had moderate-to-severe Hill-Sachs lesions and greater inferior and middle glenohumeral ligament (IGHL and MGHL) laxity.[1]

IMPORTANCE OF GLENOID BONE DEFICIENCY

Because the bony congruency of the glenohumeral joint is highly dependent upon both humeral and glenoid bone stock, the presence of glenoid bone loss may potentiate the effect of only a mild-to-moderate Hill-Sachs injury. Despite the glenoid being harder than the humeral head, traumatic bone loss to the anterior rim often accompanies a Hill-Sachs defect. Burkhart determined that anterior glenoid bone loss more than 25% of the normal width created an inverted pear shape that was inherently unstable.[2] Often, pathology of the glenoid is the most notable finding and is usually the aspect of the bone loss equation that needs to be addressed. Depending on the location and significance of the humeral defect, glenoid bone loss might be the only pathology that needs to be addressed surgically.

GLENOID TRACK CONCEPT

Stability after a Hill-Sachs injury is also dependent upon the location of the bony humeral head injury.[3] The track that the humerus glides within the glenoid has been identified as an important factor with shoulder instability.[3] When the humerus is in a position of function, Yamamoto and colleagues have demonstrated that the humeral head is seated in 84% of the glenoid cavity as the posterior rim of the glenoid abuts the cuff tendon.[3] Any anterior defect to the glenoid reduces the perch that the humeral head has upon the glenoid to less than 84%, decreasing the width of the glenoid track.[3] When a Hill-Sachs lesion rotates outside the glenoid rim and engages the anterior rim of the glenoid, an unstable position for the shoulder occurs.[19] If there is less than a normal glenoid bone stock, this ratio becomes increasingly more important as the humeral head may engage easier and become symptomatic when it wouldn't have been symptomatic if the glenoid was fully intact. Thus, the importance of the status of the glenoid in the setting of a Hill-Sachs injury cannot be overemphasized, as even small amounts of glenoid bone loss may make a humeral head Hill-Sachs deficiency much more important.

DIAGNOSTIC RADIOLOGY

A number of diagnostic plain film, ultrasound, computed tomography (CT), and magnetic resonance imaging (MRI) techniques have been described for detecting pathology of the humeral head, osseous glenoid, and labrum. The radiographic techniques most advantageous for initial evaluation of glenohumeral instability are the AP with internal and external views, axillary, axillary with exaggerated external rotation,[20] apical oblique (Garth view),[21] and West Point views.[22] The combination of these views is an important first step at effectively evaluating both the glenohumeral relationship as well as osseous pathology on both the humerus and the glenoid (Figure 18-2).

Ultrasound has been suggested as a cost-effective method for screening patients with shoulder instability for Hill-Sachs lesions. This has the advantages of allowing the patient to remain in a position of comfort and minimizing exposure to excessive radiation that accompanies CT and the multiple radiographs specific to detecting a possible Hill-Sachs lesion.[23,24] However, this practice remains to be validated for determining specific treatment.

MRI (or MR arthrogram) is advantageous as it allows for detection of soft tissue pathology that may need to be addressed during surgical intervention and can certainly be a tool to help delineate the amount of humeral and glenoid bone loss. In a double-blind, prospective study by Denti and colleagues, MRIs on 15 patients yielded a sensitivity of 60%, specificity of 100%, and accuracy of 87% compared to arthroscopy, which had a sensitivity of 80%, specificity of 100%, and accuracy of 87%.[25]

The gold standard for the evaluation of a Hill-Sachs defect remains a CT scan, with the humeral head digitally subtracted in order to critically quantify the location and size of the humeral defect. In addition, the sagittal oblique view of the glenoid should be visualized in order to look at the amount of glenoid bone loss.[26] The osseous deficits as visualized on CT scan can be precisely defined and are the most important findings for surgical decision making.

SURGICAL TREATMENT AND DECISION MAKING

In the setting of humeral bone loss (Hill-Sachs) injury, treatment can be directed at the restoration of the glenohumeral articular arc with either glenoid-based solutions, humeral-based strategies, or a combination. These can involve both arthroscopic and open repair techniques, and it is critical to have a surgical plan prior to the case in order to effectively treat the bone loss situation. Depending on the extent of pathology, the surgical procedure can include soft tissue repair, osseous autograft, or osseous allograft. It should be noted that addressing glenoid defects alone will often resolve the patient's instability.[2,27] However, there are certain situations, especially those in which the hard glenoid bone is not damaged, and with significant combined humeral and glenoid deficiencies, that humeral repair or reconstruction options should be considered (Figure 18-3).

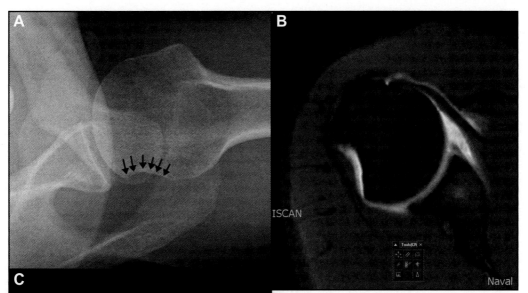

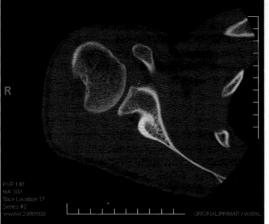

Figure 18-2. A 23-year-old man who sustained an anterior shoulder dislocation demonstrating 3 radiographic modalities for detection of the injury. (A) Plain axillary radiograph; (B) axial MR arthrogram; (C) axial CT scan.

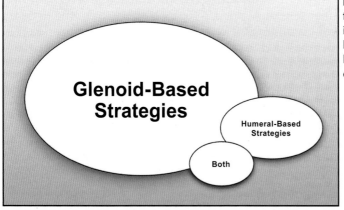

Figure 18-3. Operative strategies for management of a Hill-Sachs injury consist of primarily glenoid-based solutions, followed by either humeral solutions, and rarely a combination of both.

The concept of an engaging versus nonengaging[2] Hill-Sachs injury has been used in the past for delineating the extent of glenohumeral repair. In fact, Burkhart advocates that if the Hill-Sachs injury is engaging, a glenoid-based bone augmentation (ie, Latarjet) is sufficient for glenohumeral stability.[27] However, others advocate that, at some point, the humeral head will engage in the presence of a Hill-Sachs injury. More than a small Hill-Sachs deficiency should be augmented with a glenoid bone graft, humeral bone graft, or both.

It should be noted that the vast majority of Hill-Sachs injuries can be ignored, especially in the setting of no to minimal glenoid bone loss and without significant involvement of the humeral head. A small impaction fracture is much different from a hatchet type of fracture[17] due to the latter having a higher chance of glenoid engagement. When choosing a strategy, it should be kept in mind that Hill-Sachs deficiencies can be effectively managed with glenoid bone augmentation procedures or all-arthroscopic techniques. In the severe humeral deficiency, or combined deficiency, humeral bone graft options should be considered.

HILL-SACHS DEFICIENCY MANAGED WITH GLENOID AUGMENTATION

It should be noted that the majority of Hill-Sachs injuries can be managed with glenoid-based bone augmentation procedures.[2] Although the literature is not conclusively supportive, those patients who have presented with a Hill-Sachs injury have been successfully managed with a Latarjet procedure (or equivalent). However, it should be noted that humeral head defects are often accompanied with glenoid bone loss (Figure 18-4).

Open capsular repair without bone block remains a viable option for treating anterior instability, even with engaging Hill-Sachs defects. Pagnani performed a prospective study on 119 patients using an open capsular shift without osseous reinforcement.[28] Nearly one-third of the study population had engaging Hill-Sachs lesions, and 14% had anterior glenoid deficits with 4% having greater than 20% missing.[28] Through a deltopectoral approach, an anterior capsulotomy is used to access the anterior glenoid and identify any Bankart pathology. Depending on the osseous pathology and soft tissue laxity present, the anterior capsule is mobilized using a variety of capsulotomy incisions so that, at surgical closure, the capsule is reapproximated in a fashion that recreates the appropriate capsular tension. After a 2-year follow-up, 2% of the patients in this study had a recurrence of instability.[28] The average loss of external rotation in 90 degrees of abduction was 5 degrees.[28] Open capsular shift, as described by Pagnani, has the advantage of yielding excellent results and return to near-normal function.[28] The imbrication of the anterior capsule has the benefit of having more anterior soft tissue reinforcement; however, it could potentially be restricting and cause loss of external rotation. Ideally, this procedure could be used for athletes with high demand on the repaired structures. It could also be used as a backup for a patient who desired arthroscopic surgery, but required a conversion to an open procedure. In addition, issues with subscapularis healing have been noted, with subscapularis insufficiency described after open instability repairs.

The workhorse for the majority of Hill-Sachs injuries remains the open Latarjet procedure. There are numerous methods used to perform the Latarjet procedure, with the common denominator being a coracoid bone augmentation to the anterior glenoid. The capsule can be managed with a variety of techniques, either open or, as of recent, arthroscopically.

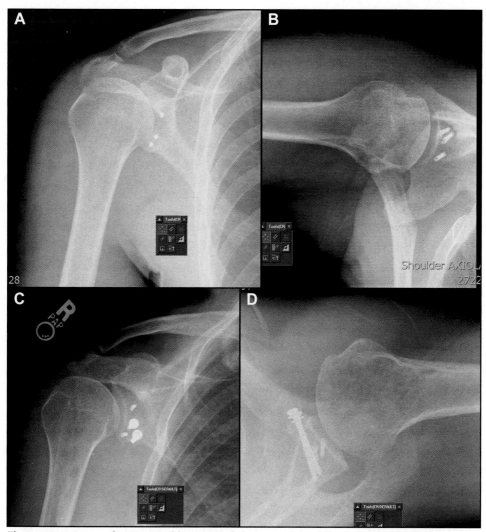

Figure 18-4. A case of a 25-year-old man who failed an initial anterior instability repair arthroscopically with 3 metal anchors. (A-C) The patient had a sizeable Hill-Sachs and approximately 15% of glenoid bone loss. (D) He was treated with a Latarjet procedure for a glenoid-based solution with the final radiograph shown after Latarjet grafting.

    The Latarjet procedure uses the coracoid process as an augment to anteroinferior glenoid bone loss that results in an inverted pear-shaped structure. The glenoid concavity and width are recreated so that a small to moderate Hill-Sachs defect does not engage the anterior glenoid rim of unstable shoulders. The coracobrachialis and short head of the biceps tendons are transferred on their bony coracoid origin to the anteroinferior glenoid, which reinforces the joint capsule at a site of potential laxity.[29] The inferior limb of the split subscapularis, likewise, is a reinforcing structure as it is tensioned when the humerus moves into abduction and external rotation.[29]

    When compared to tricortical bone grafting of the anteroinferior glenoid, the Latarjet is biomechanically superior as well. In a controlled laboratory cadaveric biomechanical study, 8 fresh frozen shoulders had "all but the rotator cuff, the middle head of the deltoid, the biceps brachii, and the coracobrachialis dissected" and mounted to a testing device.[30] The specimens were then stressed after "anteroinferior capsulotomy, anteroinferior glenoid bone defect, transplantation of a tricortical bone graft, and after the Latarjet procedure."[30] Wellman and colleagues found the Latarjet models to significantly reduce anterior translation by an average of 354% in 30 degrees of abduction and by 374% in 60 degrees of abduction, while in neutral rotation. Comparatively, the tricortical bone block did not perform as well with an average reduced translation of 179% at 30 degrees and 159% at 60 degrees.[30]

The Latarjet procedure is also well documented in its clinical success. Hovelius and colleagues conducted a study that followed 118 shoulders prospectively for 15 years. After the initial 2 years of follow-up, 1 of 118 shoulders had a recurrence of instability. At 15 years, 86% of the shoulders operated on were both stable and yielded good-to-excellent results as judged by the patient.[31] Another long-term study by Schroder and colleagues followed 52 shoulders from US Naval Academy Midshipmen for an average of 26 years. This study used the Single Assessment Numeric Evaluation (SANE), Western Ontario Shoulder Instability Index (WOSI), and Rowe tests to determine the outcomes of the procedure. The average long-term scores were as follows: SANE was evaluated as having a good/excellent score in 71.2%, fair in 11.5%, and poor in 17.3% of shoulders; WOSI was considered to have a excellent score in 57.7%, good in 11.5%, fair in 11.5%, and poor in 19.2% of shoulders; and the Rowe score had 36 excellent, 5 fair, and 11 poor results.[32] For the 52 shoulders followed, 6 had subsequent surgeries for recurrent instability.[32] The Latarjet procedure is effective in preventing instability over time; however, it has known consequences of shoulder arthrosis and loss of function with decreased external rotation.[32]

A long-term study by Allain and colleagues also found the Latarjet procedure to be effective at preventing instability, with osteoarthritis of the glenohumeral joint as a consequence.[33] Coracoid transfers that were too laterally placed and patients with pre-existing rotator cuff tears were identified as having more severe osteoarthritis at an average 14-year follow-up.[33] As a result, patients need to be free of rotator-cuff tears, and proper placement of the autograft is critical to minimize osteoarthritis in the long term.[34]

PROCEDURES ADDRESSING HUMERAL PATHOLOGY

Although the majority of Hill-Sachs injuries can successfully be managed with glenoid-based strategies, some of these injuries may require direct treatment of the Hill-Sachs defect. In general, the Hill-Sachs deformity can be addressed through both open and arthroscopic techniques. Arthroscopic techniques include filling the defect with soft tissue (usually the infraspinatus tendon),[35] percutaneous humeroplasty,[36,37] and a variety of small bone plug options.[4,38,39] Open techniques include autologous bone plugs, size-matched osteoarticular allografts, the Connolly Procedure, and rotational humeral osteotomy, although the latter has fallen out of favor.

ARTHROSCOPIC HUMERAL HEAD HILL-SACHS TECHNIQUES

The most common scenario encountered is upon the completion of an arthroscopic instability repair—a concern arises for the Hill-Sachs injury engaging the anterior

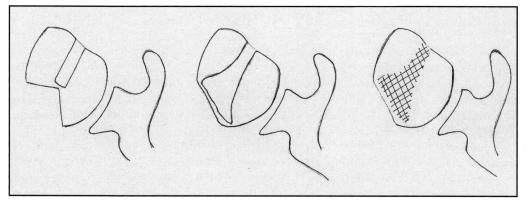

Figure 18-5. An ACL guide is depicted, which may be used to tamp an acute Hill-Sachs injury.

aspect of the glenoid during post-repair dynamic assessment. In this scenario, it has been described to "fill-in" the Hill-Sachs with the infraspinatus tendon, in a tenodesis-type fashion, which has been termed the *Remplissage procedure* by Eugene Wolf.[35] This probably works adequately for 2 reasons—it has the ability to fill the defect with viable tissue, allows the glenohumeral joint to be more centered, and restricts the anterior glenoid engagement process (Figure 18-5).

The Remplissage procedure is performed by the following steps: after a Bankart repair, the posterior port is used to directly visualize the extent of the Hill-Sachs defect, then this is used as the working port for a posterior capsulodesis.[35] The compacted defect is abraded to bleeding bone for the receipt of the infraspinatus tendon and posterior capsule that is fixated with 2 suture anchors.[35] Effectively, this procedure limits the glenoid track and prevents engagement of the Hill-Sachs defect with the anterior rim of the glenoid. In the original article, Purchase and Wolf experienced a 7% (2/24) recurrence rate of instability on follow-up, with both occurring secondary to traumatic events, with full restoration of motion.[35] The details of success are subjective as no formal postoperative questionnaire was mentioned, and the number of patients treated is limited to 24. This procedure has the advantage of being performed after a Bankart repair, using the same arthroscopic portals. Additionally, it does not expose the patient to the risk of infectious disease from cadaveric allografts.

An experimental cadaveric osseous disimpaction technique has been proposed by Kazel and colleagues by using a percutaneous bone tamp.[36] This method involves percutaneously drilling an osseous window 180 degrees from the Hill-Sachs defect, followed by using a curved bone tamp to raise the lesion to its near anatomic position. Re and colleagues have clinically applied this idea via the use of an open technique through the deltopectoral interval. The capsule is opened, the posterior humeral head defect is palpated, and an anterior cruciate ligament tibia guide is used to center the drill behind the center of the Hill-Sachs lesion.[37] A cortical window is opened with an 8-mm cannulated drill over a prepositioned K-wire.[37] Both curved and footed bone tamps are used to disimpact the defect to a near anatomic position.[37] The osseous void is then filled with cancellous bone chips prior to closure (see Figure 18-5).[37] This procedure has the advantage of restoring the humeral head to a near native topography without transpositioning soft tissue structures or using a rotational osteotomy of the humeral head. However, it does not address the problem of any osteochondral defects that could be present, and it is limited to moderate-sized defects.

OPEN HUMERAL BONY AUGMENTATION TECHNIQUES

The osseous allograft bone plug technique was introduced by Kropf and Sekiya as a novel approach to filling a moderate Hill-Sachs defect. This procedure can be performed in a stepwise approach or in combination with an anterior soft tissue repair. A vertical 6-cm incision is made over the bony defect, and the capsule is approached by splitting and retracting the infraspinatus inline with its orientation.[39] The infraspinatus is retracted, and the capsule is split over the Hill-Sachs defect.[39] A guide pin and external guide system utilized for anterior cruciate ligament reconstruction is available to facilitate placement of the guidepin in the center of the lesion. Then, cut a hole with a calibrated blade.[39] The subchondral bone is reamed to a bleeding bed in preparation for the allograft.[39] The allograft bone plug is then cut from the donor that is size-matched in diameter of the defect, yet oversized in length.[39] The allograft is inserted into the recipient site and tamped into place so that it is flush with the surrounding cartilage.[39] This procedure has the advantage of being a resurfacing technique that can be performed in stages or at the time of an anterior repair. Additionally, it can be performed with a minimal exposure, and the humeral head remains in its capsule.[39] The disadvantage is that it is limited to small to moderate lesions and has the risk of using cadaveric tissue.

Size-matched osteoarticular humeral allograft transplantation has promise as being a viable procedure for correcting large Hill-Sachs defects. A series of 18 size-matched osteoarticular allograft transplantations were performed by Miniaci and Gish.[4] The typical patient who would be a candidate for this procedure will have previously undergone and failed repair of anterior structures of the glenoid, labrum, and/or capsule. Failure was judged by having symptomatic anterior instability. The size of the defect in this series was more than 25% of the humeral head measured by CT reconstruction.[4] CT and/or MRI is ideal for planning this procedure as it gauges the size of allograft needed with 3-dimensional reconstruction (Figure 18-6).

A fresh frozen cadaver is obtained from a tissue bank and is released after appropriate viral and bacterial cultures have cleared. This leaves approximately 2 weeks from culture clearance until viable implantation, so the patient with a Hill-Sachs defect that is to be treated with a fresh allograft needs to understand the potential short notice of such a procedure in order to preserve graft viability. Although fresh grafts have been described, others have used irradiated allografts.[4]

The technique of humeral head allograft can be performed through either a deltopectoral or a deltoid-splitting approach. Our preferred method is a deltopectoral approach, and the subscapularis tendon is vertically transected. A capsulotomy is extended superiorly in line with the subscapularis tendon transaction, and a laterally based capsulotomy is made. The anteroinferior glenoid is inspected for pathology, which is addressed at this point. The final securing of the anterior structures, however, are not finalized until wound closure. The Hill-Sachs defect is exposed by externalizing the humeral head with a flat-narrow retractor. The lesion is flattened and shaped in a "chevron pattern" with a small sagittal saw. A size-matched humeral head allograft is cut and integrated into the defect by making minor adjustments in only one plane at a time. Upon congruent fit, the allograft is initially secured with K-wires and finally fixed in place (Figure 18-7). A variety of implants may be used for implantation, including cortical bone screws (3.5 mm), headless compression screws, as well as bioabsorbable and plastic screws. The success rate for the population studied was 100% with no recurrences of instability during an average 50-month follow-up.[4] This procedure is ideal for patients with large Hill-Sachs defects that are not amenable to humeroplasty (chronic injury) or bone plug allograft techniques outlined previously.

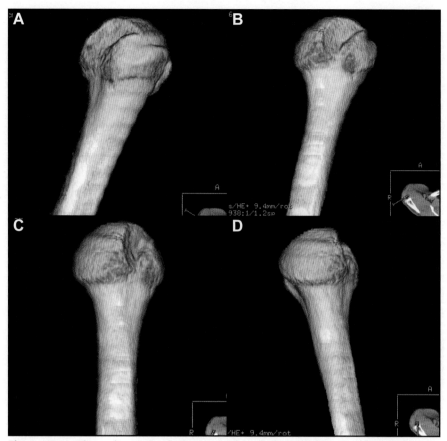

Figure 18-6. Three-dimensional CT scan with the glenoid digitally subtracted, demonstrating the typical location, orientation, and character of a Hill-Sachs lesion. This was graded as a large Hill-Sachs lesion and was eventually treated with allograft to the humeral head.

OTHER HUMERAL-BASED OPTIONS

There are metal implants that have the potential to be used for Hill-Sachs deficiency (HemiCap, Arthrosurface, Franklin, MA) and provide an easy solution for the management of patients who do not desire allograft or other bone grafting options. It should be noted that the round metal implant described above is not truly designed to fit into a Hill-Sachs deficiency, and this may prove to be problematic for obtaining a concentric fill of the Hill-Sachs injury. This is because the Hill-Sachs is not a round, cylindrical defect, but one that is linear and wedge-shaped.

The rotational humeral osteotomy, first performed in 1964 by Weber, is a procedure where an osteotomy of the surgical neck of the humerus is performed and the humeral head is rotated medially 25 degrees.[40] The osteotomy is then fixated with a blade plate, and the subscapularis tendon and anterior capsule are shortened anteriorly.[40] Fundamentally, the Hill-Sachs defect is being rotated out of the functional tract between the humeral head and the glenoid, converting an engaging lesion into a nonengaging lesion. Weber has accounted for a total of 207 of these procedures performed with 180 patients being followed.[40] During this period, the redislocation rate was 5.7%, with the nontraumatic dislocation rate being 1.1%.[40] The delayed union and nonunion rate

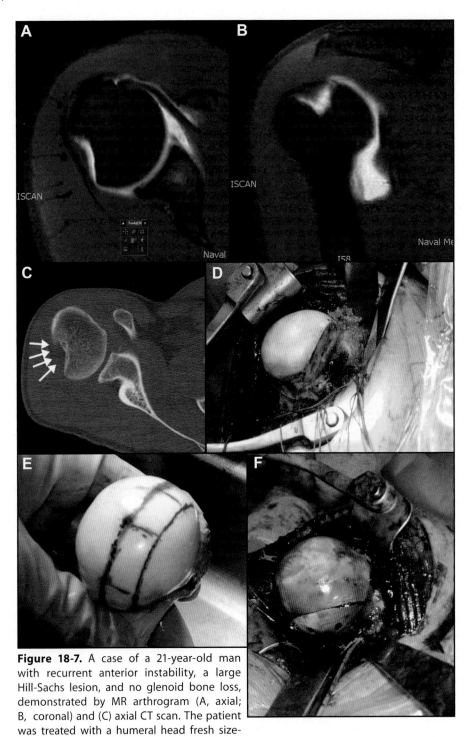

Figure 18-7. A case of a 21-year-old man with recurrent anterior instability, a large Hill-Sachs lesion, and no glenoid bone loss, demonstrated by MR arthrogram (A, axial; B, coronal) and (C) axial CT scan. The patient was treated with a humeral head fresh size-matched osteochondral allograft. (D) Through a deltopectoral approach, the Hill-Sachs lesion is exposed, and then (E-F) a fresh allograft is fixed into place with headless compression screws *(continued)*.

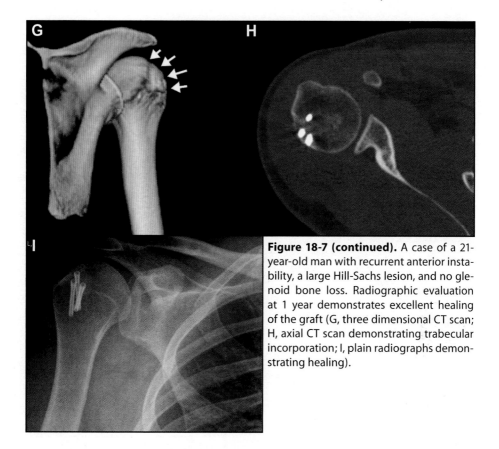

Figure 18-7 (continued). A case of a 21-year-old man with recurrent anterior instability, a large Hill-Sachs lesion, and no glenoid bone loss. Radiographic evaluation at 1 year demonstrates excellent healing of the graft (G, three dimensional CT scan; H, axial CT scan demonstrating trabecular incorporation; I, plain radiographs demonstrating healing).

combined was 2.8%, and 107 of the shoulders at follow-up had hardware removed.[40] The success rate for this procedure is comparable to the procedures described earlier. However, the disadvantages are the larger incision for the approach, a recommended hardware removal after 2 years for patients younger than 50 years, and the risk of delayed union, nonunion, and malrotation of the humeral head.[40] Given the initial success rate of more recent procedures and the risks related to rotational humeral osteotomy, this procedure has fallen out of favor for an initial approach to shoulder instability from a Hill-Sachs lesion.[40] However, in the most severe cases (usually in seizures or electric shocks), a complete humeral resurfacing or hemiarthroplasty should be considered.

HILL-SACHS DEFECTS MANAGED WITH COMBINED TECHNIQUES

Occasionally, a patient will present with severe pathology to both the posterior-lateral humerus and anteroinferior glenoid that are incompatible with a stable shoulder. The patient's history of instability might be a result of a seizure disorder, multiple traumatic dislocations, or electrocution. The combination of posterior lateral humerus and the anterior glenoid pathology will be too significant for a traditional Bankart repair or a single approach to bony pathology. The patient could have a surgical history of repair to the anterior structures with no resolution of their instability. The key is to use

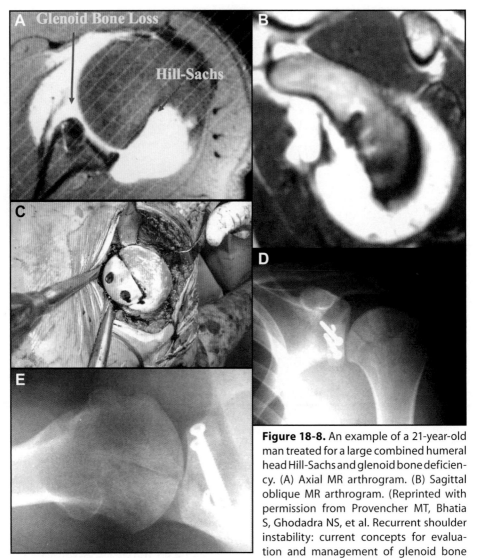

Figure 18-8. An example of a 21-year-old man treated for a large combined humeral head Hill-Sachs and glenoid bone deficiency. (A) Axial MR arthrogram. (B) Sagittal oblique MR arthrogram. (Reprinted with permission from Provencher MT, Bhatia S, Ghodadra NS, et al. Recurrent shoulder instability: current concepts for evaluation and management of glenoid bone loss. *J Bone Joint Surg Am.* 2010;92(suppl 2):133-151. (C) This was repaired with a combined approach including a fresh allograft to the humeral head fixed with biocompression screws and an iliac crest bone graft (ICBG). (D-E) Final radiographs are shown with the humeral head and ICBG at 1 year postoperatively.

current knowledge of pathophysiology to anticipate when a single approach will fail. A deficit greater than 20% to 25% of the anterior glenoid and/or a large Hill-Sachs lesion will likely be unstable and will have a risk of failing a Bankart repair without bony augmentation.[2,3,14,19] Patients with the combination of severe defects are relatively easy to predict when a single procedure will fail. The challenge arises when the humerus and glenoid together have marginal osseous deficits. Additionally, the functional goals and age of the patient are factors to consider (Figure 18-8).

The presentation of an unstable shoulder that has either a large Hill-Sachs defect or more than 25% glenoid loss in combination with minor pathology of the opposing structure will likely need a combined operation to reduce the risk of failure. The shoulder that has a large Hill-Sachs lesion and minor glenoid pathology (less than 25% of glenoid width) might need a size-matched osteoarticular allograft and an open capsular repair or Latarjet procedure. Given that both the glenoid and humeral bone augmentation are open procedures that release the subscapularis, they ideally can be performed in series under one exposure to anesthesia. Additionally, the vertical capsulotomy used for the osteoarticular allograft can be used with the T-plasty capsular shift used by Pagnani.[4,28]

The glenohumeral joint that has more than 25% of anterior osseous deficit from the anterior glenoid rim and a small to moderate, yet engaging Hill-Sachs fracture would demand a different approach. The glenoid pathology would benefit from the bony augmentation of an arthroscopic Latarjet procedure, taking care to not lateralize the coracoid autograft. As an adjunct to the Latarjet, the Hill-Sachs lesion could be decompressed with the humeralplasty described by Re and colleagues or the osseous allograft bone plugs proposed by Kropf and Sekiya.[37,39] Both of these can be performed after the completion of an arthroscopic procedure to correct the anterior structures and are intended to correct small to moderate Hill-Sachs defects that are engaging.

Various combinations of the selected procedures mentioned above can be used. Identifying overlaps in the various approaches and structures released so as to minimize the disruption of healthy native tissue is fundamental to planning combined procedures.

CONCLUSION

Although Hill-Sachs injury is a relatively common finding in recurrent anterior shoulder instability, the majority of these lesions can be largely ignored. However, as with the case in bone loss about the shoulder, larger Hill-Sachs lesions are often accompanied by various amounts of glenoid bone loss. One should be suspicious of a symptomatic Hill-Sachs deficiency in patients who present with multiple instability episodes, mechanical symptoms, an audible clunk, or examination findings of engagement of the humerus over the glenoid rim. Treatment options include both glenoid- and humeral-based strategies, including arthroscopic tenodesis of the defect with the infraspinatus (Remplissage), percutaneous humeroplasty, and a variety of glenoid and humeral bone grafting techniques (bone plugs, fresh allograft, and the Latarjet procedure). The majority of symptomatic Hill-Sachs injuries can be managed with arthroscopic Remplissage or glenoid bone grafting procedures. In the severe case, allografts or limited resurfacing or arthroplasty should be considered.

The views expressed in this chaper are those of the authors and do not reflect the official policy or position of the Department of the Navy, Department of Defense, or the US government.

REFERENCES

1. Spatschil A, Landsiedl F, Anderl W, et al. Posttraumatic anterior-inferior instability of the shoulder: arthroscopic findings and clinical correlations. *Arch Orthop Trauma Surg.* 2006;126(4):217-222.
2. Burkhart S, De Beer J. Traumatic glenohumeral bone defects and their relationship to failure of arthroscopic Bankart repairs: significance of the inverted-pear glenoid and the humeral engaging Hill-Sachs lesion. *Arthroscopy.* 2000;16(7):677-693.

3. Yamamoto N, Itoi E, Abe H, et al. Contact between the glenoid and the humeral head in abduction, external rotation, and horizontal extension: a new concept of glenoid track. *J Shoulder Elbow Surg.* 2007;16(5):649-656.
4. Miniaci A, Gish M. Management of anterior glenohumeral instability associated with large Hill-Sachs defects. *Tech Shoulder Elbow Surg.* 2004;5(3):170-175.
5. Calandra JJ, Baker CL, Uribe J. The incidence of Hill-Sachs lesions in initial anterior shoulder dislocations. *Arthroscopy.* 1989;5(4):254-257.
6. Cetik O, Uslu M, Ozsar BK. The relationship between Hill-Sachs lesion and recurrent anterior shoulder dislocation. *Acta Orthop Belg.* 2007;73(2):175-178.
7. Hintermann B, Gachter A. Arthroscopic findings after shoulder dislocation. *Am J Sports Med.* 1995;23(5):545-551.
8. Norlin R. Intraarticular pathology in acute, first-time anterior shoulder dislocation: an arthroscopic study. *Arthroscopy.* 1993;9(5):546-549.
9. Rowe CR, Patel D, Southmayd WW. The Bankart procedure: a long-term end-result study. *J Bone Joint Surg Am.* 1978;60(1):1-16.
10. Saupe N, White LM, Bleakney R, et al. Acute traumatic posterior shoulder dislocation: MR findings. *Radiology.* 2008;248(1):185-193.
11. Taylor DC, Arciero RA. Pathologic changes associated with shoulder dislocations. Arthroscopic and physical examination findings in first-time, traumatic anterior dislocations. *Am J Sports Med.* 1997;25(3):306-311.
12. Workman TL, Burkhard TK, Resnick D, et al. Hill-Sachs lesion: comparison of detection with MR imaging, radiography, and arthroscopy. *Radiology.* 1992;185(3):847-852.
13. Yiannakopoulos CK, Mataragas E, Antonogiannakis E. A comparison of the spectrum of intra-articular lesions in acute and chronic anterior shoulder instability. *Arthroscopy.* 2007;23(9):985-990.
14. Boileau P, Villalba M, Hery JY, Balg F, Ahrens P, Neyton L. Risk factors for recurrence of shoulder instability after arthroscopic Bankart repair. *J Bone Joint Surg Am.* 2006;88(8):1755-1763.
15. Richards RD, Sartoris DJ, Pathria MN, Resnick D. Hill-Sachs lesion and normal humeral groove: MR imaging features allowing their differentiation. *Radiology.* 1994;190(3):665-668.
16. Rowe CR, Zarins B, Ciullo JV. Recurrent anterior dislocation of the shoulder after surgical repair. Apparent causes of failure and treatment. *J Bone Joint Surg Am.* 1984;66:159-168.
17. Franceschi F, Longo U, Ruzzini L, Rizzello G, Maffulli N, Denaro V. Arthroscopic salvage of failed arthroscopic Bankart repair: a prospective study with a minimum follow-up of 4 years. *Am J Sports Med.* 2008;36(7):1330-1336.
18. Flatow EL, Warner JJP. Instability of the shoulder: complex problems and failed repairs. Part I. Relevant biomechanics, multidirectional instability, and severe loss of glenoid and humeral bone. *J Bone Joint Surg Am.* 1998;80(1):122-140.
19. Burkhart SS, Danaceau SM. Articular arc length mismatch as a cause of failed Bankart repair. *Arthroscopy.* 2000;16(7):740-744.
20. Rafert JA, Long BW, Hernandez EM, Kreipke DL. Axillary shoulder with exaggerated rotation: the Hill-Sachs defect. *Radiol Technol.* 1990;62(1):18-21.
21. Garth W, Slappey C, Ochs C. Roentgenographic demonstration of instability of the shoulder: the apical oblique projection. A technical note. *J Bone Joint Surg Am.* 1984;66:1450-1453.
22. Engebretsen L, Craig EV. Radiologic features of shoulder instability. *Clin Orthop Relat Res.* 1993;291:29-44.
23. Farin PU, Kaukanen E, Jaroma H, Harju A, Vaatainen U. Hill-Sachs lesion: sonographic detection. *Skeletal Radiol.* 1996;25(6):559-562.
24. Pancione L, Gatti G, Mecozzi B. Diagnosis of Hill-Sachs lesion of the shoulder. Comparison between ultrasonography and arthro-CT. *Acta Radiol.* 1997;38(4 Pt 1):523-526.
25. Denti M, Monteleone M, Trevisan C, De Romedis B, Barmettler F. Magnetic resonance imaging versus arthroscopy for the investigation of the osteochondral humeral defect in anterior shoulder instability. A double-blind prospective study. *Knee Surg Sports Traumatol Arthrosc.* 1995;3(3):184-186.
26. Kirtland S, Resnick D, Sartoris DJ, Pate D, Greenway G. Chronic unreduced dislocations of the glenohumeral joint: imaging strategy and pathologic correlation. *J Trauma.* 1988;28(12):1622-1631.
27. Burkhart SS, De Beer JF, Barth JR, Cresswell T, Roberts C, Richards DP. Results of modified Latarjet reconstruction in patients with anteroinferior instability and significant bone loss. *Arthroscopy.* 2007;23(10):1033-1041.
28. Pagnani MJ. Open capsular repair without bone block for recurrent anterior shoulder instability in patients with and without bony defects of the glenoid and/or humeral head. *Am J Sports Med.* 2008;36(9):1805-1812.
29. Lafosse L, Lejeune E, Bouchard A, Kakuda C, Gobezie R, Kochhar T. The arthroscopic Latarjet procedure for the treatment of anterior shoulder instability. *Arthroscopy.* 2007;23(11):1242.e1-5.

30. Wellmann M, Petersen W, Zantop T, et al. Open shoulder repair of osseous glenoid defects: biomechanical effectiveness of the Latarjet procedure versus a contoured structural bone graft. *Am J Sports Med.* 2009;37(1):87-94.
31. Hovelius L, Sandstrom B, Sundgre K, Saebo M. One hundred eighteen Bristow-Latarjet repairs for recurrent anterior dislocation of the shoulder prospectively followed for fifteen years: study I-clinical results. *J Shoulder Elbow Surg.* 2004;13(5):509-516.
32. Schroder D, Provencher M, Mologne T, Muldoon M, Cox J. The modified Bristow procedure for anterior shoulder instability: 26-year outcomes in Naval Academy Midshipmen. *Am J Sports Med.* 2006;34(5):778-786.
33. Allain J, Goutallier D, Glorion C. Long-term results of the Latarjet procedure for the treatment of anterior instability of the shoulder. *J Bone Joint Surg.* 1998;80(6):841-852.
34. Mochizuki Y, Hachisuka H, Kashiwagi K, Oomae H, Yokoya S, Ochi M. Arthroscopic autologous bone graft with arthroscopic Bankart repair for a large bony defect lesion caused by recurrent shoulder dislocation. *Arthroscopy.* 2007;23(6):677.e1-e.4.
35. Purchase RJ, Wolf EM, Hobgood ER, Pollock ME, Smalley CC. Hill-Sachs "Remplissage": an arthroscopic solution for the engaging Hill-Sachs lesion. *Arthroscopy.* 2008;24(6):723-726.
36. Kazel MD, Sekiya JK, Greene JA, Bruker CT. Percutaneous correction (humeroplasty) of humeral head defects (Hill-Sachs) associated with anterior shoulder instability: a cadaveric study. *Arthroscopy.* 2005;21(12):1473-1478.
37. Re P, Gallo RA, Richmond JC. Transhumeral head plasty for large Hill-Sachs lesions. *Arthroscopy.* 2006;22(7):798e1-4.
38. Knight D, Patel V. Use of allograft for the large Hill-Sachs lesion associated with anterior glenohumeral dislocation. *Injury.* 2004;35(1):96; author reply 96.
39. Kropf EJ, Sekiya JK. Osteoarticular allograft transplantation for large humeral head defects in glenohumeral instability. *Arthroscopy.* 2007;23(3):322 e1-5.
40. Weber BG, Simpson LA, Hardegger F. Rotational humeral osteotomy for recurrent anterior dislocation of the shoulder associated with a large Hill-Sachs lesion. *J Bone Joint Surg Am.* 1984;66(9):1443-1450.

19

Mini-Open and Arthroscopic Repair of the Humeral Anterior Capsular Avulsion

Drew Fehsenfeld, MD, PhD; Augustus D. Mazzocca, MS, MD; and Robert A. Arciero, MD

Instability of the shoulder is multi-factorial, involving injury to the labrum, capsule, and sometimes both. Traumatic anterior instability is most commonly associated with injury to the anteroinferior capsulolabral complex, or Bankart lesion. However, injury to the anterior capsule may also occur as a stretch injury or avulsion from the humeral insertion. In a cadaveric study, Bigliani showed the capsulolabral complex to fail at the glenoid in 40% of specimens, intrasubstance in 35%, and at the humeral attachment in 25%.[1] The latter of these injuries is known as a humeral avulsion of the glenohumeral ligament (HAGL).

The incidence of HAGL lesions has been reported to range from 2% to 9.3% in patients with recurrent shoulder instability. In a review of 547 patients with shoulder instability, Bokor and colleagues reported humeral avulsion of the lateral capsule in 7.5% of patients.[2] Wolf and colleagues found 6 of 64 shoulders (9.3%) to have a HAGL lesion present.[3] The location and character of HAGL lesions has also been reported in 71 cases.[4] The HAGL lesion is most commonly (93%) located on the anterior humerus. The anterior capsule failed as a soft tissue avulsion, bone avulsion, or at both the glenoid and humerus (floating capsule). Furthermore, these injuries may not occur in isolation and can be concurrent with a Bankart lesion.[5] Sixty-two percent of patients have associated pathology including a labral tear (25%), rotator cuff tears (23%), or a Hill-Sachs lesion (17%).[4] Failure to recognize and treat a HAGL lesion can result in persistent instability and failure of surgical stabilization.

Multiple studies have described open and arthroscopic methods of repairing the HAGL lesion. In 1942, Nicola reported on the first open repairs in traumatic anterior dislocators.[6] However, this technique requires take-down of the subscapularis tendon and the resultant postoperative risk of tendon dehiscence and muscle weakness. An alternative mini-open approach with only partial release of the inferior one-third of the subscapularis has had excellent results with no recurrent instability and maintenance of muscle strength.[7] Multiple studies have been published discussing arthroscopic techniques for HAGL repair; however, only a few have reported outcomes. Wolf and

Abrams JS. *Management of the Unstable Shoulder: Arthroscopic and Open Repair* (pp. 253-262).
© 2011 SLACK Incorporated

Figure 19-1. Anteroposterior radiograph of a shoulder showing a small bony capsular avulsion fracture at the inferomedial aspect of the humerus.

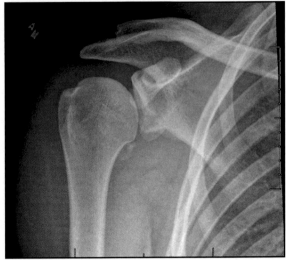

colleagues described 4 of 6 patients who were repaired arthroscopically by plicating the torn edge of the capsule to the deltopectoral fascia.[3] Kon and colleagues described 3 cases of arthroscopic repair with excellent Rowe score and no recurrent instability at 2 years.[8] Huberty and Burkhart reported on 6 patients repaired using an all-inside arthroscopic technique, who had good outcomes at more than 2 years.[9] While arthroscopic techniques have intrinsic benefits, including limited dissection and protection of the subscapularis, this approach is challenging due to the limited exposure of the anterior humeral neck and should only be attempted by the experienced arthroscopist.

PATIENT SELECTION

Patient evaluation should include standard history and physical examination for instability. While the vast majority of humeral avulsions of the glenohumeral ligament occur after violent trauma, an awareness must be maintained in all patients with instability. The likely mechanism of injury involves hyperabduction and external rotation.[6] Physical exam should include evaluation of range of motion, rotator cuff strength, and specific tests for instability, including apprehension/relocation, sulcus sign, anterior/posterior load shift, and jerk test. Unfortunately, there is no specific clinical test to delineate a HAGL lesion from other causes of instability.

Abnormal findings on plain radiographs are uncommon, but the anteroposterior view may demonstrate a small avulsion fracture at the inferomedial humeral neck as well as scalloping (Figure 19-1).[10] Magnetic resonance imaging (MRI) is recommended in all patients with instability not only to evaluate for capsular avulsion, but also injury to the labrum, rotator cuff, glenoid, and humeral head (Hill-Sachs). The capsular avulsion may be visualized on the sagittal views (Figure 19-2). Visualization of the capsule can be enhanced with the addition of intra-articular contrast. The avulsed inferior capsule may appear as a J-shaped structure with extravasation of contrast along the humeral neck (Figure 19-3). While MRI is a useful adjunct to HAGL diagnosis, the recognition of a HAGL lesion has been reported to be as low as 50%. Therefore, diagnostic arthroscopy is recommended with special attention to both the glenoid and humeral capsular attachments.

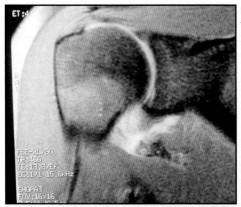

Figure 19-2. MRI of a shoulder showing coronal oblique view of a HAGL lesion.

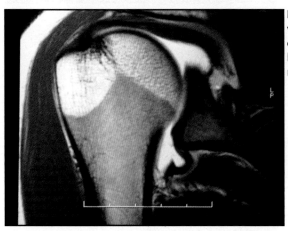

Figure 19-3. MRI arthrogram shows improved visualization of inferior capsular avulsion with extravasation of contrast along the medial humeral neck. The capsule appears retracted medially and slackened in the classic J sign.

HIGHLIGHTED SURGICAL TECHNIQUE

Mini-Open HAGL Technique

The patient is placed in the beach chair position with the extremity draped free and a bump to stabilize the scapula. The scope is introduced into the glenohumeral joint through a standard posterior portal. Diagnostic arthroscopy is performed to document the pathology, including injury to the capsule/labrum on the glenoid and humeral sides (Figure 19-4). If necessary, arthroscopic Bankart repair may be performed prior to open repair of the HAGL lesion. Performing the Bankart repair arthroscopically will allow for only partial take-down of the subscapularis during repair of the capsular avulsion.

An anterior skin incision is made extending from the axillary fold to the coracoid process. The cephalic vein is identified and taken laterally. The pectoralis and deltoid muscles are separated and retracted to expose the clavipectoral fascia. The lateral aspect of the coracobrachialis muscle is identified by the "red stripe" of muscle, and the conjoined tendon is retracted medially using a self-retainer. This exposes the subscapularis and the anterior circumflex vessels. Prior to performing the L-shaped incision in the subscapularis tendon, the axillary nerve can be identified by blunt dissection and palpation inferior and medial to the glenoid (Figure 19-5). A darrach retractor may then be used to protect the nerve during the remainder of the procedure.

Figure 19-4. Arthroscopic image of the anterior capsular avulsion from the anterior superior portal using a 30-degree scope.

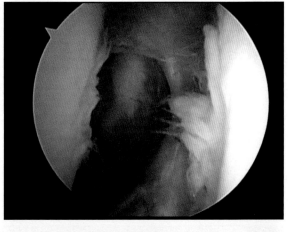

Figure 19-5. Image with the conjoined tendon retracted medially, exposing the subscapularis tendon. The axillary nerve can be seen inferior and medial to the glenoid.

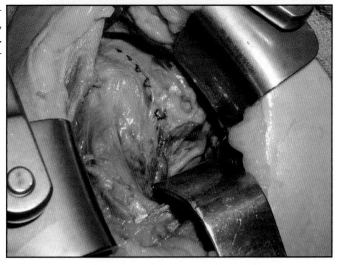

A vertical incision is then made in the lower third of the subscapularis 15 mm from the lesser tuberosity. The incision is stopped just superior to the circumflex vessels (Figure 19-6). The horizontal portion of the exposure is created by incising medially approximately 1.5 to 2 cm. The muscle is removed from the capsule using blunt Cobb or metzenbaum scissors to dissect medially. Superior retraction of the subscapularis will reveal the HAGL lesion (Figure 19-7). The injured capsule is typically located at the anteroinferior aspect of the glenohumeral joint on the humeral neck. Two to 3 suture anchors are placed along the neck of the humerus (Figure 19-8).

The sutures are then passed through the lateral capsule using a free needle in a horizontal mattress configuration. The sutures are tied, repairing the capsule to the anterior humerus (Figure 19-9). The subscapularis is then repaired anatomically. Early outcomes using this technique have been excellent, with no recurrent instability and maintenance of subscapularis strength.

Arthroscopic HAGL Repair

Arthroscopic HAGL repair has been described both in the beach chair and lateral decubitus positions.[8,11-13] Our preference is to use the lateral decubitus position because of improved joint distraction and visualization of the inferior joint.

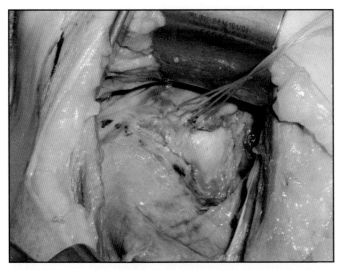

Figure 19-6. The subscapularis incised with an L-shaped incision and tagged with suture to retract it superiorly. The capsule is seen deep to the subscapularis.

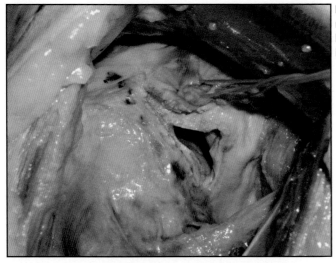

Figure 19-7. The subscapularis is retracted superiorly, and the HAGL lesion is tagged with sutures at the inferior medial humerus.

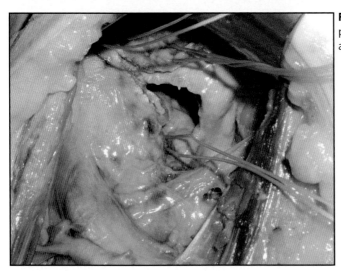

Figure 19-8. Anchors are placed perpendicular to the humerus along the anterior humeral neck.

Figure 19-9. The capsular avulsion is secured to the anterior humerus with multiple anchors, and then the sub-scapularis is repaired to the lateral insertion.

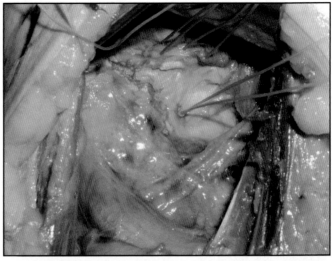

Figure 19-10. The arthroscopic set-up for HAGL repair using the lateral decubitus position. Arm is in traction with large towel bump placed in axilla.

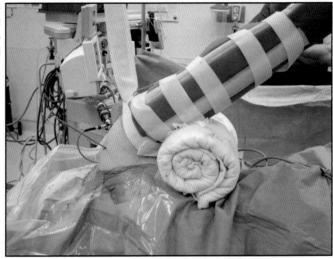

The shoulder is distracted with 7 lbs distally and 5 lbs laterally. A towel bump is placed in the axilla to improve distraction (Figure 19-10). A diagnostic arthroscopy is performed though a standard posterior portal using a 30-degree scope. The HAGL should be easily visualized at the humeral insertion (Figure 19-11). Often, the subscapularis muscle can be seen, indicating a disruption in the capsule (see Chapter 19 video). An anterosuperior portal is created using a switching stick at the superior border of the rotator interval, just below the biceps tendon and slightly lateral. An anteroinferior portal is placed just above the subscapularis tendon for anchor placement and suture management. The scope is shifted to the anterosuperior portal over the switching stick, and an 8.25-mm cannula is placed in the posterior portal. A 70-degree scope can provide improved visualization of the HAGL defect during repair. A shaver without suction is used with great care to clean the frayed edges of the avulsed capsule. The location for anchor placement is determined, and the capsule is reduced using a grasper to evaluate the appropriate tension of the inferior glenohumeral ligament. The site of repair is decorticated with a burr through the anteroinferior portal. A 5 o'clock trans-subscapular portal is often required for placement of the anchors on the anterior

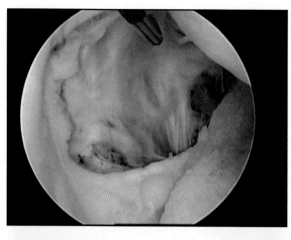

Figure 19-11. Image of HAGL with subscapularis visible beneath the capsular avulsion.

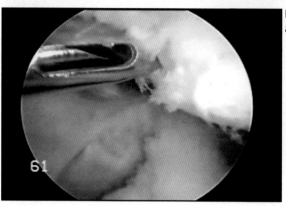

Figure 19-12. Anchors are placed along the anterior humerus at the capsular insertion.

humerus (see Chapter 19 video). The instrumentation cannula for the suture anchor is placed percutaneously through a small incision (Figure 19-12). Two to 3 anchors are sequentially placed along the insertion of the anterior humerus. As each anchor is placed, the suture limbs are shuttled through the edge of the capsular avulsion in a horizontal mattress configuration using a crescent hook suture passer (Figure 19-13, also see Chapter 19 video). The sutures are tied through the anteroinferior portal, securing the capsule to the anterior humerus (Figure 19-14).

TIPS AND PEARLS

First and foremost, successful management of the unstable shoulder requires recognition and treatment of all injured structures. The HAGL is an uncommon and therefore easily missed injury that has been shown to be associated with recurrent instability. Therefore, a high index of suspicion must be maintained. In addition, the absence of a HAGL on MRI does not definitively rule out capsular injury. Arthroscopy should be performed, focusing on evaluation of the glenoid and humeral attachments. The appearance of the subscapularis muscle on arthroscopy suggests disruption of the inferior capsule.

The open exposure of the HAGL lesion can be difficult and requires a good understanding of shoulder anatomy. The capsule and subscapularis tendon become fused near the lesser tuberosity. Incising too closely to the lesser tuberosity after the tendon

Figure 19-13. Sutures are shuttled through the free edge of the avulsed capsule.

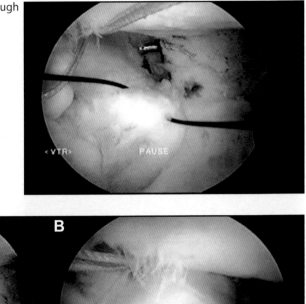

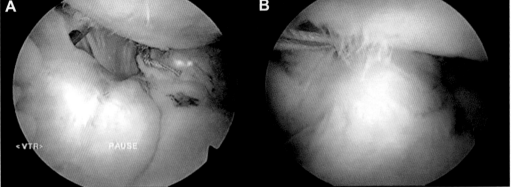

Figure 19-14. Sutures are tied through the anteroinferior portal to secure the avulsed capsule to the anterior humerus.

and capsule have united can make exposure difficult. The gap between the subscapularis and capsule should be visualized medially and dissected laterally. The inferior aspect of the subscapularis muscle inserts into the capsule and may disrupt visualization of the HAGL lesion. As discussed above, the muscle should be dissected bluntly from the capsule to expose the injured region.

Managing Complications

Complications of repairing a humeral avulsion of the glenohumeral ligament are rare. The most common complication is failure to diagnose the lesion and therefore inappropriate treatment of the patient. Untreated, a HAGL lesion does not allow tensioning of the inferior glenohumeral ligament and ultimately may result in recurrent instability. Dehiscence of the subscapularis repair is one potential complication, although this has not been observed, likely secondary to the protective effect of the intact superior two-thirds of the tendon. Due to the proximity of the approach to the musculocutaneous and axillary nerve, there is a risk of nerve injury either by stretch or laceration. Good visualization can prevent laceration; however, prolonged retraction of either nerve may result in transient numbness or weakness in the distribution of the nerve. Typically, these injuries recover with time and observation. Avoiding vigorous retraction with self-retaining instruments may decrease the risk of neuropraxia.

POSTOPERATIVE MANAGEMENT

The arm is held in neutral or slight internal rotation in a shoulder immobilizer for approximately 4 weeks. For the first 3 to 4 weeks, the patient is allowed supine well-arm assisted forward elevation. Isometric strengthening of all rotator cuff muscles and scapular stabilization exercises are initiated 2 to 3 weeks after surgery. Range of motion is progressed at 4 weeks to increase external rotation. Resistance training can be started at 6 weeks with bands, cords, or weights. At 4 months, the patient may return to all activities, including contact sports.

REFERENCES

1. Bigliani LU, Pollock RG, Soslowsky LJ, et al. Tensile properties of the inferior glenohumeral ligament. *J Orthop Res.* 1992;10(2):187-197.
2. Bokor DJ, Conboy VB, Olson C. Anterior instability of the glenohumeral joint with humeral avulsion of the glenohumeral ligament. A review of 41 cases. *J Bone Joint Surg Br.* 1999;81(1):93-96.
3. Wolf EM, Cheng JC, Dickson K. Humeral avulsion of the glenohumeral ligaments as a cause of anterior shoulder instability. *Arthroscopy.* 1995;11(5):600-607.
4. Bui-Mansfield LT, Banks KP, Taylor DC. Humeral avulsion of the glenohumeral ligaments: the HAGL lesion. *Am J Sports Med.* 2007;35:1960-1966.
5. Warner JJ, Beim GM. Combined Bankart and HAGL lesion associated with anterior shoulder instability. *Arthroscopy.* 1997;13(6):749-752.
6. Nicola T. Anterior dislocation of the shoulder. *J Bone Joint Surg Am.* 1942;24:614-616.
7. Arciero RA, Mazzocca AD. Mini-open repair technique of HAGL (humeral avulsion of the glenohumeral ligament) lesion. *Arthroscopy.* 2005;21(9):1152e1-1152e4.
8. Kon Y, Shiozak H, Sugaya H. Arthroscopic repair of a humeral avulsion of the glenohumeral ligament lesion. *Arthroscopy.* 2005;21(5):632.
9. Huberty DP, Burkart SS. Arthroscopic repair of anterior humeral avulsion of the glenohumeral ligaments. *Tech Shoulder Elbow Surg.* 2006;7(4):186-190.
10. Oberlander MA, Morgan BE, Visotsky JL. The BHAGL lesion: a new variant of anterior instability. *Arthroscopy.* 1996;12:627-633.
11. Richards DP, Burkhart SS. Arthroscopic humeral avulsion of the glenohumeral ligaments (HAGL) repair. *Arthroscopy.* 2004;20(suppl 2):134-141.
12. Spang JT, Karas SG. The HAGL lesion: An arthroscopic technique for repair of humeral avulsion of the glenohumeral ligaments. *Arthroscopy.* 2005;21(4):498-502.
13. Parameswaran AD, Provencher MT, Bach BR, Verma N, Romeo AA. Humeral avulsion of the glenohumeral ligament: injury pattern and arthroscopic repair techniques. *Orthopedics.* 2008;31(8):773-779.

**Please see video on the accompanying Web site at
http://www.slackbooks.com/unstableshouldervideos**

20

Open Surgical Approach for Posterior Stabilization

Luke S. Oh, MD and Scott P. Steinmann, MD

Posterior instability of the shoulder is not as common as anterior shoulder instability and has had a reputation for being a challenging problem to diagnose and manage. True unidirectional posterior instability in isolation is uncommon compared to posterior instability that is observed as a component of multidirectional instability. Distinguishing between physiologic laxity and instability may be challenging in patients with posterior shoulder instability because the clinical presentation may be more subtle than in cases of anterior instability. Often, a patient with posterior instability may not ever have had a history of frank dislocation and may instead present with symptoms that may be attributed to recurrent posterior subluxations. This condition is being recognized and treated more frequently among those athletes who sustain repeated posteriorly directed loads across the shoulder, such as in offensive linemen in American football.

As our awareness and level of clinical suspicion increases, accurate diagnosis and recognition of posterior instability likely is improving as well. However, even after an accurate diagnosis has been made, treatment of posterior instability in a patient with generalized laxity may not be straightforward. Often, a patulous and redundant capsule may be present either in isolation or in addition to a posterior labral tear and/or posterior bony Bankart lesion. These intra-articular findings may be observed even in athletes who were thought to have sustained a single, isolated traumatic injury. For patients who have failed nonoperative management of unidirectional posterior instability, some of these cases may be amenable to arthroscopic management, whereas others may require a formal open posterior approach to the shoulder. This chapter describes the surgical technique of open approach to the posterior shoulder.

PATIENT SELECTION

A thorough and detailed history and physical examination is essential in distinguishing isolated posterior instability with multidirectional instability. A history of

Abrams JS. *Management of the Unstable Shoulder: Arthroscopic and Open Repair* (pp. 263-274).
© 2011 SLACK Incorporated

subluxation or dislocation of other joints, family history of collagen disorders, and the absence of significant trauma should alert the clinician to the possibility of multi-directional instability. It is imperative to document any physical examination findings of generalized laxity: approximating the thumb to the volar forearm, hyperextension of the metacarpophalangeal joints beyond 90 degrees, elbow hyperextension greater than 10 degrees, knee hyperextension, and ability to touch the palm to the floor with the knees straight.

Various maneuvers for testing subluxation exist that are described elsewhere. It is important to note that patients with posterior subluxation often complain of pain rather than instability, although both may be present. It is critical to examine the contralateral shoulder, and an examination under anesthesia is an important diagnostic modality because there may be significant guarding by the patient in the office setting that renders the examination inconclusive.

In patients who have had prior surgery, it is important to note the details of the preoperative clinical presentation, intraoperative findings, and the nature of the procedure performed. It is not uncommon for patients with multidirectional instability to present with recurrence and failure of anterior stabilization surgery. If the patient had posterior stabilization surgery for isolated posterior instability, then an assessment should be made to evaluate the redundancy of the posteroinferior capsule, possible posterior glenoid erosion, and potential neurovascular deficits.

An arthroscopic approach can be used for many cases of posterior instability, but an open surgical approach to posterior instability may be considered if there is posterior bone loss, glenoid dysplasia, or failed prior surgery. Some patients may fracture the posterior edge of the glenoid during their initial dislocation or during subsequent instability episodes. This can lead to loss of bone along the posteroinferior glenoid, which is best visualized with a computed tomography (CT) scan. In this situation, a soft tissue repair may need to be supplemented with a bone block. Patients with subtle increased glenoid retroversion can be difficult to define with plain radiographs. Even with use of a CT scan, version can be difficult to determine unless 3-dimensional imaging is used. Defining true version with a 2-dimensional CT scan is unreliable due to patient positioning in the scanner with variation in the scapula gantry angle. In most cases of posterior instability, however, slight glenoid retroversion can be addressed with a soft tissue repair. Use of a bone block or even a corrective osteotomy of the glenoid should be reserved for the rare case of gross glenoid retroversion. Failed prior posterior instability surgery, either open or arthroscopic, can be successfully addressed with an arthroscopic revision procedure if imaging studies suggest a tear or attenuation of the posteroinferior glenohumeral ligament. An arthroscopic approach has the benefit of not having to dissect through previous scarred posterior tissue planes to expose the joint. A revision open approach, however, can address both a soft tissue repair and a bony augmentation if needed.

SURGICAL TECHNIQUE

The patient may be positioned in either the prone or lateral decubitus position. The Chapter 20 video demonstrates the posterior surgical approach to the shoulder with the patient in the prone position. The lateral decubitus position, however, is the preferred positioning for those cases in which a diagnostic arthroscopy is planned prior to performing an open posterior approach to the shoulder.

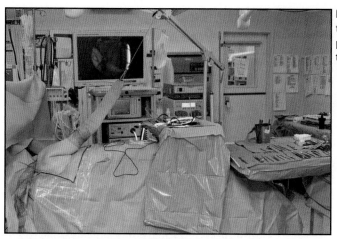

Figure 20-1. Lateral decubitus positioning for shoulder arthroscopy and possible conversion to an open posterior approach to the shoulder.

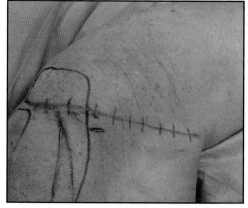

Figure 20-2. The anatomic landmarks for the skin incision: posterior aspect of the acromioclavicular joint proximally and posterior axillary fold distally.

Regardless of patient positioning, an examination under anesthesia should be performed on both shoulders to determine the direction and severity of maximal glenohumeral translation in comparison to the contralateral side. A critical component of this evaluation is to confirm the impression from the initial office assessment of whether the patient has either an isolated posterior instability or a posterior instability that is a component of multidirectional instability. Physical examination testing should be performed to assess generalized ligamentous laxity, such as presence of a shoulder sulcus sign, elbow hyperextension, hypermobility of wrist flexion, and metacarpophalangeal extension.

The patient is administered general anesthesia and is positioned on a beanbag in the lateral decubitus position. All bony prominences should be well padded, and an axillary roll may be necessary. If arthroscopy is to be performed, then a conventional shoulder holder is used to suspend the shoulder with 10-lb weights (Figure 20-1). After the arthroscopy has been completed, the arm is released from traction and placed in adduction on the side of the patient's body.

The landmarks for the skin incision are the posterior aspect of the acromioclavicular joint and the posterior axillary fold (Figure 20-2). After a long saber incision has been made, skin flaps are elevated to expose the fascia over the deltoid and trapezius muscles (Figure 20-3).

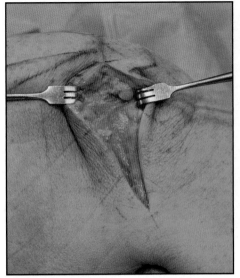

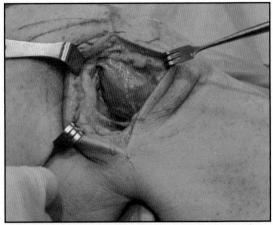

Figure 20-4. The deltoid fascia and muscle are split in line with its fibers approximately 2 to 3 cm from the posterolateral corner of the acromion. The proximal end of the muscle split is at the level of the scapular spine, and the distal end of the muscle split is approximately 5 cm from the level of the acromion in order to stay away from the axillary nerve.

Figure 20-3. Skin flaps are elevated to expose the fascia over the deltoid and trapezius muscles.

The glenohumeral joint is located approximately 2- to 3-cm medial from the posterolateral corner of the acromion. Therefore, the deltoid fascia and muscle are split in line with its fibers approximately 2 to 3 cm from the posterolateral corner of the acromion. The proximal end of the muscle split is at the level of the scapular spine, and the distal end is approximately 5 cm from the level of the acromion, which helps to stay away from the axillary nerve (Figure 20-4). The deltoid does not necessarily need to be elevated off of the acromion proximally, although doing so may improve surgical exposure. Distally, a stay suture may be placed in order to prevent propagation of the split in the deltoid fascia and muscle toward the axillary nerve.

Once the deltoid muscle is retracted using wide right-angle retractors, the underlying infraspinatus and teres minor are exposed (Figure 20-5). The infraspinatus muscle is bipennate with a fat stripe in the interval between its 2 heads (Figure 20-6). This interval between the 2 heads of the infraspinatus is at times better visualized than the interval between the infraspinatus and teres minor. Exposure of the posterior glenohumeral capsule may be performed either via a division of the 2 heads of the infraspinatus or between the infraspinatus and teres minor. Splitting the 2 heads of the infraspinatus results in exposure of the posterior capsule at the equator; however, exposure medially is limited by the location of the branches of suprascapular nerve (Figure 20-7). In order to decrease the risk of injury to the suprascapular nerve, the medial aspect of the division of the 2 heads of the infraspinatus should not extend more than 1.5 cm medial from the glenoid margin. Alternatively, if exposure of the posterior capsule is made between the infraspinatus and teres minor, the risk of injury to the suprascapular nerve is minimized and allows for a more extensile exposure (Figure 20-8). The Chapter 20 video also demonstrates a technique in which the infraspinatus is detached from its humeral insertion and retracted medially. Regardless of which of these techniques is used for the surgical exposure, the infraspinatus and the underlying posterior capsule need to be separated and carefully dissected in order to be able to mobilize the capsule for the posterior capsular shift. Medially, blunt dissection is sufficient, but sharp dissection is required laterally. Because the posterior capsule is usually thin and patulous, careful dissection is necessary, particularly at the lateral aspect when using sharp dissection.

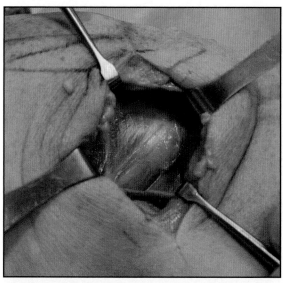

Figure 20-5. The deltoid muscle is retracted in order to expose the underlying infraspinatus and teres minor.

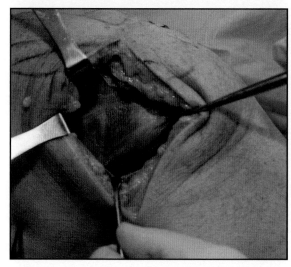

Figure 20-6. There are 2 fat stripes visible on this photograph. The superior fat stripe delineates the interval between the 2 heads of the infraspinatus, and the inferior fat stripe is the interval between the infraspinatus and teres minor. Exposure of the posterior humeral capsule may be performed either by a division of the 2 heads of the infraspinatus or at the interval between the infraspinatus and teres minor. The photos taken for this chapter demonstrate the exposure performed between the infraspinatus and teres minor, except for Figure 20-7.

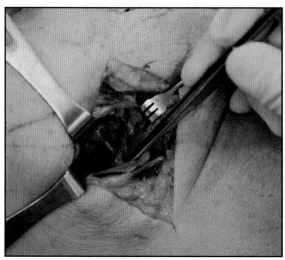

Figure 20-7. Dissection between the 2 heads of the infraspinatus results in exposure of the posterior capsule at the equator; however, exposure medially is limited by the location of the branches of suprascapular nerve. In order to decrease the risk of injury to the suprascapular nerve, the medial aspect of the division of the 2 heads of the infraspinatus should not extend more than 1.5 cm medial from the glenoid margin. This photo demonstrates the location of a branch of the suprascapular nerve in relation to the posterior capsular plication sutures.

Figure 20-8. Exposure of the posterior capsule obtained through the interval between the infraspinatus and teres minor minimizes the risk of injury to the suprascapular nerve and allows for a more extensile exposure.

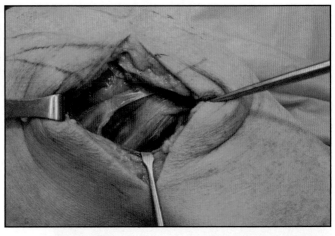

Figure 20-9. The posterior capsule is incised horizontally at the equator from the edge of the posterior glenoid labrum medially to the humeral attachment laterally.

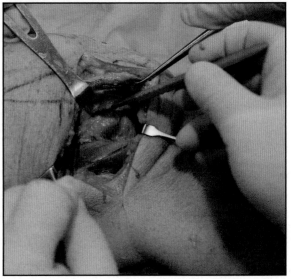

Exposure of the underlying posterior capsule is maintained by deep retractors. The capsule is divided horizontally at the equator from the edge of the posterior glenoid labrum medially to the humeral attachment laterally (Figure 20-9). The capsule may be incised superiorly and inferiorly at either the medial or lateral edge of the horizontal capsulotomy to create 2 leaflets of capsule. Surgeon preference dictates whether a medial-based or lateral-based posterior capsular shift is performed. In the majority of cases, there is not an associated reverse Bankart lesion of the posterior labrum; therefore, there is no distinct advantage of creating the T-shaped capsular incision medially versus laterally. However, if there is a posterior Bankart lesion that requires repair, then it may be preferable to create the T-shaped capsular incision medially rather than laterally and to perform a medial-based capsular shift (Figure 20-10). After abrading the posterior glenoid rim, suture anchors may be placed similar to a conventional anterior Bankart repair (Figure 20-11). The sutures are then passed through the labrum sequentially, starting from the inferior-most suture anchor. Once all sutures have been passed through the labrum, knots should be tied in the same sequential order. The posterior capsular shift is then performed by advancing the inferior capsular leaflet superiorly and medially and the superior capsular leaflet inferiorly and distally (Figure 20-12A).

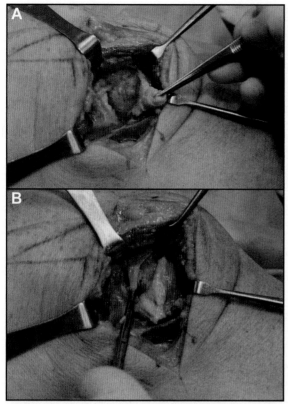

Figure 20-10. A T-shaped capsulotomy may be created either medially or laterally. In the majority of cases, there is not an associated reverse Bankart lesion of the posterior labrum; therefore, the T-shaped capsular incision may be created either medially or laterally according to surgeon preference. However, if there is a posterior Bankart lesion that requires repair, then it may be preferable to create the T-shaped capsular incision medially rather than laterally and to perform a medial-based capsular shift. (A) Inferior capsular leaflet. (B) Superior capsular leaflet.

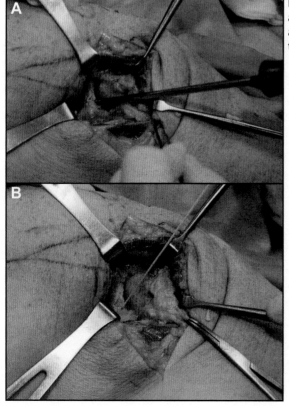

Figure 20-11. Posterior Bankart repair: After abrading the posterior glenoid rim, suture anchors may be placed similar to a conventional anterior Bankart repair.

Figure 20-12. (A) The posterior capsular shift is performed by advancing the inferior capsular leaflet superiorly and medially and then advancing the superior capsular leaflet inferiorly and distally in order to create a "vest-over-pants" capsular plication. (B) Nonabsorbable sutures are passed through the inferior leaflet, and a capsular closure is performed with the arm in 15 degrees of abduction and neutral rotation. (C) The superior capsular leaflet is advanced distally and medially and placed on the inferior capsular leaflet. Securing the superior leaflet to the inferior leaflet using nonabsorbable sutures provides added thickness to the posterior capsule.

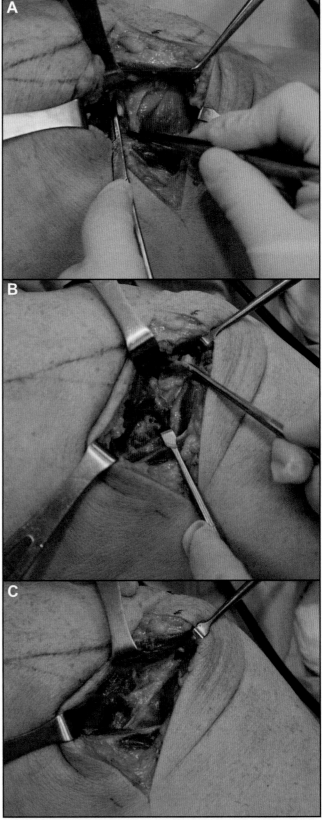

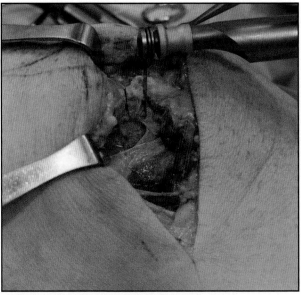

Figure 20-13. In those cases with posterior glenoid bone loss or with very thin or torn posterior capsule such as may be encountered in a revision setting after a failed capsulorrhaphy, posterior bone block may be required. A 2 x 2 cm bone graft that is approximately 1-cm thick may be obtained from the posterior scapular spine or posterior iliac crest. This figure demonstrates harvesting a bone graft from the posterior scapular spine.

Nonabsorbable sutures are passed through the inferior leaflet, and a capsular closure is performed with the arm in 15 degrees of abduction and neutral rotation (Figure 20-12B). Then, the superior capsular leaflet is advanced distally and medially and placed on the inferior capsular leaflet. Securing the superior leaflet to the inferior leaflet using nonabsorbable sutures provides added thickness to the posterior capsule (Figure 20-12C).

In those cases with posterior glenoid bone loss or with very thin or torn posterior capsule such as may be encountered in a revision setting after a failed capsulorrhaphy, posterior bone block may be required. A 2 x 2 cm bone graft that is approximately 1-cm thick may be obtained from the posterior scapular spine or posterior iliac crest (Figure 20-13). The cancellous side of the bone graft is placed on the posteroinferior aspect of the glenoid neck and is secured with 1 or 2 partially threaded screws (Figure 20-14). A burr may be used to contour the shape of the bone graft so that it remains "flush" with the remaining glenoid rim and to maintain the radius of curvature of the native glenoid.

TECHNICAL PEARLS

- Avoid a lengthy arthroscopy if one is performed prior to the open dissection. Extravasation of the arthroscopic fluid causes tissue edema and alteration of the tissue planes that will make the open dissection more difficult.

- If the decision is made to detach the deltoid from the spine of the scapula, be careful to do so subperiosteally and to meticulously repair the deltoid to the acromion via bone tunnels at the end of the procedure.

- Dissection of the infraspinatus requires correct identification of the anatomic intervals and 3 muscle bellies: the 2 heads of the infraspinatus and the teres minor. Especially in a revision setting with altered anatomy, careful dissection is critical so as to avoid neurovascular injury. Wandering too inferiorly may result in injury to the axillary nerve and posterior humeral circumflex vessels.

Figure 20-14. (A) Posterior glenoid bone loss. (B) Positioning of the posterior bone block obtained from the posterior scapular spine. The cancellous side of the bone graft is placed on the posteroinferior aspect of the glenoid neck and is positioned to maintain the contour of the posterior glenoid rim and to maintain the radius of curvature of the native glenoid. (C) Provisional fixation with a guide wire. (D) Placement of a partially threaded cannulated screw in order to secure the posterior bone block.

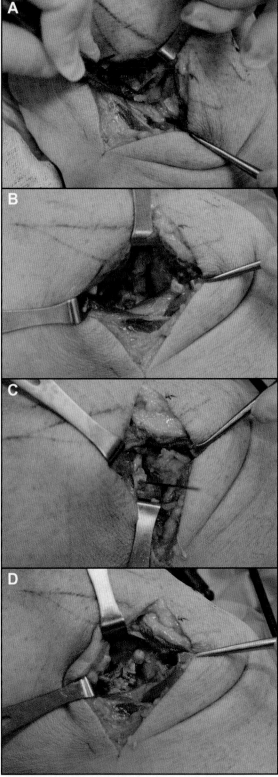

- The posterior capsule must be exposed and adequately separated from the infraspinatus in order to allow mobilization. Moreover, the T-shaped capsulotomy must also be created so as to allow sufficient advancement and shift of the capsular leaflets to eliminate the redundancy of the inferior pouch.

COMPLICATIONS

- Misdiagnosis is a common reason for failure of instability surgery, particularly the failure to recognize the difference between true isolated posterior instability and posterior instability that is part of multidirectional instability. This underscores the importance of performing an examination under anesthesia in order to confirm initial clinical impressions.

- Neurovascular injury to the suprascapular nerve may be avoided by careful dissection to only 1.5-cm medial to the glenoid rim and by avoidance of excessive traction of the infraspinatus. Risk of injury to the axillary nerve may be decreased by limiting the split of the deltoid inferiorly. A stay suture placed approximately 5 cm from the acromion helps to prevent progression of the deltoid split inferiorly.

- Recurrent instability following open capsular shift is a challenging problem. Unless a new traumatic injury has occurred, treatment should be focused on physical therapy and rehabilitation because revision surgery is often less successful than primary surgery and altered anatomy makes the technical aspect of the revision procedure more difficult.

- Voluntary dislocators have a poorer prognosis after surgery. Identification of such patients preoperatively is important in order to appropriately treat and counsel these patients.

BIBLIOGRAPHY

Bigliani LU, Pollock RG, McIlveen SJ, et al. Shift of the posteroinferior aspect of the capsule for recurrent posterior glenohumeral instability. *J Bone Joint Surg Am.* 1995;77(7):1011.

Fronek JR, Warren RF, Bowen M. Posterior subluxation of the glenohumeral joint. *J Bone Joint Surg Am.* 1989;71A(2):205.

Hawkins RJ, Janda DH. Posterior instability of the glenohumeral joint. A technique of repair. *Am J Sports Med.* 1996;24(3):275.

Hawkins RJ, Koppert G, Johnston G. Recurrent posterior instability (subluxation) of the shoulder. *J Bone Joint Surg Am.* 2984;66(2):169.

Miller S, Flatow EL. Posterior and multidirectional instability: open solutions. In Warner JJP, Ianotti JP, Flatow EL, eds. *Complex and Revision Problems in Shoulder Surgery.* Philadelphia, PA: Lippincott Williams & Wilkins; 2005.

Misamore GW, Facibene WA. Posterior capsulorrhaphy for the treatment of traumatic recurrent posterior subluxations of the shoulder in athletes. *J Shoulder Elbow Surg.* 2000;9(5):403.

Pollock RG, Bigliani LU. Recurrent posterior shoulder instability: diagnosis and treatment. *Clin Orthop.* 1993;291:85.

Tibone JE. Capsular repair for recurrent posterior instability. In Craig EV, ed. *Master Techniques in Orthopaedic Surgery: The Shoulder.* Philadelphia, PA: Lippincott Williams & Wilkins; 2004.

> **Please see video on the accompanying Web site at**
> **http://www.slackbooks.com/unstableshouldervideos**

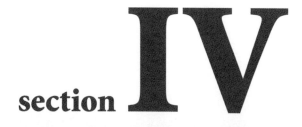

Rehabilitation of the Athlete

21

Dislocation During the Athletic Season
Treatment Options

Daniel D. Buss, MD and Aimee S. Klapach, MD

Acute traumatic anterior shoulder dislocation is a relatively common occurrence. In the high-demand athletic population, the incidence is 2-fold greater than that of the general population (1.7%).[1] The literature indicates a variety of treatment protocols for anterior shoulder instability including bracing, physical therapy, and early surgical stabilization. This chapter will review the different options for the in-season athlete with a traumatic, first-time dislocation and their respective success rates and complications.

PATIENT SELECTION

The primary goal of treating in-season shoulder dislocation is to prevent recurrent instability and to permit the athlete to complete his or her season. A first dislocation requires a full initial work-up, including post-reduction x-rays and a careful neurovascular exam. Advanced imaging such as magnetic resonance imaging (MRI), MR arthrogram, or computed tomography (CT) scanning is not mandatory but may help identify the extent of soft tissue and bony injury. Greater tuberosity fractures, full-thickness rotator cuff tears, or incomplete reduction precludes early return to sport with a brace. Patients with a history of recurrent dislocations typically do not require advanced imaging, have less acute tissue hemorrhage, and may return to play sooner than first-time dislocators. Similarly, atraumatic dislocations typically produce less soft tissue injury than traumatic dislocations; these patients may be expected to have a quicker return to play. Atraumatic dislocations should alert the examiner to underlying predisposing conditions, such as multidirectional instability, collagen disorders, or atypical glenoid morphology that may impair successful return to sport. Posterior shoulder dislocations may be successfully managed with similar principles of early range of motion and functional bracing; however, specific braces designed to limit internal rotation and posterior translation will not be discussed further in this chapter.

Abrams JS. *Management of the Unstable Shoulder: Arthroscopic and Open Repair* (pp. 277-284).
© 2011 SLACK Incorporated

Figure 21-1. Proper demonstration of pendulum exercises. Back should be flat with the involved shoulder completely relaxed. Motion should be accomplished in clockwise, counter-clockwise, anterior to posterior, and abduction to adduction.

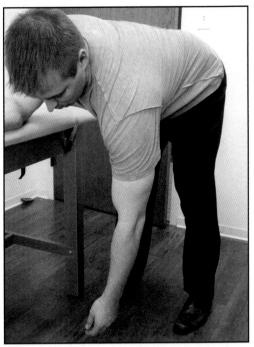

   Recurrent anterior instability rates vary by age group, with the recurrence rate as high as 94% in athletes younger than 20 years and 79% in athletes aged 20 to 30 years.[2] Conversely, the recurrence rate in active individuals older than 40 years is less than 40%.[3] Treatment may therefore be guided by age of the athlete as well as by aggressiveness of the sport. Patients involved in sports that require extreme motion of the glenohumeral joint and those in which subsequent dislocations can have catastrophic outcomes, such as pole vaulting, rock climbing, or motor cross, are best managed with either discontinuation of their sport or early surgical stabilization. Athletes in sports requiring less shoulder range of motion such as basketball, football, or soccer may be successfully braced throughout the remainder of their season. All athletes will benefit from a course of physical therapy. Initial pendulum exercises (Figure 21-1) are followed by the addition of active-assisted exercises focusing on regaining symmetrical range of motion in all directions, including external rotation. High-repetition, low-weight rotator cuff strengthening is added using free-weights, with a goal of 40 repetitions with a weight no greater than 2 lbs (Figure 21-2). Free weights allow the amount of stress to be consistent through the entire range of motion versus rubber tubing, which is at its greatest resistance when the shoulder is at its weakest point at the end-range of motion. The subscapularis is particularly important in preventing anterior dislocations.[4] Periscapular stabilization and proprioception exercises are added with gradual return to sport-specific activities (Figure 21-3). Therapy should be continued for 3 months or until the end of the athletic season.

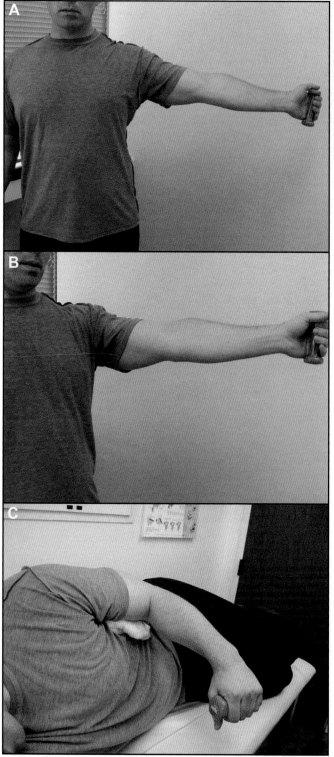

Figure 21-2. (A) Demonstrating proper abduction exercises with free weights for rotator cuff strengthening. (B) Demonstrating proper forward flexion exercises with free weights for rotator cuff strengthening. Emphasizes the supraspinatus. (C) Demonstrating external rotation exercises with free weights for rotator cuff strengthening. Emphasizes the subscapularis.

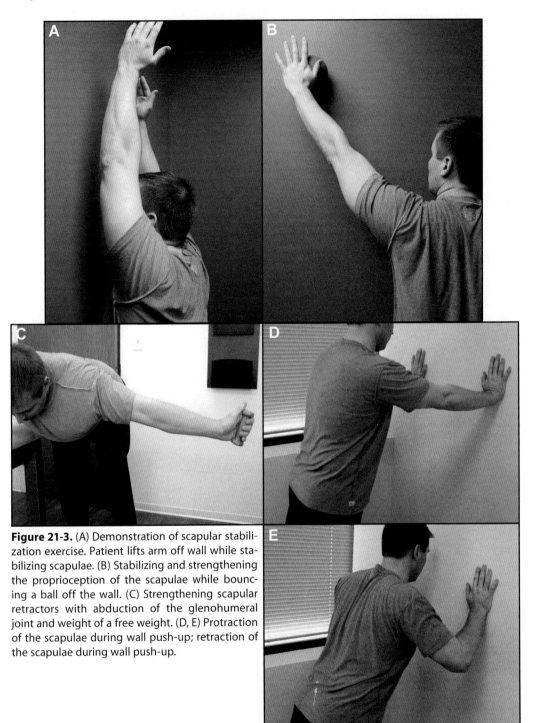

Figure 21-3. (A) Demonstration of scapular stabilization exercise. Patient lifts arm off wall while stabilizing scapulae. (B) Stabilizing and strengthening the proprioception of the scapulae while bouncing a ball off the wall. (C) Strengthening scapular retractors with abduction of the glenohumeral joint and weight of a free weight. (D, E) Protraction of the scapulae during wall push-up; retraction of the scapulae during wall push-up.

TECHNIQUES FOR MANAGING IN-SEASON ANTERIOR SHOULDER INSTABILITY

The traditional practice of immobilizing the shoulder in internal rotation following an acute traumatic dislocation has been challenged. Hovelius and colleagues reported their 25-year prospective follow-up of patients with anterior shoulder dislocation and concluded that immobilization did not improve outcomes.[5] Buss and colleagues employed early physical therapy and bracing with no period of immobilization in a series of 30 athletes, with 84% able to return to sport with completion of their season.[6] There was an average absence from competition of 10.8 days (range: 0 to 30). While 37% experienced some degree of instability throughout the remainder of their season, 53% elected to undergo surgical stabilization after the season's completion.

Itoi and colleagues immobilized the arm in external rotation for 3 weeks with a success rate of 80%.[7] Theoretically, this will reduce the labrum to its anatomic position, thereby reducing the rate of recurrence and the need for subsequent surgery. Further study and follow-up is needed before this can be recommended over other established protocols.

BRACING TECHNIQUE

A functional brace serves to decrease pain, provide stability, and reduce traumatic insult to the glenohumeral joint while the athlete completes the season. Braces may be classified based on demands of the athlete.[4] A Type I brace is used for overhead, low impact, acceleration motions, such as throwing and racket sports. Type II braces are used for overhead, low impact, deceleration positions, such as wide receivers and volleyball blockers. The Sully Brace (Saunders Group, Chaska, MN), in a category where anti-forces are created using the motion in the arm,[4] is recommended for overhead athletes (Figure 21-4).

High-impact forces require a Type III brace. Full range of motion is allowed in a Type IIIA brace, which is suitable for linebackers and defensive linemen, while sports not requiring full range of motion, such as hockey or offensive linemen, are managed with braces termed Type IIIB; an example of a Type IIIB is a Duke Wyre brace (C.D. Denison Orthopaedic Appliance Corp, Baltimore, MD; Figure 21-5).

TIPS AND PEARLS

Careful consideration of timing, age, and athletic goals must be taken into account when treating the athlete with anterior shoulder instability. Continuation of participation in high-risk sports in which further dislocations could be catastrophic, such as motor cross, pole vaulting, and rock climbing, are contraindications to nonoperative treatment. Physical therapy should be started immediately following a dislocation, beginning with pendulum exercises. Immobilization is not indicated. In general, bracing is only required during sporting activities. Custom braces are available for specific anatomic needs. Further studies are needed to address and compare the outcomes and natural history of nonoperative treatment and immediate surgical stabilization for patients with an anterior shoulder dislocation.

Figure 21-4. (A) The Sully Brace. (B, C) Type II braces are recommended for overhead, low-impact, deceleration positions.

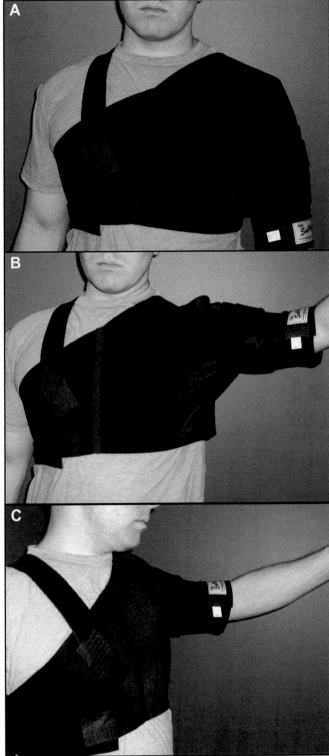

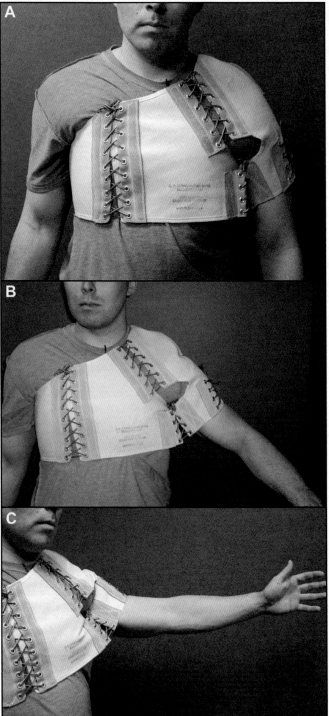

Figure 21-5. (A) The Duke Wyre Shoulder Vest. (B, C) Limitations of the Duke Wyre can help prevent further dislocations.

MANAGEMENT OF COMPLICATIONS

Recurrent multiple episodes of instability while using a brace after an adequate course of physical therapy is an indication for surgical intervention. There have been no studies indicating that delaying surgical stabilization results in further injury to the glenohumeral cartilage; however, this remains a theoretical concern, and more study on this topic is warranted.

CONCLUSION

Anterior shoulder dislocation is a common occurrence in the athletic population with a high re-dislocation rate (82% reported by Simonet and Cofield[8]). Younger age at index dislocation has a higher rate of recurrence. Arthroscopic and open surgical stabilization for anterior dislocations has proven to offer good results.[9] However, it should be noted that surgery is a season-ending event. Nonoperative management of the in-season athlete with early physical therapy and bracing is an effective technique for young athletes who are interested in returning to their sport during the athletic season.[6]

REFERENCES

1. Wang RY, Arciero RA. Treating the athlete with anterior shoulder instability. *Clin Sports Med.* 2008;27(4):631-648.
2. Rowe CR, Zarins B, Ciullo JV. Recurrent anterior dislocation of the shoulder after surgical repair. Apparent causes of failure and treatment. *J Bone Joint Surg Am.* 1984;66:159-168.
3. Reuss BL, Harding WG III, Nowicki KD. Managing anterior shoulder instability with bracing: an expanded update. *Orthopedics.* 2004;27:614-618.
4. Harding WG III, Nowicki KD, Perdue PS, Heidt RS, Stroupe AL, Cohen BK. Managing anterior shoulder instability with bracing. *J Musculoskelet Med.* 1997:54-58.
5. Hovelius L, Olofsson A, Sandstrom B, et al. Nonoperative treatment of primary anterior shoulder dislocation in patients forty years of age and younger. A prospective twenty-five-year follow-up. *J Bone Joint Surg Am.* 2008;90:945-952.
6. Buss DD, Lynch GP, Meyer CP, Huber SM, Freehill MQ. Nonoperative management for in-season athletes with anterior shoulder instability. *Am J Sports Med.* 2004;32:6.
7. Itoi E, Hatakeyama Y, Sato T, et al. Immobilization in external rotation after shoulder dislocation reduces the risk of recurrence. A randomized controlled trial. *J Bone Joint Surg Am.* 2007;89:2124-2131.
8. Simonet WT, Cofield RH. Prognosis in anterior shoulder dislocation. *Am J Sports Med.* 1984:19-24.
9. Romeo AA, Cohen BS, Carreira DS. Traumatic anterior shoulder instability. *Orthop Clin North Am.* 2001;32:399-409.

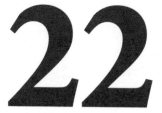

A Dynamic Approach to a Postoperative Rehabilitative Program for the Surgically Stabilized Shoulder

John M. Tokish, MD and Erick J. Kozlowski, ATC

Perhaps the most important outcome measure after shoulder instability surgery is the patient's successful return to activity. It is the one evaluation tool that assesses pain, range of motion, strength, function, and patient satisfaction into a single litmus test of success. While certainly important, the surgical treatment of the unstable shoulder is only a part of this overall goal. It is important to remember that a "stable" shoulder does not necessarily mean a functional one and that success at the highest levels requires a team approach with patients, surgeons, therapists, trainers, and coaches each bringing their particular expertise to bear to ensure an optimal outcome.

Rehabilitation after instability surgery is particularly challenging because of the delicate balance between shoulder stability and mobility. The inter-relationship between the static and dynamic stabilizers of the shoulder emphasizes the importance of optimization of both sides of this equation. This relationship is certainly damaged at the time of injury and can be further compromised while protecting the static restraint repair. Restoration of this balance does not occur by itself, especially in patients who wish to return to higher levels of function. Active retraining of the soft tissues, muscles, and neurologic patterns is critical if optimal shoulder function is to be restored.

The keys to a successful rehabilitation program include individualization, protective mobilization, and team communication. Individualization means understanding "who" a patient is, what his or her goals are, and what resources he or she has to achieve these goals. While standard protocols are certainly a helpful starting point, each patient will vary in regard to needs, resources, and goals. Table 22-1 summarizes some of the key questions each surgeon should ask for each patient in order to meet these specific needs.

Protective mobilization is critical to a successful rehabilitation program. Surgical repair of the static restraints must be protected, but there is a cost with overprotection. Stiffness, muscular tone, and neuro-proprioceptive control are all adversely

Abrams JS. *Management of the Unstable Shoulder:*
Arthroscopic and Open Repair (pp. 285-298).
© 2011 SLACK Incorporated

Table 22-1

7 KEY QUESTIONS TO GUIDING AN OPTIMAL REHABILITATION PROGRAM

1. Who is this patient?
   - Intercollegiate athlete, manual laborer, office worker (time course, return to work, and amount of time that can be devoted to rehabilitation will vary)?

2. What does "successful return" mean to this patient?
   - The rock climber and the linebacker, for example, will have different answers.

3. Is this a dominant or nondominant arm?
   - Sometimes, this will affect the chosen balance between stability and mobility.

4. What is the surgical plan?
   - Primary or revision, open versus arthroscopic, bone loss, all may affect progression and emphasis in the program.

5. "When" is this patient?
   - Intercollegiate athlete in his or her junior year may be different than a "weekend warrior."

6. What are the patient's postoperative resources?
   - Elite athlete with daily access to training staff is different than managed care patient with limited visits.

7. How is progress monitored, and how are problems communicated?
   - Individualization requires adaptation throughout healing; communication and teamwork are key.

affected with immobilization. An athlete with a stable, but stiff, atrophic, and unresponsive shoulder has a far worse prognosis than when he or she had instability alone. It is critical to understand that protection and mobilization can, and must, coexist to return the stabilized shoulder to function.

Finally, a team approach cannot be overemphasized in returning the unstable shoulder to desired activity. Orthopedic surgeons can correct anatomic pathology and understand the specific quality and limitations of the surgical repair, but do not generally understand the intricacies, manual therapies, strengthening, or proprioceptive neuromuscular facilitation. Furthermore, the surgeon has a very limited amount of actual contact after surgery with the patient compared to the rehabilitation specialist. If the patient is an athlete, it is the athletic trainer who often works with a patient's coach to establish realistic expectations on return to activity and can best determine the day-to-day pace of progression. Coaches play an important role as well by modifying workouts and providing sport-specific technique alterations to minimize dangerous positions during competition. Finally, the patient must also buy in to the active process of hard work, communication, and patience that is required to achieve a successful return. Such a team approach allows the blending of numerous disciplines in a coordinated plan to ensure not just a stable shoulder, but a functionally optimal one as well.

Table 22-2

KNOWN DETRIMENTAL EFFECTS OF IMMOBILIZATION ON BIOLOGIC TISSUES

- Decreased biomechanical performance of healing ligament
- Decreased range of motion of joint
- Decreased strength of muscles surrounding immobilized joint
- Increased pain from immobilization alone

JUSTIFICATION OF A DYNAMIC REHABILITATION PROGRAM: PREVENTING "IMMOBILIZATIONOPATHY"

One of the basic tenets of rehabilitation after shoulder stabilization is the protection of the surgically repaired tissues. While an overaggressive program can lead to recurrence of instability, it is important to note that immobilization has many detrimental effects on healing tissues (Table 22-2). First, it is well established that immobilized ligaments heal with significantly worse biomechanical properties than do mobilized ligaments.[1,2] Second, failure to mobilize the shoulder after surgery results in the formation of dense connective tissue adhesions, and such adhesions lead to decreased range of motion. Additionally, these adhesions may cut off capillary circulation so that the tissue becomes ischemic and the capacity for remobilization is diminished.[3] Third, there is evidence that immobilization itself results in hyperalgesia,[4] while early mobilization results in earlier pain relief after surgery.[5] Finally, immobilization of a joint results in significant loss of muscle strength.[6] Muscle strength decreases of 22% after 2 weeks[7] and up to 54% after 7 weeks of immobilization have been shown, which only partially resolves after remobilization.[8]

In contrast, several studies have shown that controlled mobilization of tendons and ligaments during the healing phase can prevent adhesions and reduce stiffness.[2,9] Early mobilization can prevent atrophy, and specific training programs can improve proprioception[5] after surgery.

Thus, while protection of the stabilized shoulder is important, overprotection can have severe deleterious effects. Oversight of mobilization within the envelope of protection is of paramount importance to the surgically stabilized shoulder.

PHASES AND PROGRESSION THROUGH A DYNAMIC REHABILITATION PROGRAM

Most rehabilitation programs follow a progressive approach from tissue healing and pain relief, through restoration of range of motion, strengthening, and finally toward gradual return to activity (Table 22-3). While most clinicians understand these basic phases, it is critical to note that these phases are not mutually exclusive, and that portions of each phase can be done simultaneously. Progression through each phase

Table 22-3

PROGRESSION BETWEEN PHASES BY PLATFORM, LOAD, AND NEUROMUSCULAR CHALLENGES

PHASE	POSTOPERATIVE	MOBILIZATION	ADVANCED STRENGTH	RETURN TO SPORT OR OCCUPATION
Platform	Stable	Stable or unstable with opposite load	Unstable	Sport/occupation specific
Loads	Low	Low to moderate	High	Sport/occupation specific
Neuro-muscular challenges	Controlled motion, protection	Normal kinematics, stable platform	Complete dynamic stabilization	Return to sport activity/occupation

requires specific goals to be met by the patient, and the rehabilitation specialist must have the freedom and authority to advance or decelerate a patient's progress based on these criteria. Table 22-4 summarizes these phases and criteria for advancement. It should be noted that, while general time frames can be helpful guidelines, strict adherence should be avoided, as performance-based progression is often highly variable and based on patient compliance and commitment, physiologic response to surgery, and other patient-specific factors. The only true time limits are the biologic limitations of tissue healing, which will vary based upon surgical approach and quality of tissue. For example, an anterior stabilization done through an open approach would be protected against internal rotation strengthening longer than an arthroscopic approach would because of the need to protect the subscapularis repair. Beyond these limitations, however, the pace of rehabilitation should be based more on functional achievement of specific goals than rigid time frames that are subject to variability in patient goals and resources.

Throughout this chapter, the simple push-up-plus exercise will be used to illustrate the concepts of progression through the various phases of rehabilitation and back to sport. This exercise is a good paradigm, as it demonstrates a closed chain exercise that can move from low to high loads, stable to unstable platforms, and has perturbations that are applicable in all phases of rehabilitation.

THE POSTOPERATIVE PHASE

The first phase in a dynamic progression program is the postoperative phase. The key to this phase is an understanding of what was done at surgery. Communication between the surgeon and the rehabilitation specialist is critical to ensure that the therapist understands what must be protected during early healing. Factors such as direction of instability, baseline collagen status, primary versus revision surgery, open versus arthroscopic approach, and quality of surgical repair will all play a role in determining the pace of this phase. While no definitive study exists on how long it takes for a labral lesion or capsule to heal, several studies and postoperative programs have recommended that repaired structures be protected for 4 to 6 weeks postoperatively.[10-14]

Table 22-4

REHABILITATION PHASES AFTER INSTABILITY SURGERY

I. Postoperative phase

    a. Protection: Wound(s), repaired structures (capsule-labrum, subscapularis if open)

    b. Range of motion

        i. Passive to limits of "safe zone" as defined by surgery. Joint mobilizations to minimize stiffness

        ii. Active well within safe zone to re-establish dynamic control of joint, early neuromuscular re-training

    c. Strengthening

        i. Continue preoperative core work

        ii. Scapular platform strengthening

        iii. Isometrics with protection

    d. Progression: Wound healed, repaired structures stable, pain under control, patient understands "safe zones" of active and passive motion

II. Mobilization phase

    a. Protection: Repaired structures loaded, but well below limits of repair

    b. Range of motion: Full passive and active range re-established

    c. Strengthening

        i. Repaired structures: Isometrics and dynamic stabilization exercises

        ii. Nonrepaired structures: Full strength, balance, and proprioception

    d. Progression: Full range of motion, normal rhythm of shoulder in unloaded setting, full strength and balance of nonrepaired musculature, healing of repaired tissues

III. Advanced strength phase

    a. Protection: Only against "unsafe" loaded positions of shoulder

    b. Range of motion: Completed

    c. Strengthening

        i. Reincorporate shoulder within kinetic chain

        ii. Neuromuscular and proprioceptive dynamic strength training

        iii. Muscle endurance

    d. Progression: Full strength in controlled environment, normal rhythm to shoulder in loaded setting, full confidence of patient

IV. Return to activity

    a. Protection: Limit reps, competitive situations, watch for technique breakdowns in core, scapular rhythm

    b. Progression: Gradual increase as total program becomes second nature

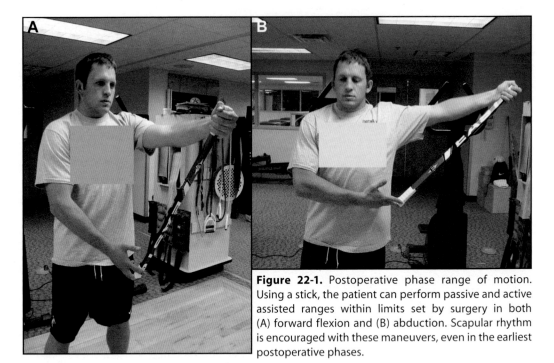

Figure 22-1. Postoperative phase range of motion. Using a stick, the patient can perform passive and active assisted ranges within limits set by surgery in both (A) forward flexion and (B) abduction. Scapular rhythm is encouraged with these maneuvers, even in the earliest postoperative phases.

Kim and colleagues, however, in a prospective randomized study, demonstrated that an accelerated rehabilitation program of immediate supervised range of motion had no increase in recurrence rate compared to those immobilized for 3 weeks.[15] The accelerated group also had less pain and earlier return of motion and functional activity. This study emphasizes that it is possible to mobilize the postoperative joint while protecting it from undue stress.

Specific Exercises in the Postoperative Phase

Once the limitations of range of motion are understood, passive motion should progress up to these limits, and active motion should begin well within the envelope of safety. Figure 22-1 demonstrates patient-controlled early motion. Initially, a stick is used for both passive- and active-assist maneuvers in both forward flexion and abduction. As the patient repeats these maneuvers, the exercise becomes less passive and more active assisted. Patients will naturally begin to fire scapular musculature in normalized firing patterns. This encourages the placement of the shoulder back within the kinetic chain as early as possible. As the patient progresses, exercises can be employed where motion is controlled by core firing, as is evidenced in Figure 22-2. Placing such an emphasis on core stabilization helps establish its primacy in kinetic function later in the postoperative course.

Strengthening is also begun immediately, and this, too, requires an understanding of the surgical details. In an arthroscopic stabilization, none of the rotator cuff musculature is violated, and therefore immediate rotator cuff strengthening is begun (Figure 22-3). In an open approach, any tendon that was compromised to allow access to the shoulder capsule must be protected. In addition, because balance and co-contraction are so critical to dynamic stabilization, we do not proceed with aggressive strengthening of the cuff until it can be strengthened in a coordinated fashion.

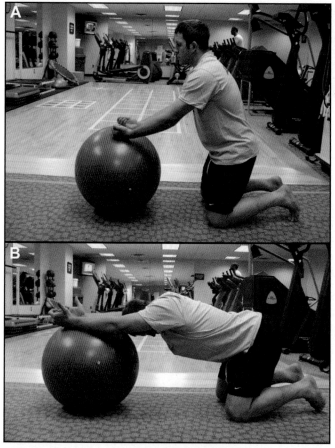

Figure 22-2. Patient-controlled passive motion. (A) A large exercise ball is used, and the patient "rolls" along this ball. (B) Range of motion is controlled by core firing, allowing dynamic core stabilization to control forward flexion.

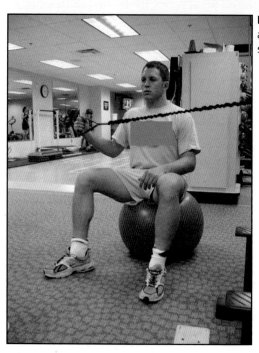

Figure 22-3. Shoulder isometric strengthening. The athlete does this exercise with attention to both shoulder form and core stabilization.

No matter which approach is used, strengthening of the scapular platform is begun immediately, with "scapular 6-packs" (Figure 22-4) emphasized very early. The scapular platform is both extremely important to postoperative function and extremely sensitive to postoperative immobilization. Atrophy of this muscle group cannot be allowed. Beginning the strengthening of this set of muscles immediately does no harm to the repaired capsular structures and encourages the early return of upper extremity rhythm and proper neuromuscular function.

Using a "push-up-plus paradigm" (Figure 22-5) can help elucidate the concepts of strengthening throughout the postoperative course. In the postoperative phase, the emphasis is on very low loads on stable platforms (see Figure 22-5A). This exercise will stimulate early co-contraction of shoulder musculature in a safe environment and will allow the beginnings of dynamic stabilization of the healing shoulder.

Finally, core strengthening should be strongly emphasized here. Given that this is the first link in the kinetic chain, core-focused training ensures that the whole kinetic chain will be ready for later incorporation of the shoulder.

Progression in the Postoperative Phase

Progression beyond the postoperative phase requires the healing of all surgical wounds and stability of healing tissues. Stability implies that tissues repaired at surgery have undergone sufficient healing to handle the loads of active range of motion and light resistance.

THE MOBILIZATION PHASE

The goals of the mobilization phase are the restoration of active and passive range of motion, re-establishment of shoulder rhythm under light loads, and progression of strength of the supporting musculature. Repaired structures are loaded in this phase progressively, but at sub-maximal levels.

Specific Exercises in the Mobilization Phase

Full range of motion is achieved during this phase, with the removal of limits on protected structures. Careful attention is paid to the restoration of proper arthrokinematics, with the rehabilitation specialist ensuring that scapulohumeral rhythm is maintained, without winging or scapular dyskinesia. Exercises like proprioceptive neuromuscular facilitation[14] are employed to accomplish this goal. Sport-specific movements with light resistance are encouraged, with the goal of allowing the athlete to re-establish normal rhythm patterns of his or her sport. Figure 22-6 is an example of one such pattern. Here, an intercollegiate wrestler in the mobilization phase uses light elastic resistance bands to simulate patterns he will use when returning to the mat. These patterns will encourage the normalization of neuromuscular recruitment that will translate into dynamic stability upon return to sport.

Strengthening in the mobilization phase proceeds with a continued emphasis on dynamic stabilization. Where the postoperative phase is characterized by single-plane isometric strengthening, this phase advances to multi-planar rhythmic stabilization. Closed-chain kinetic exercises are emphasized, as they have been shown to be optimal for strengthening around healing joints. They produce minimal translation, shear, and distraction forces due to the compressive nature of the applied load and the greater control of the resultant motions. These exercises facilitate the engagement of multiple antagonistic muscle groups and further promote dynamic stabilization.[16-18]

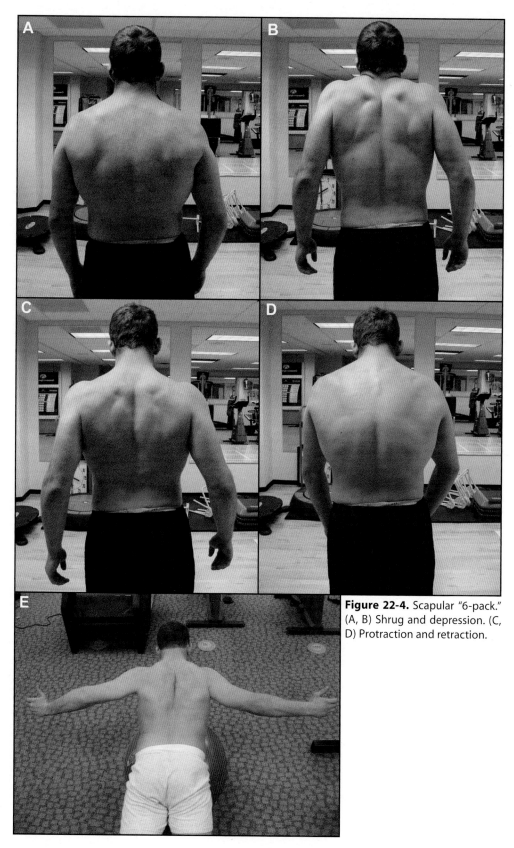

Figure 22-4. Scapular "6-pack." (A, B) Shrug and depression. (C, D) Protraction and retraction.

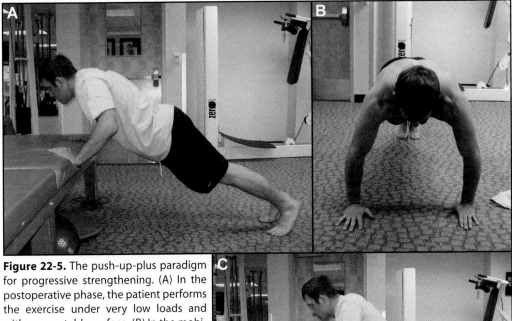

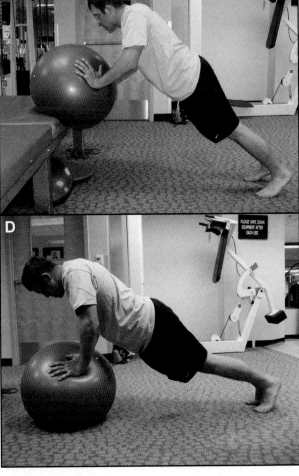

Figure 22-5. The push-up-plus paradigm for progressive strengthening. (A) In the postoperative phase, the patient performs the exercise under very low loads and with a very stable surface. (B) In the mobilization phase, exercises can be done with heavier loads on stable platforms, such as a push-up plus on the floor. (C) Another variation in the mobilization phase is to do the exercise under a lighter load, but with a less stable platform like a Swiss ball. (D) In the advanced strengthening phase, both heavy loads and unstable platforms are used to ensure maximal firing of dynamic stabilizers. Varying angles can be used to optimize function.

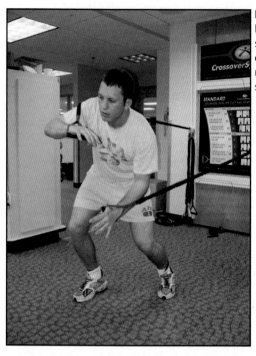

Figure 22-6. Sport-specific movement patterns. Using light resistance bands, the athlete can simulate sport-specific ranges of motion against resistance. This encourages the return of normal movement and neuromuscular firing patterns that are critical to dynamic stabilization upon return to sport.

The push-up-plus exercise can again be illustrative of progression (see Figure 22-5B and C). In this phase, the patient has a stable repair, and there is interplay between platform stability and applied load. The patient alternates between increasing loads on stable platforms (see Figure 22-5B) or lighter loads with an unstable platform (see Figure 22-5C). The addition of an unstable platform like a Swiss ball can result in increased muscle activity in the core and upper-extremity musculature.[19]

Completion of the phase occurs when healing of the surgically repaired tissues is assured, normal humeroscapular rhythm is achieved, and the patient demonstrates a confidence in multiplanar loaded motion of the shoulder.

THE ADVANCED STRENGTH PHASE

The advanced strength phase is the last phase before allowing a patient to return to competitive activity. This phase begins when there is assurance that all repaired or reconstructed structures are healed, the patient has full range of motion with no apprehension, and the patient can demonstrate normal muscle strength to manual muscle testing. The emphases in this phase are to strengthen dynamic stabilizers under realistic and activity specific loads and to train muscle endurance.

Dynamic stabilizer training in this phase advances to unstable platforms under heavy loads. Push-ups plus on a Swiss ball (see Figure 22-5D) require excellent dynamic stabilization and perturbations such as staggering hands, independent balls, and bounding, where the hands leave the ground to varied heights and positions can further enhance functional muscle strength.

It is important to note that strengthening means more than just lifting a load. Endurance training of the rotator cuff and scapular musculature is especially important in the patient with instability. As these muscles fatigue, the humeral head becomes displaced superiorly with arm movements like abduction.[20] In overhead workers or athletes, this fatigue can result in anterior subluxation, leading to painful dynamic subacromial impingement,[21] which can greatly impede return to full activity. Training for endurance is often tedious, however, and the therapist must be watchful that the athlete has no breakdowns in core form, which can imply subtle weakness further up the kinetic chain. Such weaknesses can be detrimental if missed, as they can translate into re-injury once return to full activity is allowed.

Progression Through the Advanced Strength Phase

By the end of this phase, the patient should look essentially normal in the controlled setting of the training room, with excellent strength, motion, and kinetic chain kinematics. Any subtle weakness must be addressed before allowing the patient to return to activity.

RETURN TO ACTIVITY PHASE

The return to activity phase is perhaps the most overlooked phase after shoulder stabilization. The athlete by this point no longer has pain, has full range of motion and strength, and feels "normal." His or her focus is on returning to his or her sport, and the monotony of the rehabilitation has long since set in. With this return, the athlete's attention is shifted from strict attention to form to performance of a sport-specific task. It is at this point when the therapist or athletic trainer is especially critical. The return to activity phase is also the least structured of the phases. This is because this portion of the program is highly individualized to the patient. For example, a baseball pitcher will be treated differently than a gymnast, just as a laborer will be treated differently than a swimmer.

The phase is begun with "shadow drills" specific to desired activity. For a baseball pitcher, this may mean a short and long toss program, with emphasis on accuracy. For a swimmer, it might mean return to his or her specific event, but perhaps over shorter distance. Very quickly, the athlete progresses to a point where performance is measured. This places their concentration on performance of their sport and, for the first time, takes them out of the controlled environment of the rehabilitation facility. The therapist carefully watches the "distracted" athlete for breakdowns in form or substitution. Adjustments are made as necessary to ensure performance is achieved in the setting of proper and safe kinematics.

As the athlete progresses, competition is introduced gradually, first with "one-on-one" situations and then to the "red jersey" phase. In this latter stage, the player is returned to "live" scrimmage, but repetitions are limited. It is imperative that the athletic trainer has complete authority to limit or remove a player from drills during this phase if there is any concern that distraction or fatigue might place a player in an unsafe position.

Finally, when the athlete demonstrates confidence and performance within a restored kinetic chain, full unrestricted competition is resumed. It is here that core strengthening, scapular mechanics, and both static and dynamic shoulder stability are optimized to return the patient to his or her chosen pursuit. This is the culmination of a long and sometimes tedious process and requires the expertise and dedication of an entire team of experts to optimize the most important of all outcome measures.

REFERENCES

1. Noyes FR. Functional properties of knee ligaments and alterations induced by immobilization: a correlative biomechanical and histological study in primates. *Clin Orthop Relat Res.* 1977;123:210-242.
2. Woo SL, Gomez MA, Sites TJ, Newton PO, Orlando CA, Akeson WH. The biomechanical and morphological changes in the medial collateral ligament of the rabbit after immobilization and remobilization. *J Bone Joint Surg Am.* 1987;69(8):1200-1211.
3. Kottke FJ. Therapeutic exercise to maintain mobility. In: Kottke FJ, ed. *Krusen's Handbook of Physical Medicine and Rehabilitation.* 4th ed. Philadelphia, PA: WB Saunders; 1990:436-451.
4. Terkelsen AJ, Bach FW, Jensen TS. Experimental forearm immobilization in humans induces cold and mechanical hyperalgesia. *Anesthesiology.* 2008;109(2):297-307.
5. Risberg MA, Holm I, Myklebust G, Engebretsen L. Neuromuscular training versus strength training during first 6 months after anterior cruciate ligament reconstruction: a randomized clinical trial. *Phys Ther.* 2007;87(6):737-750.
6. Farthing JP, Krentz JR, Magnus CR. Strength training the free limb attenuates strength loss during unilateral immobilization. *J Appl Physiol.* 2009;106(3):830-836.
7. Urso ML, Clarkson PM, Price TB. Immobilization effects in young and older adults. *Eur J Appl Physiol.* 2006;96(5):564-571.
8. Christensen B, Dyrberg E, Aagaard P, et al. Effects of long-term immobilization and recovery on human triceps surae and collagen turnover in the Achilles tendon in patients with healing ankle fracture. *J Appl Physiol.* 2008;105(2):420-426.
9. Gelberman RH, Woo SL, Lothringer K, Akeson WH, Amiel D. Effects of early intermittent passive mobilization on healing canine flexor tendons. *J Hand Surg (Am).* 1982;7(2):170-175.
10. Hattrup SJ, Cofield RH, Weaver AL. Anterior shoulder reconstruction: prognostic variables. *J Shoulder Elbow Surg.* 2001;10(6):508-513.
11. Shall LM, Cawley PW. Soft tissue reconstruction in the shoulder. Comparison of suture anchors, absorbable staples, and absorbable tacks. *Am J Sports Med.* 1994;22(5):715-718.
12. Warner JJ, Miller MD, Marks P. Arthroscopic Bankart repair with the Suretac device. Part II: experimental observations. *Arthroscopy.* 1995;11(1):14-20.
13. Warner JJ, Miller MD, Marks P, Fu FH. Arthroscopic Bankart repair with the Suretac device. Part I: clinical observations. *Arthroscopy.* 1995;11(1):2-13.
14. Wilk KE, Arrigo C. Current concepts in the rehabilitation of the athletic shoulder. *J Orthop Sports Phys Ther.* 1993;18(1):365-378.
15. Kim SH, Ha KI, Jung MW, Lim MS, Kim YM, Park JH. Accelerated rehabilitation after arthroscopic Bankart repair for selected cases: a prospective randomized clinical study. *Arthroscopy.* 2003;19(7):722-731.
16. Bynum EB, Barrack RL, Alexander AH. Open versus closed chain kinetic exercises after anterior cruciate ligament reconstruction. A prospective randomized study. *Am J Sports Med.* 1995;23(4):401-406.
17. Lephart SM, Henry TJ. The physiological basis for open and closed kinetic chain rehabilitation for the upper extremity. *J Sports Rehab.* 1996;5:71-87.
18. Shelbourne KD, Nitz P. Accelerated rehabilitation after anterior cruciate ligament reconstruction. *Am J Sports Med.* 1990;18(3):292-299.
19. Lehman GJ, MacMillan B, MacIntyre I, Chivers M, Fluter M. Shoulder muscle EMG activity during push up variations on and off a Swiss ball. *Dyn Med.* 2006;5:7.
20. Wickiewicz TH, Otis JC, Warren RF. Glenohumeral kinematics in a muscle fatigue model: a radiographic study. *Orthop Trans.* 1995;18:126.
21. Kvitne RS, Jobe FW. The diagnosis and treatment of anterior instability in the throwing athlete. *Clin Orthop Relat Res.* 1993(291):107-123.

Financial Disclosures

Dr. Jeffrey S. Abrams is a consultant for ConMed Linvatec Medical, Arthrocare Corporation, Wright Medical, Cayenne Medical, KFx Medical, Ingen Technologies Inc, and Core Medical. He owns stock or stock options in Arthrocare Corporation, Cayenne Medical, KFx Medical, and Ingen Technologies Inc. He has lectured for DePuy Mitek. He receives royalties from ConMed Linvatec Medical, Arthrocare Corporation, and Springer Publications. He is a board member of Arthroscopy Association of North America; Vice President, Executive Committee, American Shoulder and Elbow Surgeons.

Dr. Richard L. Angelo is a consultant for Depuy/Mitek.

Dr. Robert A. Arciero receives educational and research grants from Arthrex, is a consultant for Biomet, and receives an honoraria for teaching.

Dr. Matthew Bollier has no financial or proprietary interest in the materials presented herein.

Dr. Simon Boyle has no financial or proprietary interest in the materials presented herein.

Dr. Marcus S. Briones has no financial or proprietary interest in the materials presented herein.

Dr. Robert T. Burks is a consultant with Arthrex.

Dr. Daniel D. Buss discloses financial relationships with Wright Medical Technology, Inc; Disc Dynamics; Minnesota Twins; Medica Physician Advisory Board; United Healthcare Advisory Board; Abbott Northwestern Hospital.

Dr. Joseph P. DeAngelis serves as a consultant to Connective Orthopaedics, Woburn, MA. He has received research support in the form of a Restricted Grant from Zimmer, Inc, Warsaw, IN, and his research is funded by a grant from Major League Baseball, Inc.

Dr. Michael J. DeFranco has no financial or proprietary interest in the materials presented herein.

Dr. Drew Fehsenfeld has no financial or proprietary interest in the materials presented herein.

Dr. John H. Flint has no financial or proprietary interest in the materials presented herein.

Dr. Tistia Gaston has no financial or proprietary interest in the materials presented herein.

Dr. J. Douglas Haltom has no financial or proprietary interest in the materials presented herein.

Dr. Laurence D. Higgins has no financial or proprietary interest in the materials presented herein.

Dr. Aimee S. Klapach has no financial or proprietary interest in the materials presented herein.

Erick J. Kozlowski has no financial or proprietary interest in the materials presented herein.

Dr. John E. Kuhn receives research support from Arthrex Corporation, he has family members who own stock in Pfizer Corporation, and he is an editor for the *Journal of Shoulder and Elbow Surgery.*

Dr. Laurent Lafosse has no financial or proprietary interest in the materials presented herein.

Dr. William J. Mallon has no financial or proprietary interest in the materials presented herein.

Dr. Guido Marra has no financial or proprietary interest in the materials presented herein.

Dr. Augustus D. Mazzocca is a consultant for and receives research support from Arthrex Inc.

ENS Sean McIntire has no financial or proprietary interest in the materials presented herein.

Dr. Peter J. Millett is a consultant and receives royalties from Arthrex; is a consultant for Arthrocare; has stock options from Game Ready; has stock in VuMedi; and receives research support from Ossur, Smith & Nephew, Arthrocare, Arthrex, Siemens, and OrthoRehab.

Dr. Gary W. Misamore has no financial or proprietary interest in the materials presented herein.

Dr. Todd C. Moen has no financial or proprietary interest in the materials presented herein.

Dr. Monica Morman has no financial or proprietary interest in the materials presented herein.

Dr. Gordon W. Nuber has no financial or proprietary interest in the materials presented herein.

Travis G. O'Brien has no financial or proprietary interest in the materials presented herein.

Dr. Luke S. Oh, has no financial or proprietary interest in the materials presented herein.

Dr. Michael J. Pagnani has no financial or proprietary interest in the materials presented herein.

Dr. William Peace has no financial or proprietary interest in the materials presented herein.

Dr. Matthew T. Provencher has no financial or proprietary interest in the materials presented herein.

Dr. Matthew Rose has no financial or proprietary interest in the materials presented herein.

Dr. Richard Ryu receives honoraria from Mitek for lectures and is a paid consultant for Medbridge.

Dr. Anshu Singh has no financial or proprietary interest in the materials presented herein.

Dr. Daniel J. Solomon has not disclosed any relevant financial relationships.

Dr. Scott P. Steinmann is a consultant for Arthrex and Wright. He is also a consultant for and receives a royalty from DePuy.

Dr. Jason Sullivan has no financial or proprietary interest in the materials presented herein.

Dr. Raymond Thal receives royalties from DePuy Mitek, Inc.

Dr. John M. Tokish has no financial or proprietary interest in the materials presented herein.

Dr. Jianhua Wang has no financial or proprietary interest in the materials presented herein.

Dr. Jon J. P. Warner has no financial or proprietary interest in the materials presented herein.

Dr. Mark T. Wichman has no financial or proprietary interest in the materials presented herein.

Dr. Bojan Zoric is a consultant for Smith and Nephew

Index

adhesions, 287

advanced strength phase, of rehabilitation, 289, 295-296

allografts, osteoarticular, for Hill-Sachs lesions, 244, 246, 248-249

analgesia, local application of, chondrolysis due to, 54, 192

anchors
for Bankart repair, 52
for humeral anterior capsular avulsion repair, 258-259
impingement of, 190-192
knotless suture, 59-75
repair of, 186-189
for SLAP tear repair, 177
for subscapularis repair, 212-213

anesthesia
awake monitored, 35
for Bankart repair, 47
for beach chair position, 34, 35
for capsular shift, 217
for first-time dislocation repair, 119
for glenoid rim deficiency bone graft, 224
for lateral decubitus position, 24
for posterior stabilization, 265
for split pectoralis major transfer, 213
for subscapularis repair, 211

anterior labroligamentous periosteal sleeve avulsion lesion, 61, 129

anterior plication sutures, 83-84

anterior portals
for Bankart repair, 48
in lateral decubitus position, 29
for subscapularis repair, 212

anteroinferior portal, 120-123
for Bankart repair, 49
for humeral anterior capsular avulsion repair, 259
for multidirectional instability repair, 93-94
for revision surgery, 185

anterolateral portal, for subscapularis repair, 212

anterosuperior portal, 5, 120-123
for Bankart repair, 48, 50-51
for humeral anterior capsular avulsion repair, 258
for multidirectional instability repair, 93-94
for SLAP tear repair, 176

apprehension
in bone loss, 145
in Hill-Sachs lesion, 236
in laxity, 7
in recurrent instability, 183

arthritis, degenerative, after revision surgery, 192

arthroscopic techniques
Bankart repair, 45-57, 155-169
beach chair position for. See beach chair position
for bone loss assessment, 135-147
diagnostic. See diagnostic arthroscopy
for dislocation
anterior, 9-11, 155-169
in elite athlete, 127-133
first-time, 9-11, 113-125
for Hill-Sachs lesions, 238-240, 242-243
for humeral anterior capsular avulsion, 253-261

for humeral posterior capsular avulsion, 106-107
for hyperlaxity, 8
knotless suture anchor, 59-75
Latarjet graft, 155-169
lateral decubitus position for, 23-33
for multidirectional instability, 89-99
for posterior instability, 101-109, 264
posterior plication sutures in, 77-87, 105-106
for recurrent instability, 13-15
rehabilitation after. *See* rehabilitation
revision, 181-195
for soft tissue repair, 149-153
for subscapularis repair, 211-216
for superior labral tears, 171-180
arthrotomy
for anterior glenoid rim deficiency, 223-233
for capsular deficiency, 216-222
for glenohumeral instability, 199-207
for subscapularis repair, 209-216
athletes
Bankart repair for, 45-57
dislocation in
during athletic season, 277-284
in middle-aged person, 16-18
treatment decisions for, 9-10, 127-133
Latarjet procedure for, 157
multidirectional instability in, 96
posterior plication sutures for, 85-87
rehabilitation program for, 285-297
revision surgery for, 193-194
SLAP tears in, 171-180
axillary fold, I portal in, 160
axillary pouch portal, in lateral decubitus position, 29
axillary roll, 24-25
axillary view, for bone loss, 137

Bankart lesion, 113-126, 135-141
pathoanatomy of, 4
posterior plication sutures for, 85-86
recurrent, 184
Bankart repair, 11, 135-141, 199-207
arthroscopic, 45-57
with capsular plication, 152
failure of, 155-156
open, 184
for posterior stabilization, 104-105, 268-270
for recurrent instability, 184
revision of, 157
beach chair position, 34-43
for anterior glenoid rim deficiency repair, 225
for humeral anterior capsular avulsion repair, 255, 256
La Jolla, 27

for multidirectional instability repair, 93
for recurrent instability, 184
for split pectoralis major transfer, 213
for subscapularis tear repair, 211
Bernageau view, for bone loss, 137
biceps tendon pathology
after SLAP tear repair, 179
subscapularis repair and, 211-212
BioKnotless Suture Anchor, 59-60, 71-75
blood pressure measurement, in lateral decubitus position, 20
bone block, for glenoid rim deficiency, 223-233
bone graft
for anterior glenoid rim deficiency, 223-233
complications of, 152
for Hill-Sachs lesion, 16
vs. Latarjet procedure, 157-158
for posterior stabilization, 271-272
preparation of, 227
for revision surgery, 184-185
tricortical, 241-242
bone loss, 135-147
glenoid. *See* glenoid, bone loss in
humeral head, 141-144, 156-157. *See also* Hill-Sachs lesions
imaging for, 145-146
Latarjet procedure for, 156-157
measurement of, 150-151, 184
pathophysiology of, 4-5
physical examination for, 144-145
recurrent instability in, 11-13
soft tissue repair for, 149-154
bone plug, for Hill-Sachs lesions, 244
bone tamps, for Hill-Sachs lesions, 243
"bony apprehension test," for bone loss, 145
"Bony Bankart" fragment, 136
braces
for anterior dislocation, 9, 281-283
after revision surgery, 193
brachial plexus strain, in improper positioning, 41
Bristow procedure, 15
modified, vs. Latarjet procedure, 158
Buford complex, 171-172

Calandra classification, of Hill-Sachs lesions, 237
capsule
deficiency of, 216-221
detachment of, from humeral head, 45-57
incision in, in Bankart repair, 201-204
pathoanatomy of, 3-6
repair of, 204, 206
shift procedures for, 204, 206, 221
for multidirectional instability, 92
posterior, 268-270

stretch of, in knotless suture anchor, 61-62
tears of, 184
capsulolabral complex, 113
capsulorrhaphy, electrothermal, 93
carotid kinking, prevention off, 39
Chia wires, in Latarjet procedure, 163-164
chondrolysis
after Bankart repair, 54
after revision surgery, 192
"circle" method, for computed tomography, 139
"cliff sign," in bone loss, 137
competition, return to, 296
complications
of anterior dislocation repair, 131
of Bankart repair, 54, 56, 206
of bone graft, 152
of capsular reconstruction, 220-221
of first-time dislocation repair, 125
of glenoid rim deficiency repair, 232
of humeral anterior capsular avulsion repair, 260
of knotless suture anchors, 70-71
of labrum reconstruction, 220-221
of Latarjet procedure, 167
of lateral decubitus position, 31-32
of multidirectional instability repair, 96-97
of operating positions, 41
of posterior stabilization, 273
of revision surgery, 192
revision surgery for. *See* revision surgery
of SLAP tear repair, 178
computed tomography
for bone loss, 137-139, 149-150
for first-time dislocation, 114-115
for Hill-Sachs lesions, 238-239, 246
for humeral head bone loss, 143
for posterior instability, 103, 264
for recurrent instability, 11-12
concavity-compression mechanism, 4
Connolly procedure, for Hill-Sachs lesion, 188-189
coracoacromial ligament, in bone graft, 223-233
coracohumeral ligament
in bone graft, 223-233
shortening of, for rotator interval closure, 78-81
coracoid, osteotomy of, for Latarjet procedure, 164-165
coracoid graft
complications of, 152
fixation of, 164-166
for glenoid rim deficiency, 223-233
harvesting of, 161-164
transfer of, 164

coracoid ligament, detachment of, in Latarjet procedure, 160
core stabilization exercises, 290-292
cysts, periglenoid, with SLAP tears, 173

decubitus position, lateral. *See* lateral decubitus position
diagnostic arthroscopy
for Bankart lesion, 47
for bone loss, 140-141, 144
for Hill-Sachs lesions, 238
for humeral anterior capsular avulsion, 255
for posterior instability, 103
for revision surgery, 185-186
dislocation
anterior
in athletic season, 277-284
in elite athlete, 127-133
first-time, 9-11, 113-126
recurrent, 11-16
in athletic season, 277-284
Bankart lesion in, 135-141
Bankart repair for, 45-57
capsular deficiency in, 216-222
in elite athlete, 127-133
first-time
anterior, 9-11
treatment options for, 113-126
Hill-Sachs lesions in, 141-144, 235-251
humeral anterior capsular avulsion in, 253-261
in middle-aged athlete, 16-18
posterior, 263-273
recurrent, Bankart repair for, 45-57
subscapularis tears in, 209-216
drilling
of coracoid, 162-163, 166
for knotless suture anchor, 63-64
Duke Wyre brace, 281, 283

Eden-Hybinette procedure, for glenoid rim deficiency, 223-233
electrothermal capsulorrhaphy, 93
endurance training, 295-296
exercise. *See* rehabilitation
external rotation exercises, 193, 279

Flatow-Warner classification, of Hill-Sachs lesions, 237
forward flexion exercises, 279
fractures
glenoid. *See* Bankart lesion
humeral head. *See* Hill-Sachs lesions
Franceschi classification, of Hill-Sachs lesions, 236-237

Gagey test, for bone loss, 145
Gerber method, for computed tomography, 139
glenohumeral joint, motion of, 4
glenohumeral ligaments
    closure of, 79-81
    pathoanatomy of, 3-6
    preparation of, for knotless suture anchors, 61-62
glenoid
    bone graft for, 240-242
    bone loss in, 135-141
        bone graft for, 184-185
        Latarjet procedure for, 156-157
        soft tissue repair for, 149-154
    deficiency of, in Hill-Sachs lesions, 237
    fracture of. *See* Bankart lesion
    "inverted-pear," 12-13, 130
    labrum of. *See* labrum
    pathoanatomy of, 3-6
    preparation of, for knotless suture anchor, 63-64
    rim of, deficiency of, bone graft for, 223-233
    version measurement, 141
glenoid track concept, 237-238
graft
    bone. *See* bone graft
    coracoid. *See* coracoid graft
    Latarjet. *See* Latarjet procedure
    tendon
        for capsular reconstruction, 218-221
        for labrum reconstruction, 218

H portal, for Latarjet procedure, 161-162
HAGL. *See* humeral avulsion glenohumeral ligament lesion
"hatchet fracture," 237
head position, 39
healing, immobilization effects on, 287
Hill-Sachs lesions, 141-144, 235-251
    arthroscopic techniques for, 238-240, 242-243
    biomechanics of, 236-236
    classification of, 236-236
    combined techniques for, 247-249
    diagnosis of, 238
    engaging, 12-16
        bone graft for, 184-185
        bone loss measurement in, 150-151
        Latarjet procedure for, 159
        vs. nonengaging, 240
        symptoms of, 236
    glenoid deficiency in, 237
    glenoid track concept and, 237-238

mechanisms of, 235-236
metal implants for, 245
open techniques for, 238, 240-242, 244, 246
pathoanatomy of, 5
physical examination for, 236
posterior plication sutures for, 85-86
revision surgery for, 188-189
rotational osteotomy for, 245, 247
humeral anterior capsular avulsion, 253-261
    arthroscopic technique for, 256, 258-259
    incidence of, 253
    mini-open technique for, 255-257
humeral avulsion glenohumeral ligament lesion
    Bankart repair for, 45-57
    Latarjet procedure for, 157
    posterior, 106-107
humeral head
    bone loss in, 141-144, 156-157
    injury of. *See* Hill-Sachs lesions
    pathoanatomy of, 3-6
    procedures involving, for Hill-Sachs lesions, 243-247
    rotational osteotomy of, 245, 247
    stabilization of, for glenoid rim deficiency, 223-233
hyperlaxity, 6-8, 79-81

I portal, for Latarjet procedure, 160, 163-164
iliac graft
    complications of, 152
    for glenoid rim deficiency, 223-233
immobilization
    detrimental effects of, 287
    for in-season injuries, 281
    after multidirectional instability repair, 97
infraspinatus, exposure of, for posterior stabilization, 266-267
instability
    incidence of, 3
    vs. laxity, 90
    pathoanatomy of, 3-6
Instability Severity Index, 13-14
interval, rotator. *See* rotator interval
"inverted-pear" glenoid, 12-13, 130

J portal, for Latarjet procedure, 161
jerk test, for posterior instability, 102

kidney rest, for beach chair position, 36
Kim test, for posterior instability, 103
Kinsa knotless suture anchors, 60, 67-68, 71-75
knotless suture anchors, 59-75
    BioKnotless, 59-60, 71-75
    comparison of, 71-75
    complications of, 70-71
    designs for, 59-60

Kinsa type, 60, 67-68, 71-75
materials for, 71-73
Opus-style, 60, 68, 71-75
patient selection for, 59-60
postoperative management of, 71
PushLock, 60, 68, 71-75
techniques for, 61-68, 74-75

La Jolla beach chair position, 27
labrum
anatomy of, 171-172
biomechanics of, 172-173
fixation of, 177-178
mechanisms of injury of, 173-174
pathoanatomy of, 3-6, 173
reconstruction of, 218
repair of, 176-177
revision surgery involving, 186-187
SLAP tears of, 171-180
Latarjet procedure
arthroscopic, 155-169
complications of, 167
vs. free bone graft, 157-158
indications for, 156-157
vs. modified Bristow procedure, 158
postoperative management of, 167-168
principles of, 155-156
technique for, 158-166
for Hill-Sachs lesions, 240-242
for recurrent instability, 15-16
for revision surgery, 184-185
Latarjet-Patte procedure, for glenoid rim deficiency, 223-233
lateral decubitus position, 23-33
advantages of, 30
for Bankart repair, 47
complications of, 31-32
for first-time dislocation repair, 119
for humeral anterior capsular avulsion repair, 256
modifications of, 26-27
patient selection for, 23-24
portal placement in, 28-29
for posterior stabilization, 264-265
set-up for, 24-26
traction with, 27-28
lateral portal, in lateral decubitus position, 29
laxity
congenital, 5-7
definition of, 7
excessive, 6-8
rotator interval closure for, 79-81
symptoms of, 7
treatment of, 8
leg positioning, for lateral decubitus position, 25-26

liberator, for suture anchor repair, 186-187
load and shift test
for laxity, 7
for posterior instability, 103
in recurrent instability, 183
loose shoulder joint syndrome, 90
low posterolateral portal, in lateral decubitus position, 28-29

McConnell arm positioner, 41
magnetic resonance arthrography
for bone loss, 139
for first-time dislocation, 114-115
for Hill-Sachs lesions, 246
for humeral head bone loss, 143
for hyperlaxity, 7
for multidirectional instability, 90
for SLAP tears, 174
for subscapularis tears, 211
magnetic resonance imaging
for anterior dislocation, 9
for Bankart lesion, 200
for capsular deficiency, 217
for Hill-Sachs lesions, 238-239
for humeral anterior capsular avulsion, 254
for laxity, 7
for posterior instability, 103
for recurrent instability, 11-12
for subscapularis tears, 211
manual lock McConnell arm positioner, 41
metal implants, for Hill-Sachs lesions, 245
mini-open technique, for humeral anterior capsular avulsion, 255-257
mobilization phase, of rehabilitation, 289, 292-294
multidirectional instability, 7, 89-99
diagnosis of, 90
pathoanatomy of, 89-90
rotator interval closure for, 79-81
treatment of, 8, 91-97
types of, 89

needles, for labral fixation, 177
nerve injury
in Bankart repair, 56
in glenoid rim deficiency bone graft procedure, 232
in multidirectional instability repair, 96
position-related, 41
in posterior stabilization, 273
prevention of, in traction, 27-28
nonoperative treatment
for dislocation, 17
anterior, 127-128
in athletes, 127-128

during athletic season, 277-284
first-time, 9, 116-118
for hyperlaxity, 8
for multidirectional instability, 91
for posterior instability, 103
for recurrent instability, 182-183
nonunion, of coracoid graft, 167

open capsular shift, for multidirectional instability, 92
open techniques
for anterior glenoid rim deficiency, 223-233
Bankart repair, 184, 199-207
for capsular deficiency, 216-222
for dislocation, in elite athlete, 127-133
for glenohumeral instability, 199-207
for Hill-Sachs lesions, 238-242, 244-249
for humeral anterior capsular avulsion, 253-261
for hyperlaxity, 8
for multidirectional instability, 92, 95-96
for posterior stabilization, 263-273
for recurrent instability, 13-16
rehabilitation after. *See* rehabilitation
for rotator interval closure, 78
for soft tissue repair, 149-153
for subscapularis repair, 209-216
Opus-style knotless suture anchors, 60, 68, 71-75
osseous disimpaction technique, for Hill-Sachs lesions, 243
osteoarthritis, after revision surgery, 192
osteoarticular allograft transplantation, for Hill-Sachs lesions, 244, 246, 248-249
osteotomy
coracoid, for Latarjet procedure, 164-165
rotational humeral, for Hill-Sachs lesions, 245, 247

partial articular sided tendon avulsion (PASTA) lesion, 87
pectoralis transfer, for subscapularis tear, 213-216
pendulum exercises, 278
percutaneous bone tamp, for Hill-Sachs lesions, 243
plication
posterior, 81-87, 105-106
rotator interval, 78-81
portals
for Bankart repair, 48-51
for first-time dislocation repair, 119-123
for humeral anterior capsular avulsion repair, 258-259
for Latarjet procedure, 159-166

for lateral decubitus position, 28-29
for multidirectional instability repair, 93-94
for posterior instability repair, 103-107
for revision surgery, 185-186
for SLAP tear repair, 176
for subscapularis repair, 212
posterior instability, 101-109, 263-273
posterior plication sutures, 81-87, 105-106
posterior portals
in lateral decubitus position, 28-29
for multidirectional instability repair, 93-94
for revision surgery, 185
for SLAP tear repair, 176
for subscapularis repair, 212
posteromedial portal, in lateral decubitus position, 29
postoperative phase, of rehabilitation, 288-294
Prolene sutures, 65, 68-69
protraction and retraction exercise, 293
PushLock knotless suture anchors, 60, 68, 71-75
push-up-plus exercises, 294-295
push-ups, 295-296

radiography
for anterior dislocation, 9
for bone loss, 137
for capsular deficiency, 217
for first-time dislocation, 114
for Hill-Sachs lesions, 238-239
for humeral anterior capsular avulsion, 254
for humeral head bone loss, 143
for hyperlaxity, 7
for multidirectional instability, 90
for recurrent instability, 11-12
for revision surgery, 183-184
for subscapularis tears, 211
range of motion exercises, 292, 294-295
recurrent instability
anterior, 11-16
anterior glenohumeral, 223-233
during athletic season, 277-284
Bankart repair for, 45-57
bone loss in, 135-147, 149-154
after first-time dislocation repair, 113-126
after Latarjet procedure, 167
after multidirectional instability repair, 96-97
posterior plication sutures for, 85-87
after posterior stabilization, 273
after revision surgery, 192
revision surgery for. *See* revision surgery
rotator interval closure for, 79-81
in SLAP tear repair, 178
soft tissue repair for, 149-154

rehabilitation, 285-297
    after anterior dislocation repair, 131-132
    after Bankart repair, 54-55, 207
    after capsular reconstruction, 220
    after first-time dislocation repair, 125
    after glenoid rim deficiency bone graft procedure, 232
    after humeral anterior capsular avulsion repair, 261
    justification of, 287
    keys to success in, 285-286
    after labrum reconstruction, 220
    after Latarjet procedure, 167-168
    for laxity, 8
    after multidirectional instability repair, 97
    after pectoralis tendon transfer, 215-216
    phases and progression of, 287-288
        advanced strength, 289, 295-296
        mobilization, 289, 292, 293-294
        postoperative, 288-294
        return to activity, 289, 296
    after posterior instability repair, 108
    for recurrent instability, 182-183
    after revision surgery, 190, 193-194
    after subscapularis repair, 213
    team approach to, 285-286
Remplissage technique
    for Hill-Sachs lesions, 188-189, 243
    for recurrent instability, 16, 152
resistance band exercises, 292
resistive exercise, after revision surgery, 193
return to activity phase, of rehabilitation, 289, 296
revision surgery, 181-195
    arthroscopic, 183-184, 185-189
    of Bankart repair, 157
    bone grafting in, 184-185
    complications of, 192
    Latarjet procedure for, 157
    nonoperative, 182-183
    open Bankart repair, 184
    pain after, 190-191
    patient selection for, 182
    rehabilitation after, 193-194
rotational humeral osteotomy, for Hill-Sachs lesions, 245, 247
rotator cuff muscles
    dysfunction of, 4
    tears of, in middle-aged athletes, 16-18
rotator interval
    anatomy of, 78
    closure of, 8
        in Bankart repair, 52, 55
        for multidirectional instability, 94, 96
        plication sutures for, 78-81
        in revision surgery, 189

    opening of, in Latarjet procedure, 159-160
    pathoanatomy of, 3-6
Rowe classification, of Hill-Sachs lesions, 236

scapular platform, strengthening exercises for, 292-293
scapular stabilization exercise, 278, 280
screw fixation
    for glenoid bone block, 229-230
    for Latarjet procedure, 166
    for osteoarticular allograft, 244, 246
    for posterior stabilization, 272
Severity Index Score, 13-14
"shadow drills," 296
shoulder instability. *See* instability
shrug and depression exercise, 293
SLAP (superior labral tears from anterior to posterior) tears, 171-180, 188
soft tissue
    injury of, Latarjet procedure for, 157
    repair of, with bone loss, 149-154
spine alignment, for beach chair position, 36, 38
split pectoralis major transfer, for subscapularis tear, 213-216
Spyder arm positioner, 41-42
"squeaky" shoulder, 190
stick exercises, 290
stiffness
    after revision surgery, 190-192
    after SLAP tear repair, 178-179
strength, measurement of, 183
strengthening exercises, 54, 193, 290-292
Sub Cap Channeler, 163
subclavian portal, in lateral decubitus position, 29
subscapularis tendon
    incision in, in Bankart repair, 201-204
    injury of, in glenoid rim deficiency bone graft procedure, 232
    repair of, 204, 206
    splitting of, in Latarjet procedure, 160-161
    tears of, 209-216
sulcus sign, in multidirectional instability, 90
Sully Brace, 281-282
superior labral tears from anterior to posterior (SLAP tears), 171-180, 188
superior medial portal, in lateral decubitus position, 29
suprascapular nerve, protection of, in posterior stabilization, 266
sutures
    anchors for. *See* anchors
    for Bankart repair, 52-53, 55
    for glenoid rim deficiency bone graft procedure, 230

impingement of, 190-192

knotless, anchor design and techniques for, 59-75

for multidirectional instability repair, 94

for posterior plication, 81-87, 105-106

for posterior stabilization, 268-271

for rotator interval closure, 78-81

for SLAP tear repair, 177-178

for subscapularis repair, 212-213

Swiss ball exercises, 291, 294-295

switching stick, 258

tamps, for Hill-Sachs lesions, 243

tendon graft

for capsular reconstruction, 218-221

for labrum reconstruction, 218

teres minor, exposure of, for posterior stabilization, 266-267

top hats, for Latarjet procedure, 163

traction, 27-28

transplantation, osteoarticular, for Hill-Sachs lesions, 244, 246, 248-249

trans-subscapular portal, for humeral anterior capsular avulsion repair, 258-259

tricortical bone graft, for Hill-Sachs lesions, 241-242

triple block effect

in glenoid rim deficiency, 223

in Latarjet procedure, 156

ultrasound, for Hill-Sachs lesions, 238

utility loop, for knotless suture anchor, 64, 69

"vest-over-pants" capsular plication, 270

weight training, 278-279

West Point view, for bone loss, 137

Wissinger rod, 48

wrist padding, 27-28

x-ray. *See* radiography

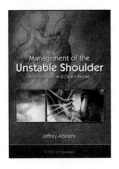
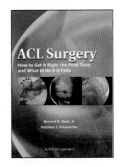

Attention Industry Partners!

Whether you are interested in buying multiple copies of a book, chapter reprints, or looking for something new and different — we are able to accommodate your needs.

MULTIPLE COPIES

At attractive discounts starting for purchases as low as 25 copies for a single title, SLACK Incorporated will be able to meet all of your needs.

CHAPTER REPRINTS

SLACK Incorporated is able to offer the chapters you want in a format that will lead to success. Bound with an attractive cover, use the chapters that are a fit specifically for your company. Available for quantities of 100 or more.

CUSTOMIZE

SLACK Incorporated is able to create a specialized custom version of any of our products specifically for your company.

Please contact the Marketing Communications Director for further details on multiple copy purchases, chapter reprints or custom printing at 1-800-257-8290 or 1-856-848-1000.

*Please note all conditions are subject to change.

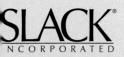

SLACK®
INCORPORATED

Health Care Books and Journals • 6900 Grove Road • Thorofare, NJ 08086

1-800-257-8290
Fax: 1-856-848-6091
E-mail: orders@slackinc.com
CODE: 328

www.slackbooks.com